MCQs in Oral Pathology and Oral Medicine with Comments for Under and Post-Graduates

Adel M Abdel-Azim, BDS, MDSc, PhD
Professor and Former Chairman of
Oral Pathology Department,
Faculty of Dentistry, Ain Shams University

Ahmed A Abdel-Azim, BDS, MD, PhD
Oral Medicine Consultant and Lecturer of Oral Medicine

theWay

2022

Second Edition, 2022

theWay Publishing

A Print Replica (e-book) of this book is also available at Amazon

ISBN 978-1-7341882-5-7

Email address: adelmam55@gmail.com

Other books by the same authors:

Oral and Maxillofacial Pathology: A Study Guide

Oral and Maxillofacial Pathology: Tips and Tricks

Oral Pathology for Dental Hygienists and Assistants: Your Way to Success

PREFACE

Most students find oral pathology and oral medicine the most challenging courses they have taken so far during their long medical studies. The course content is extensive and usually intermingled with oral subjects, and it is required to know the material at a very high level of detail. In this book, we will be providing real and actual questions, and we hope to take away some of the stress of wondering what the level of questioning will be like.

This book acts as a companion to the other author's books, particularly "Oral and Maxillofacial Pathology: Tips and Tricks" and the textbook "Oral and Maxillofacial Pathology: A Study Guide".

The present book's MCQs are "multiple choice" in nature, with some "true/false" questions thrown in for good measure. Each question will begin with a statement or stem, which will be followed by a set of sentences. You must indicate which is the most correct answer(s) and also whether you believe each statement is true or false. You will find the page with the correct answer at the end of each stem. In the e-book version of this book, you can click on the answer to go directly to it. Each phrase in the group is independent of the others, and a question can contain any number of true or incorrect phrases. The main aim is to gain as many points of knowledge as possible.

We do not claim exclusive approval for the book. Much of the material has been collected from periodicals, journals, books, review articles, discussions, personal communications, and past undergrad, postgraduate, and board exams.

There will undoubtedly be inaccuracies, minor flaws, omissions, and oversimplifications. We are expecting that the remaining information will be sufficient to elicit fresh insights and lines of inquiry into the fields of oral pathology and medicine. We gave it a little of our heart and soul. So, we are hoping that this task will be quite educational. We continue to welcome comments from my students and colleagues to further improvements in future editions.

If you have comments on or error corrections to this documentation, please send them to the author mail: adelmam55@gmail.com

How to Use This Book

Choose **one or more** of the most appropriate answers. Some questions may have **more than one** correct answer. You have to choose all the correct answers as best as you can.

Questions starting with the sign ♣ may have zero, one or several correct answers. Other questions have a single correct answer.

Do not forget to see chapter Multi Span Questions on page (359) and chapter Oral Pathology and Medicine for Saudi Board on page (395).

The correct answer with the explanation, if available, is found at the end of the question. You can click on the answer in the **electronic version** to go forth and back.

When doing MCQs, read the questions carefully and read what is written and not what you expect to read. For example, there are often little things in them to trip you up, like double negatives. Rest assured, we have tried to keep them minimally incorporate into the questions in this book. Another tip is to look for questions that include words like "always" and "never," as these are often false. Each question usually has the same amount of marks, so it is essential to do the whole paper. As with most things, the only way to get good at MCQs is to practice them, and this book will provide you with an opportunity to do that. Each question has accurate answers listed on separate pages and a short explanation about the questions to help your revision. This book is intended to help you practice MCQs to prepare for examinations in oral pathology or oral medicine and is suitable for both undergraduates and postgraduate students. We hope you find it helpful and wish you every success in your forthcoming studies.

In the actual exam, it is essential to understand how the questions will be graded. If negative marking is utilized, for example, you will earn a mark for each correct answer and have a mark deducted for each incorrect answer. This is crucial to understand because guessing in this type of test will result in a loss of marks. It is feasible to think of replies without losing marks if there is no negative grading.

Contents

CHAPTER 1
INTRODUCTION TO DEVELOPMENTAL DISEASES

Developmental diseases are those resulting from a disturbance in normal development and growth of an individual. They may be manifested at birth (*congenital*) or appear later on life (*tarda*). The etiologic factors responsible for the causation of developmental diseases may be hereditary or environmental (acquired). See table (1.1) for the different terms used in the field of developmental diseases.

1.1 MCQs Questions

Choose **one or more** of the most appropriate answers. Some questions may have **more than one** correct answer. You have to choose all the correct answers as best as you can.

Questions using the sign ♣ may have zero, one or several correct answers. Other questions have a single correct answer.

1. Expressivity in genetics is [1]:
   (a) The random segregation of genes during meiosis
   (b) The ability of the gene to be expressed in each generation
   (c) The degree to which a phenotype is expressed by individuals having a particular genotype which may result from interactions between some genes
   (d) Crossing-over of genes during mitosis
   Answer for Q 1 on page 19

Table 1.1: The difference between some genetic terms

Always Remember

- ✦ Not all congenital diseases are hereditary
- ✦ All congenital diseases are developmental
- ✦ Not all developmental diseases are congenital

Note

2. Penetrance in genetics is [1]:
   (a) The ability of the gene to express itself in every generation
   (b) The phenotype might not occur as often as the genotype
   (c) The tendency of the gene to skip expression in some generations
   (d) All of the above

   Answer for Q 2 on page 20

3. ♣ An example of an autosomal dominant genetic disease with incomplete expressivity is:
   (a) Marfan syndrome
   (b) Treacher Collins syndrome
   (c) Facial fibrous dysplasia
   (d) Cherubism

   Answer for Q 3 on page 20

4. ♣ An example of an autosomal dominant genetic disease with incomplete penetrance is:
   (a) Pierre Robin Syndrome sequence
   (b) Treacher Collins syndrome
   (c) Osteogenesis imperfecta
   (d) Cherubism

   Answer for Q 4 on page 20

5. ♣ An example of Lyon hypothesis (Lyonization) in oral pathology is:
   (a) Some cases of dentinogenesis imperfecta
   (b) Some cases of amelogenesis imperfecta
   (c) Hereditary ectodermal dysplasia
   (d) Regional odontodysplasia

   Answer for Q 5 on page 20

6. Hemophilia is more common in males because it is a:
   (a) Recessive character carried by Y-chromosome
   (b) Dominant character carried by Y-chromosome
   (c) Dominant trait carried by X-chromosome
   (d) Recessive trait carried by X-chromosome

   Answer for Q 6 on page 20

7. In Down's syndrome of a male child, the sex complement is:
   - (a) XO
   - (b) XY
   - (c) XX
   - (d) XXY

   Answer for Q 7 on page 20

8. Which terms refers to a defect present at birth?
   - (a) anomaly
   - (b) congenital defect
   - (c) developmental defect
   - (d) inherited defect

   Answer for Q 8 on page 20

9. In human beings 45 chromosomes/ single X/XO abnormality causes:
   - (a) Down's syndrome
   - (b) Klinefelter's syndrome
   - (c) Turner's syndrome
   - (d) Edward's syndrome

   Answer for Q 9 on page 21

10. Down's syndrome is due to:
    - (a) Crossing over
    - (b) Linkage
    - (c) Sex-linked inheritance
    - (d) Non-disjunction of chromosomes

    Answer for Q 10 on page 21

11. A child's blood group is "O". The parent's blood groups cannot be:
    - (a) A and B
    - (b) A and A
    - (c) AB and O
    - (d) B and O

    Answer for Q 11 on page 21

12. In humans, each cell normally contains only one of the pairs of chromosomes:

    (a) 11 pairs

    (b) 23 pairs

    (c) 32 pairs

    (d) 46 pairs

    Answer for Q 12 on page 21

13. Inter-generational transmission to offspring can occur as a result of parental exposures to:

    (a) war

    (b) natural disasters

    (c) hunger

    (d) all of these

    Answer for Q 13 on page 21

14. A form of vitamin D-resistant rickets, known as hypophosphatemia, is inherited as an X-linked dominant trait. If a male with hypophosphatemia marries a normal female, which of the following predictions concerning their potential progeny would be **true**?

    (a) All of their sons would inherit the disease

    (b) All of their daughters would inherit the disease

    (c) About 50% of their sons would inherit the disease

    (d) About 50% of their daughters would inherit the disease

    (e) None of their daughters would inherit the disease

    Answer for Q 14 on page 21

15. Which of the following is the most likely explanation for a high rate of crossing-over between two genes?

    (a) The two genes are far apart on the same chromosome.

    (b) The two genes are both located near the centromere.

    (c) The two genes are sex-linked.

    (d) The two genes code for the same protein.

    (e) The two genes are on different chromosomes.

    Answer for Q 15 on page 21

16. Some strains of the bacterium Streptococcus pyogenes secrete poisonous substances called exotoxins. The gene encoding the exotoxins are thought to have originated in bacteriophages, which are viruses

that infect bacteria. Which of the following is the most likely mechanism by which the S. pyogenes acquired the ability to produce exotoxins?

(a) Bacteriophages engulfed cellular debris from dead bacteria.

(b) Bacteriophages in the environment activated bacterial cell division.

(c) Bacteriophage DNA became integrated in the bacterial chromosome.

(d) Bacteriophage proteins were absorbed into bacterial cells by endocytosis.

Answer for Q 16 on page 21

17. All developmental diseases are:

(a) Hereditary

(b) Congenital

(c) Appears later on life

(d) None of the above

Answer for Q 17 on page 21

18. The tendency of an offspring to resemble its parent is known as:

(a) Variation

(b) Heredity

(c) Resemblance

(d) Inheritance

Answer for Q 18 on page 21

19. Who is known as the "Father of Genetics"?

(a) Morgan

(b) Mendel

(c) Watson

(d) Bateson

Answer for Q 19 on page 22

20. The alternate form of a gene is:

(a) Alternate type

(b) Recessive character

(c) Dominant character

(d) Allele

Answer for Q 20 on page 22

21. The genotypic ratio of a monohybrid cross is:

    (a) 1:2:1

    (b) 3:1

    (c) 2:1:1

    (d) 9:3:3:1

    Answer for Q 21 on page 22

22. The crossing of F1 to either of the parents is known as:

    (a) Test cross

    (b) Back cross

    (c) F1 cross

    (d) All of the above

    Answer for Q 22 on page 22

23. Which of the following statements is **true** regarding the "law of segregation"?

    (a) Law of segregation is the law of purity of genes

    (b) Alleles separate from each other during gametogenesis

    (c) Segregation of factors is due to the segregation of chromosomes during meiosis

    (d) All of the above

    Answer for Q 23 on page 22

24. Homozygosity and heterozygosity of an individual can be determined by:

    (a) Back cross

    (b) Self-fertilization

    (c) Test cross

    (d) All of the above

    Answer for Q 24 on page 22

25. An exception to Mendel's law is:

    (a) Independent assortment

    (b) Linkage

    (c) Dominance

    (d) Purity of gametes

    Answer for Q 25 on page 22

26. Pea plants were used in Mendel's experiments because:
    (a) They were cheap
    (b) They had contrasting characters
    (c) They were available easily
    (d) All of the above

Answer for Q 26 on page 22

27. The smallest unit of genetic material which produces a phenotypic effect on mutation is:
    (a) Muton
    (b) Gene
    (c) Recon
    (d) Nucleic acid

Answer for Q 27 on page 22

28. Alleles are:
    (a) Alternate forms of genes
    (b) Linked genes
    (c) Chromosomes that have crossed over
    (d) Homologous chromosomes

Answer for Q 28 on page 22

29. When the activity of one gene is suppressed by the activity of a non-allelic gene, it is known as:
    (a) Pseudo-dominance
    (b) Hypostasis
    (c) Epistasis
    (d) Incomplete dominance

Answer for Q 29 on page 22

30. Cystic fibrosis is:
    (a) Sex-linked recessive disorder
    (b) Autosomal dominant disorder
    (c) Autosomal recessive disorder
    (d) Sex-linked dominant disorder

Answer for Q 30 on page 22

31. 9:7 ratio in the F2 generation represents:
   (a) Incomplete dominance
   (b) Co-dominance
   (c) Epistasis[1]
   (d) Complementary interaction

   Answer for Q 31 on page 22

32. A small amount of lethal mutation is always present in the population due to:
   (a) Positive selection
   (b) Negative selection
   (c) Frequency-dependent selection
   (d) Mutation-selection balance

   Answer for Q 32 on page 23

33. If a plant with genotype AaBb is self-fertilized, the probability of getting AABB genotype will be (A and B are not linked):
   (a) $\frac{1}{2}$
   (b) $\frac{1}{4}$
   (c) $\frac{1}{8}$
   (d) $\frac{1}{16}$

   Answer for Q 33 on page 23

34. How many phenotypes can occur in the human blood group ABO with alleles IA IB i?
   (a) 2
   (b) 3
   (c) 4
   (d) 1

   Answer for Q 34 on page 23

35. The geometrical device that helps to find out all the possible combinations of male and female gametes is known as:
   (a) Bateson Square
   (b) Mendel Square
   (c) Punnett Square
   (d) Mendel's Cube

   Answer for Q 35 on page 23

[1] Epistasis is the interaction of genes that are not alleles, in particular, the suppression of the effect of one gene by another. The suppressed gene is said to be hypostatic, and the other is said to be hyperstatic.

36. Which term represents a pair of contrasting characters?
    (a) Heterozygous
    (b) Homozygous
    (c) Codominant genes
    (d) Allelomorphs

Answer for Q 36 on page 23

37. Gene for sex determination is:
    (a) Shh
    (b) SRY
    (c) AZF
    (d) HOX

Answer for Q 37 on page 23

38. A hemophilia patient has married a normal woman, then his:
    (a) Daughters are carriers
    (b) Sons are all affected
    (c) Daughter are affected
    (d) All are normal

Answer for Q 38 on page 23

39. Which of the following is the carrier of genetic information?
    (a) Proteins
    (b) Amino acids
    (c) Carbohydrates
    (d) DNA

Answer for Q 39 on page 23

40. 2. On which of the following chromosomal disorders are based on?
    (a) Mutant allele and their defective products
    (b) Imbalance in chromosome number and chromosome arrangement
    (c) Mutant allele and chromosome arrangement
    (d) Mutant allele and imbalance in chromosome number

Answer for Q 40 on page 23

41. In which year, Down's syndrome was described?

    (a) 1866

    (b) 1986

    (c) 1898

    (d) 1968

    Answer for Q 41 on page 23

42. Which of the following is not a characteristic feature of Down's syndrome?

    (a) Very tall

    (b) Small round head

    (c) Furrowed tongue

    (d) Partially open mouth

    Answer for Q 42 on page 23

43. Only mental development is retarded in the case of Down's syndrome:

    (a) True

    (b) False

    (c) Not sure

    Answer for Q 43 on page 23

44. Which of the following is the most prominent characteristic feature of Down's syndrome?

    (a) Congenital heart disease

    (b) Short stature

    (c) Broad palm with palm crease

    (d) Underdeveloped gonads

    Answer for Q 44 on page 23

45. Which of the following is **not** a feature of the tongue of the person suffering from Down's syndrome?

    (a) Furrowed tongue

    (b) Big tongue

    (c) Wrinkled tongue

    (d) Straight tongue

    Answer for Q 45 on page 23

46. What is the genotype of the person suffering from Klinefelter's syndrome?
    (a) 44+ XXX
    (b) 42+ XXX
    (c) 44+ XXY
    (d) 42+ XXY

Answer for Q 46 on page 24

47. Which of the following is incorrect with respect to Klinefelter's syndrome?
    (a) The fusion of an abnormal egg with normal sperm
    (b) The fusion of a normal egg with an abnormal sperm
    (c) The fusion of a normal egg with a normal sperm
    (d) An additional copy of X-chromosome

Answer for Q 47 on page 24

48. There are no loops on the finger-tips of the people suffering from Down's syndrome:
    (a) True
    (b) False
    (c) Not sure

Answer for Q 48 on page 24

49. Which of the following is not the character of a person suffering from Klinefelter's syndrome?
    (a) Short stature
    (b) Breast development
    (c) Small testes
    (d) Female type pubic hair pattern

Answer for Q 49 on page 24

50. Which of the following is not the character of the person suffering from Turner's syndrome?
    (a) Short stature
    (b) Poor breast development
    (c) Well-developed ovaries
    (d) No menstruation

Answer for Q 50 on page 24

51. Which of the following is a representation of a recessive trait?
    (a) Achondroplasia
    (b) Blue eyes
    (c) Huntington disease
    (d) Brown eyes

    Answer for Q 51 on page 24

52. Which of the following is the representation of a dominant trait?
    (a) Widow's peak
    (b) Tongue non-roller's
    (c) Fused ear lobes
    (d) Tay-Sach's disease

    Answer for Q 52 on page ??

53. What is the inheritance of characters by plasmagenes known as?
    (a) Extrafield inheritance
    (b) Maternal inheritance
    (c) Extrachromosomal inheritance
    (d) Maternal inheritance

    Answer for Q 53 on page 24

54. Extrachromosomal inheritance is usually carried through:
    (a) Mitochondria
    (b) Chloroplasts
    (c) Cellular parasites e.g., viruses or bacterial
    (d) All of the above

    Answer for Q 54 on page 24

55. Which of the following is an incorrect statement with respect to organelle inheritance?
    (a) Iojap inheritance in maize
    (b) Inheritance of poky
    (c) Plastid inheritance in Mirabilis jalapa
    (d) Coiling of shells

    Answer for Q 55 on page 24

56. Which of the following is a type of autosomal recessive genetic disorder?
   (a) Hemophilia
   (b) Skeletal dysplasia
   (c) Sickle cell anemia
   (d) None of the above

   Answer for Q 56 on page 24

57. Which of the following disorder is also called the Royal disease?
   (a) Color blindness
   (b) Hemophilia
   (c) Sickle cell anemia
   (d) Alzheimer's disease

   Answer for Q 57 on page 24

58. Which of the following disorder is an example of point mutation?
   (a) Sickle cell anemia
   (b) Down's syndrome
   (c) Night blindness
   (d) Thalassemia

   Answer for Q 58 on page 24

59. If the father in a family has a disease while the mother is normal, the daughters only are inherited by this disease and not the sons. Name this type of disease?
   (a) Autosomal recessive
   (b) Autosomal dominant
   (c) Sex-linked recessive
   (d) Sex-linked dominant

   Answer for Q 59 on page 24

60. Which of the following genotypes and phenotypes in a man may be the correct result of aneuploidy in sex chromosomes?
   (a) 22 pairs + Y females
   (b) 22 pairs + XY females
   (c) 22 pairs + XXY females
   (d) 22 pairs + XXXY females

   Answer for Q 60 on page 24

61. What will be the condition of the progeny if the father is normal, while the mother has one gene for hemophilia and one gene for color blindness on one of the X chromosomes?

    (a) Only daughters are hemophiliac and color blind

    (b) Both sons and daughters will be hemophiliac and color blind

    (c) 50 per cent hemophiliac and color blind sons and 50% normal sons

    (d) 50 per cent hemophiliac color blind daughters and 50% color blind daughters

    Answer for Q 61 on page 24

62. Cystic fibrosis is an autosomal recessive genetic disorder. What are the chances that the child would have the disease if any one of the parents (either mother or father) is a carrier of the faulty cystic fibrosis gene (Cc)?

    (a) 100 per cent

    (b) 50 per cent

    (c) 25 per cent

    (d) 0 per cent

    Answer for Q 62 on page 25

63. Alpha-1 anti-trypsin deficiency is an autosomal recessive genetic disorder. What are the chances that any of the offspring **do not** express the disease characteristics if both parents are genotype (Aa)?

    (a) 100 per cent

    (b) 75 per cent

    (c) 50 per cent

    (d) 25 per cent

    Answer for Q 63 on page 25

64. Which of the following is a trait of X-linked recessive?

    (a) Albinism

    (b) Hemophilia

    (c) Huntington's disease

    (d) None of these answers are correct

    Answer for Q 64 on page 25

65. The mode of inheritance for the trait – Fragile X syndrome is:

    (a) X linked dominant

    (b) X linked recessive

    (c) Autosomal dominant

    (d) Autosomal recessive

    Answer for Q 65 on page 25

66. All genes in sex chromosomes are sex linked:
    (a) True
    (b) False

    Answer for Q 66 on page 25

67. An X linked recessive gene would appear to:
    (a) Be expressed in both males and females equally
    (b) Skip generations
    (c) Be lethal
    (d) Gradually degrade

    Answer for Q 67 on page 25

68. A Y linked gene:
    (a) Is carried by mother
    (b) Is expressed only when homozygous
    (c) Can be transmitted from the mother to her sons
    (d) Expressed only in men

    Answer for Q 68 on page 25

69. Genes which are present in the homologous region of X and Y chromosomes are called:
    (a) Autosomal
    (b) Sex linked
    (c) Partially sex linked
    (d) Unlinked

    Answer for Q 69 on page 25

70. Choose the different one of the following:
    (a) Color blindness
    (b) Hemophilia
    (c) Duchenne muscular dystrophy
    (d) Enamel hypoplasia

    Answer for Q 70 on page 25

71. X linked dominant trait tends to be milder in heterozygous females. State if it is true or false:
    (a) True
    (b) False

    Answer for Q 71 on page 25

72. In a family of four, including a normal mother, a normal father, a colorblind son, and a normal son; who do you think has the defective X gene other than the affected son?
    (a) The mother
    (b) The father
    (c) The normal son
    (d) The effected son only
    Answer for Q 72 on page 25
73. A colorblind mother and a normal father give birth to a Klinefelter child with normal vision. Where do you think the non-disjunction has taken place?
    (a) 1st meiotic division of mother
    (b) 2nd meiotic division of the father
    (c) 2nd meiotic division of mother
    (d) 1st meiotic division of father
    Answer for Q 73 on page 25
74. If colorblindness was a dominant trait, which of the following would not be **true**?
    (a) It would be expressed in heterozygous females
    (b) It would be expressed in males
    (c) It would never be turned off
    (d) It would not skip generations
    Answer for Q 74 on page 25
75. What is the probability that the son of a color blind father would be color blind?
    (a) 0
    (b) $\frac{1}{4}$
    (c) $\frac{1}{2}$
    (d) 1
    Answer for Q 75 on page 25
76. Y linked inheritance is:
    (a) Criss cross inheritance[2]
    (b) Straight inheritance
    (c) Loop inheritance
    (d) Jumping inheritance
    Answer for Q 76 on page 25
77. Which of the following is wrong?
    (a) Y chromosome lacks dosage compensation
    (b) X linked genes are inherited as criss cross
    (c) Y linked gene like Hemophilia passes from father to son
    (d) X linked recessive genes are carried by females
    Answer for Q 77 on page 25

[2]The criss cross inheritance is the transmission of a gene from father to the daughter or from mother to the son. This pattern of inheritance of genes is also called skip generations because the character is inherited to the second generation through the carrier of the first generation.

78. Which of the following is a Y linked gene?
    (a) Amelogenesis imperfecta
    (b) Hemophilia
    (c) Hypertrichosis with hairy ear pinna trait
    (d) Phenyl ketone urea

    Answer for Q 78 on page 25

79. Which of the following is partially sex linked?
    (a) Complete colorblindness
    (b) Hypertrichosis
    (c) Faulty tooth enamel
    (d) Hemophilia

    Answer for Q 79 on page 26

80. A **turner** affected child born to normal parents is hemophilia affected. Where did the non-disjunction occur?
    (a) Mother
    (b) Father
    (c) Zygote
    (d) Grand mother

    Answer for Q 80 on page 26

81. The chromosomal theory of inheritance was proposed by?
    (a) Mendel
    (b) Watson and Crick
    (c) Darwin
    (d) Sutton and Boveri

    Answer for Q 81 on page 26

82. Which of the following doesn't agree with the chromosomal theory of inheritance?
    (a) The genes are located on the chromosome
    (b) The genes on the same chromosome are always passed together
    (c) The genes are located linearly on the chromosomes
    (d) The distance between two genes can be mapped

    Answer for Q 82 on page 26

83. If there is a non-disjunction in the X chromosome, the progeny being XXY, what will be the constitution of the chromosome(s) in the gamete?

   (a) X and Y

   (b) X and XY

   (c) XX and Y

   (d) XXY with no separation

   Answer for Q 83 on page 26

84. The chromosomal theory of inheritance violates which of the following laws?

   (a) Law of dominance

   (b) Law of segregation

   (c) Law of independent assortment

   (d) None

   Answer for Q 84 on page 26

85. You observe a genetic trait which is a common occurrence in the male of a particular pedigree, this is possibly a:

   (a) X linked

   (b) Y linked

   (c) X linked recessive

   (d) Y linked dominant

   Answer for Q 85 on page 26

86. The genetic constitution of an individual is his/her:

   (a) Phenotype

   (b) Heritability

   (c) Genotype

   (d) None of the above

   Answer for Q 86 on page 26

87. If both the copies of gene in a chromosome are identical the individual is described as:

   (a) Heterozygous

   (b) Homozygous

   (c) Alleles

   (d) Pleiotropic[3]

Answer for Q 87 on page 26

[3]A gene that exhibits multiple phenotypic expression by affecting the expression of two or more other genes.

88. If a trait or a disease manifests itself when the affected person carries only one copy of gene responsible along with one normal allele in somatic chromosome, the mode of inheritance is:
    (a) Dominant
    (b) X linked
    (c) Recessive
    (d) None of the above

    Answer for Q 88 on page 26

89. Y-linked inheritance:
    (a) Is also termed Holandric inheritance
    (b) Can be transmitted from the mother to her daughters
    (c) Can be transmitted from the mother to her sons
    (d) More widespread than X-linked inheritance

    Answer for Q 89 on page 26

90. Mitochondrial inheritance:
    (a) Are more widespread than nuclear inheritance
    (b) Cannot be transmitted from mother to her offspring
    (c) Can be transmitted from mother to her offspring
    (d) Are also termed holandric inheritance

    Answer for Q 90 on page 26

91. Genetic heterogeneity is a term used to describe:
    (a) Different genetic mechanisms that produce different phenotypes
    (b) Different genetic mechanisms that produce the same or similar phenotypes
    (c) The ability of the gene to express itself in every generation thus can skip some generations
    (d) The ability of the gene to express its full features in all generations

    Answer for Q 91 on page 26

1.2 Answers with Comments:

1. The correct answer is **C** – Expressivity is the degree to which a phenotype is expressed by individuals having a particular genotype which may result from interactions between some genes. In other words, it may refer to the degree of the expression of a specific gene by individuals having a certain phenotype.

   Back to Q 1 on page 1

2. The correct answer is **D** – Penetrance could be defined as the ability of genes to penetrate (express) through every generation. Sometimes a dominant gene fails to produce any detectable effect and a dominant trait may then miss a generation. This is an example of reduced penetrance, a term used when some individuals with the appropriate genotype fail to express it.

   Back to Q 2 on page 2

3. The correct answer is **AB** – the features of Marfan syndrome vary widely; some people have only mild symptoms, such as being tall and thin with long, slender fingers, whereas others also experience life-threatening complications involving the heart and blood vessels. Although the features of Marfan syndrome are highly variable, all people with this disorder have a dominant mutation in the gene coding for fibrillin 1, (FBN1) [1].

   Back to Q 3 on page 2

4. The correct answer is **CD** – A specific example of incomplete penetrance is the human bone disease osteogenesis imperfecta (OI). The majority of people with this disease have a dominant mutation in one of the two genes that produce type 1 collagen, COL1A1 or COL1A2. Collagen is a tissue that strengthens bones and muscles and multiple body tissues. However, this disease doesn't affect everyone who has COLIA1 and COLIA2 mutations in the same way. In fact, some people can carry the mutation but have no symptoms. Thus, families can unknowingly transmit the mutation from one generation to the next through someone who carries the mutation but does not express the OI phenotype. Cherubism also follows the same pattern [1].

   Back to Q 4 on page 2

5. The correct answer is **BC** – In addition to the amelogenesis imperfecta, some cases of hereditary ectodermal dysplasia show also the same phenomenon.

   Back to Q 5 on page 2

6. The correct answer is **D** – Hemophilia is more common in males than females because it is a recessive trait carried by X-chromosome. Hemophilia A is the most common form of X-linked genetic disease that prevents normal blood clotting when blood vessels are severed. In severe cases, an affected person can bleed to death from an injury, bruise, or cut. Hemophilia A, in particular, is caused by the absence of a protein called an antihemophilic factor or factor VIII that is required for blood clotting.

   Back to Q 6 on page 2

7. The correct answer is **B** – In Down's syndrome (trisomy 21) of a male child, the sex complement is normal (XY). The disease is a relatively common birth defect resulting from the presence of an extra chromosome number 21 (three instead of two number 21 chromosomes, or trisomy 21). This chromosome abnormality adversely affects both the physical and intellectual development of the individual. It is also the first syndrome to be described in humans.

   Back to Q 7 on page 3

8. The correct answer is **B** – Any disease presents at birth is termed congenital.

   Back to Q 8 on page 3

9. The correct answer is **C** – In human beings, 45 chromosomes/single X or XO abnormality results in Turner's syndrome. Individuals having a single X chromosome 2A + XO (45) have female sexual differentiation, but ovaries are rudimentary and the female is sexually underdeveloped. This condition's other associated phenotypes are webbed neck, short stature, broad chest, lack of secondary sexual characteristics, and sterility. Thus, any unbalance in the copies of the sex chromosomes usually disrupt the genetic information necessary for normal sexual development.

   Back to Q 9 on page 3

10. The correct answer is **D** – See Answer 7.

    Back to Q 10 on page 3

11. The correct answer is **C** – O blood group of a child cannot be obtained from the parents having blood group O x AB. The parents blood groups may be A x O, A x B, B x O, B x A, O x A and O x B.

    Back to Q 11 on page 3

12. The correct answer is **B** – Each human cell except the ova and sperms contains 23 pair of chromosomes equaling a total of 46 alleles. The ova and the sperms contains the half number.

    Back to Q 12 on page 4

13. The correct answer is **D** – war, natural disasters and hunger results in migration of many troops and families leading to the new formation of genetic pools with transmission of new genes from one population to another.

    Back to Q 13 on page 4

14. The correct answer is **B** – As the disease is dominant, and the females inherit X chromosomes from their father only, all the daughters will exhibit the disease.

    Back to Q 14 on page 4

15. The correct answer is **A** – Crossing-over usually affects genes far apart on the chromosomes.

    Back to Q 15 on page 4

16. The correct answer is **C** – For the organism to be capable for secreting the protein, the macrophage's DNA should be incorporated in its genome.

    Back to Q 16 on page 5

17. The correct answer is **D** – Developmental disease can be congenital or appears later on life and also can be hereditary, due to environmental factors or of multifactorial nature (ie environmental with hereditary predisposition.

    Back to Q 17 on page 5

18. The correct answer is **B** – All developmental diseases may be hereditary or not, congenital or not.

Back to Q 18 on page 5

19. The correct answer is **B** – Hereditary is the ability to pass traits from one generation to the other. Mendel is the father of modern genetics.

Back to Q 19 on page 5

20. The correct answer is **D** – No explanation is available for this answer.

Back to Q 20 on page 5

21. The correct answer is **A** – No explanation is available for this answer.

Back to Q 21 on page 5

22. The correct answer is **B** – No explanation is available for this answer.

Back to Q 22 on page 6

23. The correct answer is **D** – No explanation is available for this answer as all of the above is true.

Back to Q 23 on page 6

24. The correct answer is **C** – No explanation is available for this answer.

Back to Q 24 on page 6

25. The correct answer is **B** – No explanation is available for this answer.

Back to Q 25 on page 6

26. The correct answer is **B** – No explanation is available for this answer.

Back to Q 26 on page 7

27. The correct answer is **A** – No explanation is available for this answer.

Back to Q 27 on page 7

28. The correct answer is **A** – No explanation is available for this answer.

Back to Q 28 on page 7

29. The correct answer is **C** – Epistasis is a circumstance where the expression of one gene is modified (e.g., masked, inhibited or suppressed) by the expression of one or more other genes. The suppressed gene is said to be hypostatic, and the other is said to be hyperstatic. An example of epistasis is the interaction between hair color and baldness. A gene for total baldness would be epistatic (hyperstatic) to one for blond hair or red hair. The hair-color genes are hypostatic to the baldness gene. The baldness phenotype supersedes genes for hair color, and so the effects are non-additive.

Back to Q 29 on page 7

30. The correct answer is **C** – No explanation is available for this answer. Remember almost all metabolic disturbances are recessive.

Back to Q 30 on page 7

31. The correct answer is **C** – No explanation is available for this answer. Epistasis is the interaction of genes that are not alleles, in particular, the suppression of the effect of one gene by another. The suppressed gene is said to be hypostatic, and the other is said to be hyperstatic.

    Back to Q 31 on page 8

32. The correct answer is **D** – No explanation is available for this answer.

    Back to Q 32 on page 8

33. The correct answer is **D** – No explanation is available for this answer.

    Back to Q 33 on page 8

34. The correct answer is **C** – No explanation is available for this answer.

    Back to Q 34 on page 8

35. The correct answer is **C** – The Punnett square is a square diagram that is used to predict the genotypes of a particular cross or breeding experiment. It is named after Reginald C. Punnett, who devised the approach in 1905.

    Back to Q 35 on page 8

36. The correct answer is **D** – No explanation is available for this answer.

    Back to Q 36 on page 9

37. The correct answer is **B** – No explanation is available for this answer.

    Back to Q 37 on page 9

38. The correct answer is **A** – No explanation is available for this answer.

    Back to Q 38 on page 9

39. The correct answer is **D** – No explanation is available for this answer.

    Back to Q 39 on page 9

40. The correct answer is **B** – No explanation is available for this answer.

    Back to Q 40 on page 9

41. The correct answer is **B** – No explanation is available for this answer.

    Back to Q 41 on page 10

42. The correct answer is **B** – No explanation is available for this answer.

    Back to Q 42 on page 10

43. The correct answer is **B** – No explanation is available for this answer.

    Back to Q 43 on page 10

44. The correct answer is **B** – No explanation is available for this answer.

    Back to Q 44 on page 10

45. The correct answer is **B** – No explanation is available for this answer.

Back to Q 45 on page 10

46. The correct answer is **B** – No explanation is available for this answer.

Back to Q 46 on page 11

47. The correct answer is **B** – No explanation is available for this answer.

Back to Q 47 on page 11

48. The correct answer is **B** – No explanation is available for this answer.

Back to Q 48 on page 11

49. The correct answer is **B** – No explanation is available for this answer.

Back to Q 49 on page 11

50. The correct answer is **B** – No explanation is available for this answer.

Back to Q 50 on page 11

51. The correct answer is **B** – No explanation is available for this answer.

Back to Q 51 on page 12

52. The correct answer is **B** – No explanation is available for this answer.

Back to Q 52 on page 12

53. The correct answer is **B** – No explanation is available for this answer.

Back to Q 53 on page 12

54. The correct answer is **B** – No explanation is available for this answer.

Back to Q 54 on page 12

55. The correct answer is **B** – No explanation is available for this answer.

Back to Q 55 on page 12

56. The correct answer is **B** – No explanation is available for this answer.

Back to Q 56 on page 13

57. The correct answer is **B** – No explanation is available for this answer.

Back to Q 57 on page 13

58. The correct answer is **B** – No explanation is available for this answer.

Back to Q 58 on page 13

59. The correct answer is **B** – No explanation is available for this answer.

Back to Q 59 on page 13

60. The correct answer is **B** – No explanation is available for this answer.

Back to Q 60 on page 13

61. The correct answer is **B** – No explanation is available for this answer.

Back to Q 61 on page 14

62. The correct answer is **B** – No explanation is available for this answer.

    Back to Q 62 on page 14

63. The correct answer is **B** – No explanation is available for this answer.

    Back to Q 63 on page 14

64. The correct answer is **B** – No explanation is available for this answer.

    Back to Q 64 on page 14

65. The correct answer is **B** – No explanation is available for this answer.

    Back to Q 65 on page 14

66. The correct answer is **B** – No explanation is available for this answer.

    Back to Q 66 on page 15

67. The correct answer is **B** – No explanation is available for this answer.

    Back to Q 61 on page 15

68. The correct answer is **B** – No explanation is available for this answer.

    Back to Q 68 on page 15

69. The correct answer is **B** – No explanation is available for this answer.

    Back to Q 69 on page 15

70. The correct answer is **B** – No explanation is available for this answer.

    Back to Q 70 on page 15

71. The correct answer is **B** – No explanation is available for this answer.

    Back to Q 71 on page 15

72. The correct answer is **B** – No explanation is available for this answer.

    Back to Q 72 on page 16

73. The correct answer is **B** – No explanation is available for this answer.

    Back to Q 73 on page 16

74. The correct answer is **B** – No explanation is available for this answer.

    Back to Q 74 on page 16

75. The correct answer is **B** – No explanation is available for this answer.

    Back to Q 75 on page 16

76. The correct answer is **B** – No explanation is available for this answer.

    Back to Q 76 on page 16

77. The correct answer is **B** – No explanation is available for this answer.

    Back to Q 77 on page 16

78. The correct answer is **B** – No explanation is available for this answer.

Back to Q 78 on page 17

79. The correct answer is **B** – No explanation is available for this answer.

Back to Q 79 on page 17

80. The correct answer is **B** – No explanation is available for this answer.

Back to Q 80 on page 17

81. The correct answer is **B** – No explanation is available for this answer.

Back to Q 81 on page 17

82. The correct answer is **B** – No explanation is available for this answer.

Back to Q 82 on page 17

83. The correct answer is **B** – No explanation is available for this answer.

Back to Q 83 on page 18

84. The correct answer is **B** – No explanation is available for this answer.

Back to Q 84 on page 18

85. The correct answer is **B** – No explanation is available for this answer.

Back to Q 85 on page 18

86. The correct answer is **B** – No explanation is available for this answer.

Back to Q 86 on page 18

87. The correct answer is **B** – No explanation is available for this answer.

Back to Q 87 on page 18

88. The correct answer is **A** – Dominant trait is the trait expressing itself while in heterozygous state i.e., the two alleles are different.

Back to Q 88 on page 19

89. The correct answer is **A** – Yes Y-linked inheritance is termed holandric inheritance.

Back to Q 89 on page 19

90. The correct answer is **C** – Yes mitochondrial genes can be transmitted from the mother to her offspring. The sperm contains no mitochondria or at least tiny fragments of its DNA.

Back to Q 90 on page 19

91. The correct answer is **B** – Genetic heterogeneity refers to the existence of cases with similar phenotypes but with differing genetic mechanisms.

Back to Q 91 on page 19

Chapter 2

Developmental Disturbances of Hard Tooth Structure

Tooth development (***odontogenesis***) comprises the following physiologic processes; Stimulation of certain cells to multiply (initiation and proliferation); Establishment of tooth pattern (morpho differentiation); differentiation of cells to perform special functions (histo-differentiation); Formation of dentin and enamel matrix (apposition); Influx of mineral salts and their subsequent crystallization (mineralization and maturation); Emergence of the crown into the oral cavity (eruption).

2.1 MCQs Questions

Choose **one or more** of the most appropriate answers. Some questions may have **more than one** correct answer. You have to choose all the correct answers as best as you can.

1. Ghost teeth is the term given to:
   (a) dentinogenesis imperfecta
   (b) regional odontodysplasia
   (c) dentinal dysplasia I
   (d) dentinal dysplasia II
   Answer for Q 1 on page 52
2. Amalgam staining of teeth is considered:
   (a) Extrinsic stain
   (b) Bacterial stain
   (c) Intrinsic stain
   (d) Foreign body
   Answer for Q 2 on page 52

3. What are the most important genes name that might influence number of teeth?

    (a) Pax9 genes

    (b) Hedgehog genes[1]

    (c) P53 genes

    (d) Tabby genes

    Answer for Q 3 on page 52

4. Double teeth are an anomaly most commonly found in:

    (a) permanent incisors

    (b) permanent canines

    (c) primary incisors and canines

    (d) primary molars

    Answer for Q 4 on page 53

5. Enamel hypoplasia is presented with all **except**:

    (a) Reduction in volume of matrix

    (b) pits and grooves on the enamel surface

    (c) enamel with fewer prisms

    (d) incomplete calcification

    Answer for Q 5 on page 53

6. What is the most important genes name that might influence number of teeth?

    (a) MSX1 genes

    (b) Tabby genes

    (c) P53 genes

    (d) Col genes

    Answer for Q 6 on page 53

7. Pituitary dwarfism might show:

    (a) Gemination

    (b) Fusion

    (c) Concrescence

    (d) Microdontia

    Answer for Q 7 on page 53

---

[1]Hedgehog is a protein encoded for by the SHH genes. The protein is named after the video game character Sonic the Hedgehog. These are versatile signaling molecules involved in a wide spectrum of biological events including cell differentiation, proliferation, and survival and aging.

8. Shovel-shaped incisors usually associated with:
   (a) Talon cusp
   (b) Dens evaginatus
   (c) Dens invaginatus
   (d) Internal resorption

   Answer for Q 8 on page 53

9. The following defect has problem in elaborating organic matrix in enamel is called:
   (a) Hypoplastic amelogenesis imperfecta
   (b) Hypocalcified amelogenesis imperfecta
   (c) Hypomaturation amelogenesis imperfecta
   (d) Dentin dysplasia

   Answer for Q 9 on page 53

10. A 20-years-old patient came to your clinic with golden brown teeth, he has blue sclera, his mother has the blue sclera as well. He has:
   (a) Dentin dysplasia type I
   (b) Dentin dysplasia type II
   (c) Dentinogenesis imperfecta Type I
   (d) Dentinogenesis imperfecta Type II

   Answer for Q 10 on page 53

11. 32-year-age female patient came to you with slight mobility of the anterior teeth, upon radiographic examination revealed that some roots of her teeth are completely missing or very short, the most appropriate diagnosis is:
   (a) Dentin dysplasia type I
   (b) Dentin dysplasia type II
   (c) Dentinogenesis imperfecta Type I
   (d) Dentinogenesis imperfecta Type II

   Answer for Q 11 on page 53

12. Otodental syndrome (otodental dysplasia) is usually associated with:
   (a) Microdontia
   (b) Macrodontia
   (c) Hypodontia
   (d) Hyperdontia

   Answer for Q 12 on page 53

13. Hypomineralized enamel is characterized with following **except**:
    (a) Enamel appears white and opaque
    (b) tooth may appear pigmented buff, yellow, or brown quickly chipped and worn away
    (c) organic matrix of hypomineralized enamel remains acid-soluble
    (d) failure of the ameloblasts to fully calcify enamel

    Answer for Q 13 on page 53

14. Which of the following is considered as an acquired disorder?
    (a) Gemination
    (b) Fusion
    (c) Concrescence
    (d) None of the above

    Answer for Q 14 on page 54

15. All of the following are the features seen in congenital syphilis **except**:
    (a) infection of the tooth germ by spirochetes
    (b) Hutchinson's incisors
    (c) hypomineralized changes in the enamel
    (d) Moon's molars

    Answer for Q 15 on page 54

16. Causes of hypercementosis can be all **except**:
    (a) Paget's disease
    (b) periapical inflammation
    (c) cleidocranial dysplasia
    (d) mechanical stimulation

    Answer for Q 16 on page 54

17. Otodental syndrome (otodental dysplasia) is usually associated with macrodontia affecting:
    (a) Canines
    (b) Premolars
    (c) Upper lateral incisors
    (d) Lower central incisors

    Answer for Q 17 on page 54

18. In fusion of the teeth, we have:
    (a) Normal number of teeth
    (b) More number of teeth
    (c) Less number of teeth
    (d) Large teeth
    (e) None of the above is correct

    Answer for Q 18 on page 54

19. To guard against teeth pigmentation, it is necessary to avoid the prescribing tetracyclines between the age groups from:
    (a) 4 months to 7 years
    (b) 1 year to 3 years
    (c) 4 months to 10 months
    (d) 7 months to 5 years
    (e) Zero to 12 years

    Answer for Q 19 on page 54

20. Look for the following image and try to diagnose the case: (Source of the image: Su, Jm et al. [2]):

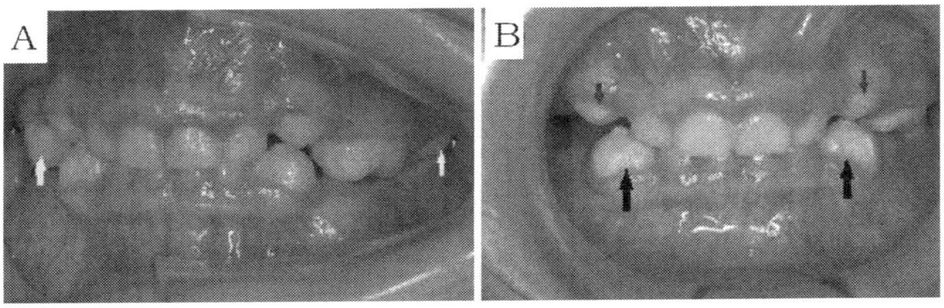

    (a) Regional odontodysplasia
    (b) Cleidocranial dysplasia
    (c) Otodental syndrome
    (d) Hereditary ectodermal dysplasia

    Answer for Q 20 on page 54

21. A union of the roots of adjacent teeth through the cementum is referred to as:
    (a) Concrescence
    (b) Fusion
    (c) Gemination
    (d) Dilaceration

    Answer for Q 21 on page 54

22. The term dilaceration refers to:
   (a) A deformity of a tooth consisting of a sharp bend in the root
   (b) Abrasions on two surfaces of a single tooth
   (c) A root or tooth that is split into two
   (d) A tooth that is fractured at two or more places

   Answer for Q 22 on page 55

23. The term dilaceration refers to:In otodental syndrome (otodental dysplasia) globodontia means:
   (a) Notched incisal edge of the upper central incisors
   (b) Globe shaped and enlarged canines and molar teeth
   (c) Moon's molars
   (d) Mulberry molars

   Answer for Q 23 on page 55

24. One of the following conditions is characterized by peg-shaped incisors which taper towards the incisal edge:
   (a) Congenital syphilis
   (b) Rickets
   (c) Osteomalacia
   (d) Supernumerary teeth

   Answer for Q 24 on page 55

25. Developing ameloblasts are affected by the ingestion of high fluoride content in drinking water resulting in:
   (a) Turner's tooth
   (b) Hutchinson's tooth
   (c) Mottled enamel
   (d) Moon's molars

   Answer for Q 25 on page 55

26. Teeth that erupt within 30 days of birth are called:
   (a) Natal teeth
   (b) Neonatal teeth
   (c) Primary teeth
   (d) Prenatal teeth

   Answer for Q 26 on page 55

27. Otodental syndrome (otodental dysplasia) is usually associated with macrodontia affecting:
   (a) Molars
   (b) Premolars
   (c) Upper lateral incisors
   (d) Lower central incisors

   Answer for Q 27 on page 55

28. A permanent tooth with local hypoplastic deformity in crown is called:
   (a) Turner's tooth
   (b) Taurodontism
   (c) Enameloma
   (d) Ghost teeth

   Answer for Q 28 on page 55

29. True generalized microdontia is characterized by:
   (a) Small teeth with large jaws
   (b) Small teeth with small jaws
   (c) Smaller teeth than normal
   (d) Large teeth with small jaws

   Answer for Q 29 on page 55

30. Gemination of teeth occur due to:
   (a) division of a single tooth bud after calcification
   (b) division of a single tooth bud before calcification
   (c) fusion of two teeth before calcification
   (d) fusion of two teeth after calcification

   Answer for Q 30 on page 55

31. A deep pit lined by enamel seen in the lingual surface of maxillary lateral incisor is most likely to be:
   (a) Dens in dente
   (b) Enamel hypoplasia
   (c) Talon's cusp
   (d) Occlusal enamel drop

   Answer for Q 31 on page 55

32. Ghost teeth is seen in which of the following?
    (a) Dens in dente
    (b) Regional odontodysplasia
    (c) Dentin dysplasia
    (d) Dentinogenesis imperfecta

    Answer for Q 32 on page 55

33. Absence of pulp chambers is seen in:
    (a) Craniofacial dysostosis
    (b) Dentinogenesis imperfecta
    (c) Amelogenesis imperfecta
    (d) Any of the above

    Answer for Q 33 on page 55

34. Dentinogenesis imperfecta differs from amelogenesis imperfecta in that, the former is:
    (a) A hereditary disturbance
    (b) The result of excessive fluoride ingestion
    (c) The result of faulty enamel matrix formation
    (d) Characterized by calcification of pulp chambers and the root canals of the teeth

    Answer for Q 34 on page 55

35. The most common supernumerary tooth form is:
    (a) Tuberculated
    (b) Conical
    (c) Screw shaped
    (d) Incisor shaped

    Answer for Q 35 on page 55

36. Most common missing tooth in the permanent dentition is:
    (a) Maxillary canine
    (b) Maxillary first molar
    (c) Mandibular second premolar
    (d) Upper lateral incisor

    Answer for Q 36 on page 55

37. Hypoplastic defects in permanent central, lateral incisors, canines and first molars **only** are likely to result due to:
    (a) Severe illness or other factors during teeth development
    (b) Hereditary causes
    (c) Obscure causes
    (d) Osteogenesis imperfecta

    Answer for Q 37 on page 55

38. Dentinogenesis imperfecta is:
    (a) Autosomal dominant
    (b) Autosomal recessive
    (c) Sex linked recessive
    (d) Not an inheritable trait

    Answer for Q 38 on page 56

39. Clinical evidence of dentinogenesis imperfecta is:
    (a) Defective enamel and dentin
    (b) Defective dentin and obliterated pulp chamber
    (c) Increased rate of caries
    (d) Oligodontia

    Answer for Q 39 on page 56

40. False about total anodontia:
    (a) May involve both the deciduous and the permanent dentition
    (b) In false anodontia, tooth doesn't undergo full development
    (c) May involve a single tooth
    (d) In total anodontia, all teeth are missing

    Answer for Q 40 on page 56

41. False about total anodontia:Turner's tooth is seen in:
    (a) Enamel hypoplasia due to hypocalcemia
    (b) Enamel hypoplasia due to birth injuries
    (c) Enamel hypoplasia due to congenital syphilis
    (d) Enamel hypoplasia due to local infection or local trauma

    Answer for Q 41 on page 56

42. Supernumerary are:
    (a) Not similar morphologically to normal teeth
    (b) Similar morphologically to normal teeth
    (c) Teeth showing signs of enamel hypoplasia
    (d) Teeth which are larger than normal (macrodontia)

    Answer for Q 42 on page 56

43. Dental anomaly of teeth associated with defective bone formation is seen in:
    (a) Amelogenesis imperfecta
    (b) dentinogenesis imperfecta
    (c) Odontodysplasia
    (d) Osteitis deformans

    Answer for Q 43 on page 56

44. Fusion of teeth is more common in:
    (a) Molar area
    (b) Incisor area
    (c) Premolar area
    (d) Anywhere in the dental arch

    Answer for Q 44 on page 56

45. A four-year-old child has a smaller number of teeth and lateral incisors with bifurcated roots with two root canals. This condition is called:
    (a) Dilaceration
    (b) Concrescence
    (c) Gemination
    (d) Fusion

    Answer for Q 45 on page 56

46. Microdontia is seen most commonly affecting:
    (a) Maxillary lateral incisor
    (b) Mandibular second premolar
    (c) Mandibular central incisor
    (d) Mandibular first premolar

Answer for Q 46 on page 56

47. Taurodontism is characterized by:
    (a) Hypercementosis
    (b) Enlarged tooth trunk and short roots
    (c) Obliterated pulp chambers with secondary dentin deposition
    (d) Rootless teeth with thin shell of enamel

    Answer for Q 47 on page 56

48. Mottled enamel is due to:
    (a) Vitamin A deficiency
    (b) Excess of fluoride in drinking water
    (c) Vitamin D deficiency
    (d) Teratogens

    Answer for Q 48 on page 56

49. Anodontia affects the growth of:
    (a) Maxilla
    (b) Mandible
    (c) Alveolar bone
    (d) Cranium

    Answer for Q 49 on page 56

50. Delayed eruption of at least part of the dentition is a recognized feature of all of the following **except**:
    (a) Rickets[2]
    (b) Congenital hyperthyroidism
    (c) Cleidocranial dysplasia
    (d) Cherubism

    Answer for Q 50 on page 56

51. Which of the following dental sequel is likely in child with a history of generalized growth failure (failure to thrive) in the first 6 months of life?
    (a) Retrusive maxilla
    (b) Enamel hypoplasia
    (c) Retrusive mandible
    (d) Dentinogenesis imperfecta

    Answer for Q 51 on page 56

---

[2] Is the deficiency of calcium, phosphorus or vitamin D

52. A 4-year-old child has a normal complement of primary teeth, but they are gray and exhibit extensive occlusal and incisal wear. Radiographic examination indicates extensive deposits of secondary dentin in these teeth. This condition is most likely:
    (a) Neonatal hypoplasia
    (b) Amelogenesis imperfecta
    (c) Cleidocranial dysplasia
    (d) Dentinogenesis imperfecta

    Answer for Q 52 on page 56

53. A developmental abnormality characterized by the presence of fewer than the usual number of teeth is:
    (a) Anodontia
    (b) Oligodontia
    (c) Microdontia
    (d) Dens in dente

    Answer for Q 53 on page 56

54. Most commonly submerged tooth (ankylosed) is:
    (a) Mandibular primary first molar
    (b) Mandibular primary second molar
    (c) Maxillary primary first molar
    (d) Maxillary primary second molar

    Answer for Q 54 on page 57

55. A dens in dente is caused by:
    (a) An abnormal proliferation of pulp tissue
    (b) Denticle formation within the pulp tissue
    (c) A deep invagination of the enamel organ during formation
    (d) A supernumerary tooth bud enclaved within a normal tooth

    Answer for Q 55 on page 57

56. The most frequently missing permanent teeth are:
    (a) First premolars
    (b) Second premolars
    (c) Maxillary lateral incisors
    (d) Mandibular lateral incisors

    Answer for Q 56 on page 57

57. Hutchinson's incisors are present in:
    (a) Congenital syphilis
    (b) Tertiary syphilis
    (c) Secondary syphilis
    (d) Acquired syphilis

    Answer for Q 57 on page 57

58. Odontodysplasia is most common in:
    (a) Mandibular premolar
    (b) Mandibular canine
    (c) Mandibular third molar
    (d) Maxillary central and lateral incisor

    Answer for Q 58 on page 57

59. In children the most frequently missing permanent teeth are:
    (a) First premolars
    (b) Second premolars
    (c) Maxillary lateral incisors
    (d) Mandibular lateral incisors

    Answer for Q 59 on page 57

60. Which of the following is **not** hereditary?
    (a) Amelogenesis imperfecta
    (b) Cleidocranial dysostosis
    (c) Regional odontodysplasia
    (d) Dentinogenesis imperfecta

    Answer for Q 60 on page 57

61. The second most common supernumerary tooth is:
    (a) Mesiodens
    (b) Distal to third molar in maxilla
    (c) Distal to mandibular third molar
    (d) Paramolars

    Answer for Q 61 on page 57

62. Turner's hypoplasia most commonly affects:
    (a) Deciduous maxillary anteriors
    (b) Deciduous mandibular anteriors
    (c) Permanent maxillary anteriors
    (d) Permanent mandibular anteriors

Answer for Q 62 on page 57

63. Shell teeth are more common in this variant of dentinogenesis imperfecta:
    (a) Type I
    (b) Type II
    (c) Type III
    (d) Type III and I

Answer for Q 63 on page 57

64. Complete obliteration of pulp is seen in all **except**:
    (a) Type I dentinogenesis imperfecta
    (b) Type II dentinogenesis imperfecta
    (c) Type III dentinogenesis imperfecta
    (d) Dentin Dysplasia

Answer for Q 64 on page 57

65. Which of the following is **unlikely** to cause enamel hypoplasia?
    (a) Rickets
    (b) Fluoride
    (c) Congenital syphilis
    (d) Cleidocranial dysostosis

Answer for Q 65 on page 57

66. Mulberry molars are characteristic features of:
    (a) Severe fluorosis
    (b) Trauma at the time of birth
    (c) Congenital Syphilis
    (d) Due to chronic suppurative abscess in overlying gingival tissue

Answer for Q 66 on page 57

67. Talon's cusp is characteristic of which syndrome?

    (a) Edward's syndrome

    (b) Klinefelter's syndrome[3]

    (c) Rubinstein-Taybi Syndrome[4]

    (d) Down's Syndrome

    Answer for Q 67 on page 57

68. Thistle tube appearance of pulp chamber is a feature of (see the associated image below):

    (a) Coronal dentin dysplasia particularly type II

    (b) Regional odontodysplasia

    (c) Dentinogenesis imperfecta

    (d) Amelogenesis imperfecta

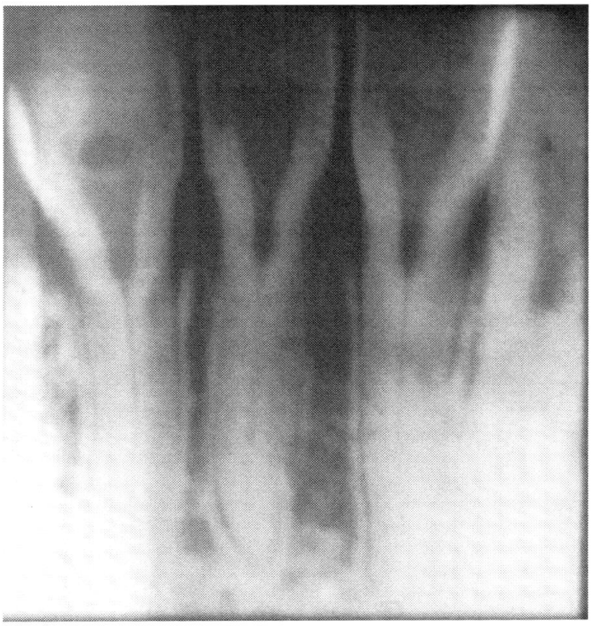

Answer for Q 68 on page 57

69. Which of the following conditions is characterized by abnormally large pulp chambers?

    (a) Amelogenesis imperfecta

    (b) Regional odontodysplasia

    (c) Dentinogenesis imperfecta

    (d) Dentinal dysplasia type I

    Answer for Q 69 on page 57

[3] A male with an extra X chromosome to be XXY

[4] Characterized by short stature, moderate to severe intellectual disability, distinctive facial features, and dental anomalies.

70. Which of the following teeth is most likely to be congenitally missing?
    (a) Maxillary lateral incisor
    (b) Mandibular canine
    (c) Mandibular second premolar
    (d) Maxillary first premolar

    Answer for Q 70 on page 57

71. Which of the following dentitions shows the highest frequency of occurrence of supernumerary teeth?
    (a) Maxillary deciduous dentition
    (b) Maxillary permanent dentition
    (c) Mandibular deciduous dentition
    (d) Mandibular permanent dentition

    Answer for Q 71 on page 58

72. The most common inheritance pattern of dentinogenesis imperfecta is:
    (a) Homozygous
    (b) Autosomal dominant
    (c) Recessive
    (d) X-linked recessive

    Answer for Q 72 on page 58

73. Large pulp chambers are characteristic of all the following conditions **except**:
    (a) Shell teeth
    (b) Taurodontism
    (c) Dentin dysplasia
    (d) Dentinogenesis imperfecta

    Answer for Q 73 on page 58

74. Dens in dente is commonly seen in:
    (a) Premolars
    (b) Paramolars
    (c) Lateral incisors
    (d) Maxillary canine

    Answer for Q 74 on page 58

75. Taurodontism is usually seen in:
    (a) Mesiodens
    (b) Incisor with talon/cusp
    (c) Mandibular first molar
    (d) Maxillary premolars

    Answer for Q 75 on page 58

76. Which one of the following is the cause of dilacerations?
    (a) Trauma to the tooth germ during root development
    (b) Abnormal displacement of tooth germ during root development
    (c) Abnormal proliferation of enamel epithelium during tooth development
    (d) Abnormal displacement of ameloblasts during tooth formation

    Answer for Q 76 on page 58

77. Dentinal union of two embryologically developing teeth is referred as:
    (a) Gemination
    (b) Twinning
    (c) Concrescence
    (d) Fusion

    Answer for Q 77 on page 58

78. In hypodontia, the most commonly affected tooth is:
    (a) Permanent third molar
    (b) Permanent second premolar
    (c) Permanent lateral incisor
    (d) Permanent Canine

    Answer for Q 78 on page 58

79. Submerged teeth (ankylosed) are:
    (a) Ankylosed teeth
    (b) Unerupted teeth
    (c) Impacted teeth
    (d) Intruded teeth

    Answer for Q 79 on page 58

80. The histological appearance of "lava flowing around boulders in dentin dysplasia" suggests:

    (a) Attempt to repair the defective dentin

    (b) Abrupt arrest to dentin formation in crown

    (c) Abnormal dentin formation in disorganized fashion

    (d) Cascades of dentin to form root

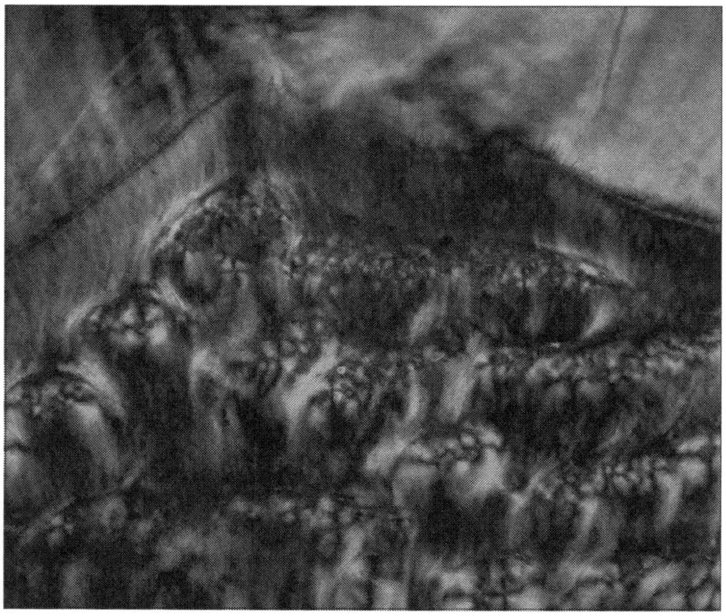

Answer for Q 80 on page 58

81. A four-year-old child with one tooth less than the normal dentition shows a large tooth with two crowns and two root canals. The anomaly is:

    (a) Dilaceration

    (b) Fusion

    (c) Concrescence

    (d) Gemination

Answer for Q 81 on page 58

82. A 6-year-old patient with extra cusp on maxillary central incisor is associated with all **except**:

    (a) Mohr's syndrome

    (b) Sturge-Weber syndrome

    (c) Rubinstein Taybi Syndrome

    (d) Proteus Syndrome

Answer for Q 82 on page 58

83. Taurodontism is seen in:
   (a) Klinefelter's syndrome
   (b) Sturge-Weber syndrome
   (c) Down syndrome
   (d) Turner syndrome

Answer for Q 83 on page 58

84. A girl suffering from browning of teeth, wearing of enamel but not cavitory. OPG shows obliteration of pulp with narrowing of canal and deposition of secondary dentin, she gave the history that out of her four brothers, 2 are suffering from the same disease. She is suffering from:
   (a) Amelogenesis imperfecta
   (b) Dentinogenesis imperfecta
   (c) Fluorosis
   (d) Odontodysplasia

Answer for Q 84 on page 58

85. Developmental hereditary enamel defects are most commonly seen in:
   (a) Primary dentition
   (b) Secondary dentition
   (c) Both primary and secondary dentition
   (d) None of the above

Answer for Q 85 on page 58

86. A 7-year-old child has yellowish discolored spot of maxillary central incisor. His mother mentioned a history of injury to deciduous tooth three years back with recurrent infections and swelling. The diagnosis is:
   (a) Turner's hypoplasia
   (b) Generalized dental fluorosis
   (c) Syphilitic hypoplasia
   (d) Rickets hypomineralization

Answer for Q 86 on page 58

87. Marked reduction in amount of dentin, widening of predentin layer, presence of large area of interglobular dentin and irregular pattern of dentin is seen in:
    (a) Hypocalcified dentin
    (b) Odontodysplasia
    (c) Dentin dysplasia
    (d) Dentinogenesis imperfecta

    Answer for Q 87 on page 59

88. Amelogenesis imperfecta is a disorder of:
    (a) Ectoderm
    (b) Mesoderm
    (c) Endoderm
    (d) Ecto and Mesoderm

    Answer for Q 88 on page 59

89. Hypodontia is mainly found in all, **except**:
    (a) Papillon-Lefevre syndrome
    (b) Osteopetrosis
    (c) Cleidocranial dysostosis
    (d) Ectodermal dysplasia

    Answer for Q 89 on page 59

90. Supernumerary tooth, tooth within tooth is most commonly seen in:
    (a) Mandibular second premolar
    (b) Maxillary lateral incisors
    (c) Mandibular incisors
    (d) Mandibular central and lateral incisors

    Answer for Q 90 on page 59

91. Osteogenesis imperfecta is often associated with one of the following dental abnormalities
    (a) Amelogenesis imperfecta
    (b) Dentinogenesis imperfecta
    (c) Regional odontodysplasia
    (d) Environmental enamel hypoplasia

    Answer for Q 91 on page 59

92. The clinical findings of opalescent teeth, blue sclera and multiple bone fractures in a patient are more suggestive of
    (a) Cleidocranial dysplasia
    (b) Osteopetrosis
    (c) Osteoporosis
    (d) Osteogenic imperfecta

    Answer for Q 92 on page 59

93. Which term refers to the developmental anomaly that arises when a single tooth germ attempts to divide and results in the incomplete formation of two teeth?
    (a) Fusion
    (b) Gemination
    (c) Concrescence
    (d) Dilaceration

    Answer for Q 93 on page 59

94. Which term refers to a developmental anomaly in which teeth exhibit elongated, large pulp chamber and short root?
    (a) Dentinogenesis imperfecta
    (b) Amelogenesis imperfecta
    (c) Concrescence
    (d) Taurodontism

    Answer for Q 94 on page 59

95. Which of the following is the cause of concrescence?
    (a) Crowding of teeth
    (b) Hereditary
    (c) Fluoride intake
    (d) Enamel hypoplasia

    Answer for Q 95 on page 59

96. Tetracycline taken during development is deposited in:
    (a) Enamel rods
    (b) Incremental lines of dentin
    (c) Enamel tufts
    (d) Enamel surface

    Answer for Q 96 on page 59

97. Delayed shedding of deciduous teeth and delayed eruption of permanent teeth are seen in:

(a) Facial hemihypertrophy

(b) Streeter's syndrome (hereditary ectodermal dysplasia)

(c) Cleidocranial dysplasia

(d) Congenital syphilis

Answer for Q 97 on page 59

98. A trauma to a tooth during development may lead to:

(a) Dilacerations

(b) Hutchinson's incisors

(c) Supernumerary teeth

(d) Talon cusp

Answer for Q 98 on page 59

99. Turner's teeth are a condition caused by Enamel hypoplasia due to:

(a) Hypocalcemia

(b) Birth injury

(c) Congenital syphilis

(d) Local infection or trauma

Answer for Q 99 on page 59

100. "Screw driver" shaped incisors with notched incisal edge are seen in:

(a) Amelogenesis imperfect

(b) Dentinogenesis imperfect

(c) Cleidocranial dysplasia

(d) Congenital syphilis

Answer for Q 100 on page 59

101. Complete obliteration of the pulp chamber by pulp stones occurs in:

(a) Amelogenesis imperfecta

(b) Shell tooth

(c) Dentinogenesis imperfecta

(d) Microdontia

Answer for Q 101 on page 59

102. In hypoplastic type of amelogenesis imperfecta there is a defect in:
   (a) Formation of enamel matrix
   (b) Maturation of Hydroxyapatite crystals
   (c) Mineralization of enamel matrix
   (d) Mineralization and maturation of Hydroxyapatite crystals

   Answer for Q 102 on page 59

103. Congenital syphilis is:
   (a) Acquired non developmental disease
   (b) Acquired developmental disease
   (c) Developmental hereditary disease
   (d) Results from chromosomal abnormalities

   Answer for Q 103 on page 60

104. Hypoplastic teeth due to local infection or trauma are known as :
   (a) Fournier's molars
   (b) Hutchinson's teeth
   (c) Mulberry molars
   (d) Turner's teeth

   Answer for Q 104 on page 60

105. Multiple unerupted supernumerary teeth are seen in:
   (a) Craniofacial dysostosis
   (b) Cleidocranial dysplasia
   (c) Pierre-Robin syndrome
   (d) Treacher Collins syndrome

   Answer for Q 105 on page 60

106. The stigmata of congenital syphilis **do not** include:
   (a) Cleft lip
   (b) Eighth nerve deafness
   (c) Interstitial keratitis
   (d) Rhagades

   Answer for Q 106 on page 60

107. Shell tooth may be a characteristic feature of:

(a) Amelogenesis imperfecta

(b) Dentinogenesis imperfecta

(c) Dental fluorosis

(d) Dentinal dysplasia

Answer for Q 107 on page 60

108. Gemination may be observed as a dental manifestation in one of the following syndromes:

(a) Cleidocranial dysplasia

(b) Gardener syndrome

(c) Pierre Robin syndrome

(d) Streeter's syndrome (hereditary ectodermal dysplasia)

Answer for Q 108 on page 60

109. Initiation and positioning of tooth bud is determined by:

(a) MSX1 gene

(b) MSX2 gene

(c) PAX9 Gene

(d) None of the above

Answer for Q 109 on page 60

110. Tetracycline taken during development is deposited in:

(a) Bone

(b) Dentin

(c) Enamel

(d) All of the above

Answer for Q 110 on page 60

111. The most commonly inherited form of amelogenesis imperfecta is:

(a) Autosomal dominant pattern

(b) Autosomal recessive pattern

(c) X-linked pattern

(d) Y-linked pattern

Answer for Q 111 on page 60

112. The coexistence of amelogenesis imperfecta and anterior open bite can be due to:

(a) A pleiotropic action of the AI genes, influencing the growth of the craniofacial skeleton.

(b) Alterations in the eruption mechanism

(c) Local mechanical interference by the tongue to guard against thermal stimuli

(d) All of the above

(e) None of the above

Answer for Q 112 on page 60

113. Microdontia can occur as a part of some of the following genetic diseases:

(a) Ectodermal dysplasia

(b) Down syndrome

(c) Focal dermal hypoplasia syndrome

(d) Congenital hypopituitarism

(e) All of the above

Answer for Q 113 on page 60

114. Complications affecting partially erupted teeth are:

(a) Pericoronitis

(b) Formation of apical cysts

(c) Induction of malignant tumors

(d) Induction of osteomyelitis

(e) Formation of odontogenic tumors

Answer for Q 114 on page 60

115. All of the following can cause macrodontia **except**:

(a) XYY male

(b) Pituitary dwarfism

(c) Otodental syndrome

(d) Pituitary gigantism

(e) Facial hemihypertrophy

Answer for Q 115 on page 60

116. A 15-year-old boy came to your clinic complaining of severe attrition of his teeth. Clinical examination revealed loss of enamel with wearing of the teeth crowns to the gum margins with loss of vertical di-

mension. Radiographic examination revealed obliteration of the pulp with relatively short roots. The most possible diagnosis for this case is:

(a) Amelogenesis imperfecta

(b) Regional odontodysplasia

(c) Dentinogenesis imperfecta

(d) Dilaceration

Answer for Q 116 on page 60

117. In the above mentioned case (Q 116), the suggested etiology will be:

(a) Environmental causes

(b) Autosomal dominant

(c) X-linked recessive

(d) Chromosomal abnormalities

Answer for Q 117 on page 60

118. A 12-year-old girl was referred to your clinic complaining of delayed eruption of the upper left central incisor, lateral incisor and canine. There was no history of tooth or genetic anomalies in the family. The child's general health was good and no congenital or acquired disease was reported. Radiographic examination revealed shadows of malformed unerupted teeth in the affected quadrant. The most possible diagnosis for this case is:

(a) Amelogenesis imperfecta

(b) Regional odontodysplasia

(c) Dentinogenesis imperfecta

(d) Congenital syphilis

Answer for Q 118 on page 60

2.2 Answers with Comments:

1. The correct answer is **A** – Regional odontodysplasia radiographically appears as ghost of teeth and hence the term ghost teeth was given.

Back to Q 1 on page 27

2. The correct answer is **A** – Amalgam in this case is considered as an external stain as it is a stain not found naturally within the human body as for example bilirubin.

Back to Q 2 on page 27

3. The correct answer is **A.** Tooth development is a complex process which involves a combination of genetic, epigenetic, and environmental factors. Many genes are involved in the process of odontogenesis. The most notable ones are PAX9 and MSX1 genes.

Back to Q 3 on page 28

4. The correct answer is **C** – Double teeth is the term applied to cases of fusion and gemination. Double teeth are more common in the primary than in the permanent dentition, the prevalence in different series ranging from 0.5–2.5 percent for the primary and 0.1–0.2 percent for the permanent dentitions. The incisors (and also the canines in the primary dentition) are most frequently affected, and the condition may be bilaterally symmetrical. In the primary dentition, the majority of cases involve the anterior mandibular teeth.

Back to Q 4 on page 28

5. The correct answer is **D** – In enamel hypoplasia, the defect is mainly in matrix formation. The ameloblasts fail to produce a standard volume of the matrix, but any produced matrix generally becomes as fully mineralized as normal enamel. Enamel hypoplasia presents clinically as pits, grooves, or fissures in the enamel surface or as a general decrease in the thickness of the whole enamel. The defective enamel has fewer prisms than normal, and they may run in abnormal directions. In some cases, no prism structure can be seen (loss of prismatic structure, so-called prismless enamel).

Back to Q 5 on page 28

6. The correct answer is **A.** Tooth development is a complex process which involves a combination of genetic, epigenetic, and environmental factors. Many genes are involved in the process of odontogenesis. The most notable ones are PAX9 and MSX1 genes.

Back to Q 6 on page 28

7. The correct answer is **D.** In pituitary dwarfism all body organs are small.

Back to Q 7 on page 28

8. The correct answer is **B.** No explanation is available for this answer.

Back to Q 8 on page 29

9. The correct answer is **A.** Hypoplastic enamel results from insufficient matrix formation.

Back to Q 9 on page 29

10. The correct answer is **C.** No explanation is available for this answer.

Back to Q 10 on page 29

11. The correct answer is **A.** No explanation is available for this answer.

Back to Q 11 on page 29

12. The correct answer is **B.** No explanation is available for this answer.

Back to Q 12 on page 29

13. The correct answer is **C** – Hypomineralized enamel results from a failure of the ameloblasts to fully calcify the previously formed matrix, and in general, such enamel appears clinically as white and opaque. After the eruption, it may become pigmented buff, yellow, or brown, fast chipped and worn away.

    Back to Q 13 on page 29

14. The correct answer is **C** – Concrescence is a disorder in which the roots of one or more teeth are fused by cementum alone after the formation of the crowns. The proposed cause is the crowding of teeth in the jaw. This is most frequently seen in the permanent dentition where the roots of teeth develop close together (for example, between maxillary second and third molars) or following hypercementosis associated with chronic inflammation.

    Back to Q 14 on page 30

15. The correct answer is **C** – The mineralization process in congenital syphilis is not the primary issue. This disease produces characteristic hypoplastic changes and malformation in the enamel of permanent incisors and first molars due to infection of the tooth germ by Spirochetes. The distal and mesial surfaces of the incisors converge towards the incisal edges rather than toward the cervical margin, giving the characteristic "screwdriver" appearance, and the incisal edges are usually notched (Hutchinson's incisors). These peculiar changes are most evident in the maxillary central incisors. The occlusal surfaces and occlusal thirds of the crowns of the first molars are covered by small cuspules of enamel (Moon's molars or mulberry molars).

    Back to Q 15 on page 30

16. The correct answer is **C** – Hypoplasia and aplasia of cementum are rare. In cleidocranial dysplasia, there is a lack of cellular cementum following the deposition of acellular cementum.

    Back to Q 16 on page 30

17. The correct answer is **A.** No explanation is available for this answer.

    Back to Q 17 on page 30

18. The correct answer is **C.** Fusion is associated with decrease in number of teeth by one, except if one of the fused teeth is a supernumerary one.

    Back to Q 18 on page 30

19. The correct answer is **E**: It is essential to avoid tetracyclines from day zero to about 12 years of age if severe clinical discoloration of both primary and permanent dentition is to be avoided. Avoid tetracyclines from 4 months to about 12 years of age if severe clinical discoloration of the permanent dentition is to be avoided [3].

    Back to Q 19 on page 31

20. The correct answer is **C**: No explanation is available for this answer.

    Back to Q 20 on page 31

21. The correct answer is **A**: No explanation is available for this answer.

    Back to Q 21 on page 31

22. The correct answer is **A**: No explanation is available for this answer.

    Back to Q 22 on page 32

23. The correct answer is **B**: No explanation is available for this answer, Source: [2].

    Back to Q 23 on page 32

24. The correct answer is **D**: No explanation is available for this answer.

    Back to Q 24 on page 32

25. The correct answer is **C**: No explanation is available for this answer.

    Back to Q 25 on page 32

26. The correct answer is **B**: No explanation is available for this answer.

    Back to Q 26 on page 32

27. The correct answer is **A**: No explanation is available for this answer.

    Back to Q 27 on page 32

28. The correct answer is **A**: No explanation is available for this answer.

    Back to Q 28 on page 33

29. The correct answer is **C**: No explanation is available for this answer.

    Back to Q 29 on page 33

30. The correct answer is **B**: No explanation is available for this answer.

    Back to Q 30 on page 33

31. The correct answer is **A**: No explanation is available for this answer.

    Back to Q 31 on page 33

32. The correct answer is **B**: No explanation is available for this answer.

    Back to Q 32 on page 33

33. The correct answer is **B**: No explanation is available for this answer.

    Back to Q 33 on page 34

34. The correct answer is **D**: No explanation is available for this answer.

    Back to Q 34 on page 34

35. The correct answer is **B**: No explanation is available for this answer.

    Back to Q 35 on page 34

36. The correct answer is **D**: No explanation is available for this answer.

    Back to Q 36 on page 34

37. The correct answer is **A**: No explanation is available for this answer.

Back to Q 37 on page 34

38. The correct answer is **A**: No explanation is available for this answer.

Back to Q 38 on page 35

39. The correct answer is **B**: No explanation is available for this answer.

Back to Q 39 on page 35

40. The correct answer is **B**: In false anodontia, the tooth develops normally but fails to erupt.

Back to Q 40 on page 35

41. The correct answer is **D**: No explanation is available for this answer.

Back to Q 41 on page 35

42. The correct answer is **A**: No explanation is available for this answer.

Back to Q 42 on page 35

43. The correct answer is **B**: No explanation is available for this answer.

Back to Q 43 on page 36

44. The correct answer is **B**: No explanation is available for this answer.

Back to Q 44 on page 36

45. The correct answer is **D**: No explanation is available for this answer.

Back to Q 45 on page 36

46. The correct answer is **A**: No explanation is available for this answer.

Back to Q 46 on page 36

47. The correct answer is **B**: No explanation is available for this answer.

Back to Q 47 on page 36

48. The correct answer is **B**: No explanation is available for this answer.

Back to Q 48 on page 37

49. The correct answer is **C**: No explanation is available for this answer.

Back to Q 49 on page 37

50. The correct answer is **B**: No explanation is available for this answer.

Back to Q 50 on page 37

51. The correct answer is **D**: No explanation is available for this answer.

Back to Q 51 on page 37

52. The correct answer is **D**: No explanation is available for this answer.

Back to Q 52 on page 37

53. The correct answer is **B**: No explanation is available for this answer.

Back to Q 53 on page 38

54. The correct answer is **A**: No explanation is available for this answer.

Back to Q 54 on page 38

55. The correct answer is **C**: No explanation is available for this answer.

Back to Q 55 on page 38

56. The correct answer is **C**: No explanation is available for this answer.

Back to Q 56 on page 38

57. The correct answer is **A**: No explanation is available for this answer.

Back to Q 57 on page 38

58. The correct answer is **D**: No explanation is available for this answer.

Back to Q 58 on page 39

59. The correct answer is **C**: No explanation is available for this answer.

Back to Q 59 on page 39

60. The correct answer is **C**: No explanation is available for this answer.

Back to Q 60 on page 39

61. The correct answer is **D**: No explanation is available for this answer.

Back to Q 61 on page 39

62. The correct answer is **C**: No explanation is available for this answer.

Back to Q 62 on page 39

63. The correct answer is **C**: No explanation is available for this answer.

Back to Q 63 on page 40

64. The correct answer is **A**: No explanation is available for this answer.

Back to Q 64 on page 40

65. The correct answer is **A**: No explanation is available for this answer.

Back to Q 65 on page 40

66. The correct answer is **C**: No explanation is available for this answer.

Back to Q 66 on page 40

67. The correct answer is **C**: No explanation is available for this answer.

Back to Q 67 on page 40

68. The correct answer is **A**: No explanation is available for this answer.

Back to Q 68 on page 41

69. The correct answer is **C**: Some variants of dentinogenesis imperfecta (shell tooth) is characterized by wide pulp chamber.

Back to Q 69 on page 41

70. The correct answer is **A**: No explanation is available for this answer.

Back to Q 70 on page 42

71. The correct answer is **B**: No explanation is available for this answer.

Back to Q 71 on page 42

72. The correct answer is **B**: No explanation is available for this answer.

Back to Q 72 on page 42

73. The correct answer is **D**: No explanation is available for this answer.

Back to Q 73 on page 42

74. The correct answer is **C**: No explanation is available for this answer.

Back to Q 74 on page 42

75. The correct answer is **C**: No explanation is available for this answer.

Back to Q 75 on page 42

76. The correct answer is **A**: No explanation is available for this answer.

Back to Q 76 on page 43

77. The correct answer is **D**: No explanation is available for this answer.

Back to Q 77 on page 43

78. The correct answer is **C**: No explanation is available for this answer.

Back to Q 78 on page 43

79. The correct answer is **A**: No explanation is available for this answer.

Back to Q 79 on page 43

80. The correct answer is **C**: No explanation is available for this answer.

Back to Q 80 on page 43

81. The correct answer is **B**: No explanation is available for this answer.

Back to Q 81 on page 44

82. The correct answer is **C**: No explanation is available for this answer.

Back to Q 82 on page 44

83. The correct answer is **A**: No explanation is available for this answer.

Back to Q 83 on page 45

84. The correct answer is **B**: No explanation is available for this answer.

Back to Q 84 on page 45

85. The correct answer is **C**: No explanation is available for this answer.

Back to Q 85 on page 45

86. The correct answer is **A**: No explanation is available for this answer.

Back to Q 86 on page 40

87. The correct answer is **D**: No explanation is available for this answer.

Back to Q 87 on page 45

88. The correct answer is **A**: No explanation is available for this answer.

Back to Q 88 on page 46

89. The correct answer is **A**: No explanation is available for this answer.

Back to Q 89 on page 46

90. The correct answer is **B**: No explanation is available for this answer.

Back to Q 90 on page 46

91. The correct answer is **B**: No explanation is available for this answer.

Back to Q 91 on page 46

92. The correct answer is **C**: No explanation is available for this answer.

Back to Q 92 on page 46

93. The correct answer is **B**: No explanation is available for this answer.

Back to Q 93 on page 47

94. The correct answer is **D**: No explanation is available for this answer.

Back to Q 94 on page 47

95. The correct answer is **A**: No explanation is available for this answer.

Back to Q 95 on page 47

96. The correct answer is **B**: No explanation is available for this answer.

Back to Q 96 on page 47

97. The correct answer is **C**: No explanation is available for this answer.

Back to Q 97 on page 47

98. The correct answer is **A**: No explanation is available for this answer.

Back to Q 98 on page 48

99. The correct answer is **D**: No explanation is available for this answer.

Back to Q 99 on page 48

100. The correct answer is **D**: No explanation is available for this answer.

Back to Q 100 on page 48

101. The correct answer is **C**: No explanation is available for this answer.

Back to Q 101 on page 48

102. The correct answer is **A**: No explanation is available for this answer.

Back to Q 102 on page 48

103. The correct answer is **B**: No explanation is available for this answer.

Back to Q 103 on page 49

104. The correct answer is **D**: No explanation is available for this answer.

Back to Q 104 on page 49

105. The correct answer is **B**: No explanation is available for this answer.

Back to Q 105 on page 49

106. The correct answer is **A**: No explanation is available for this answer.

Back to Q 106 on page 49

107. The correct answer is **B**: No explanation is available for this answer.

Back to Q 107 on page 49

108. The correct answer is **A**: No explanation is available for this answer.

Back to Q 108 on page 50

109. The correct answer is **C**: No explanation is available for this answer.

Back to Q 109 on page 50

110. The correct answer is **D**: No explanation is available for this answer.

Back to Q 110 on page 50

111. The correct answer is **A**: About 5% of amelogenesis imperfecta cases are caused by mutations in the AMELX gene and are inherited in an X-linked pattern.

Back to Q 111 on page 50

112. The correct answer is **D**: No explanation is available for this answer.

Back to Q 112 on page 50

113. The correct answer is **E**: No explanation is available for this answer.

Back to Q 113 on page 51

114. The correct answer is **A**: No explanation is available for this answer.

Back to Q 114 on page 51

115. The correct answer is **B**: No explanation is available for this answer.

Back to Q 115 on page 51

116. The correct answer is C: No explanation is available for this answer.

Back to Q 116 on page 51

117. The correct answer is B: No explanation is available for this answer.

Back to Q 117 on page 52

118. The correct answer is B: No explanation is available for this answer.

Back to Q 118 on page 52

Chapter 3
Developmental Disturbances of Soft Tissues

In this chapter, questions relevant to the developmental disturbances affecting the soft tissues and hard tissues except teeth that is related to oral and paraoral structures.

3.1 MCQs Questions

Choose **one or more** of the most appropriate answers. Some questions may have **more than one** correct answer. You have to choose all the correct answers as best as you can.

1. Which of the following conditions is **NOT** an ectopic condition?
   (a) Fordyce's granules
   (b) Latent bone cyst
   (c) White spongy nevus
   (d) Lingual thyroid nodule
   Answer for Q 1 on page 82
2. Transverse facial cleft is due to failure of fusion between:
   (a) maxillary and mandibular processes
   (b) maxillary and medial nasal processes
   (c) medial nasal and lateral nasal processes
   (d) maxillary and lateral nasal processes
   Answer for Q 2 on page 82
3. All the following are considered as ectopic conditions **except**:
   (a) Fordyce's granules
   (b) torus palatinus
   (c) enamel pearl
   (d) lingual thyroid nodule
   Answer for Q 3 on page 82

4. Loss of tongue papillae occurs in:
   (a) black hairy tongue
   (b) lingual thyroid nodule
   (c) median rhomboid glossitis
   (d) tongue hypermobility

   Answer for Q 4 on page 82

5. Bohn's nodules are
   (a) same as enamel pearls
   (b) imperfection in the tooth bud
   (c) seen in vitamin D deficiency
   (d) small keratin cysts of newborn infant

   Answer for Q 5 on page 82

6. Psoriasiform mucositis is the term that is sometimes used to describe benign migratory glossitis. This is because:
   (a) Frequent presence of suprabasilar clefts
   (b) Frequent presence of subepithelial dense lymphocytic band
   (c) Frequent presence of Munro abscess in the epithelium
   (d) Frequent presence of Munro abscess in the epithelium

   Answer for Q 6 on page 82

7. Inflammation of the lips is referred to as:
   (a) Stomatitis
   (b) Glossitis migrican
   (c) Cheilitis
   (d) Vincent Angina
   (e) Sialadenitis

   Answer for Q 7 on page 82

8. Early closure of sutures is a common feature of:
   (a) Pierre Robin syndrome
   (b) Melkersson Rosenthal syndrome
   (c) Down syndrome
   (d) Crouzon syndrome

   Answer for Q 8 on page 82

9. Paralysis of the tongue is referred to as:
   (a) Ankyloglossia
   (b) Glossoplegia
   (c) Macroglossia
   (d) Pyroglossia
   (e) Geographic tongue

   Answer for Q 9 on page 82

10. Failure of the tuberculum impar to retract prior to fusion of the lateral halves of the tongue results in:
    (a) Median rhomboid glossitis
    (b) Cleft (bifid) tongue
    (c) Geographic tongue
    (d) Scrotal tongue
    (e) Sarcoma of tongue

    Answer for Q 10 on page 82

11. Macrognathia could be associated with the following conditions **except**:
    (a) Acromegaly
    (b) Facial hemihypertrophy
    (c) Paget's disease
    (d) Pierre-Robin syndrome

    Answer for Q 11 on page 82

12. Geographic tongue is characterized by:
    (a) atrophy of fungiform and persistence of filiform papilla
    (b) atrophy of foliate and persistence of circumvallate papilla
    (c) atrophy of foliate and persistence of filiform papilla
    (d) atrophy of filiform and persistence of fungiform papilla

    Answer for Q 12 on page 82

13. The Melkersson-Rosenthal syndrome is characterized by facial paralysis, Cheilitis granulomatosa, and:
    (a) Black Hairy tongue
    (b) Scrotal tongue
    (c) Geographic tongue
    (d) Bifid tongue
    (e) White Hairy tongue

    Answer for Q 13 on page 82

14. The main difference between Apert and Crouzon syndrome is:
    (a) pseudocleft of palate
    (b) premature suture closure
    (c) fused fingers
    (d) hypoplasia of the maxilla

    Answer for Q 14 on page 82

15. Cleft lip and cleft palate main **features**:
    (a) The cleft lip results from failure of fusion of the maxillary process with the median nasal process.
    (b) Flattening of the nostril is a feature
    (c) The nasal septum may be abnormally thick.
    (d) The deformities result from teratogenic or genetic factors operating in the second month of fetal life.
    (e) Bifid uvula is a minor form.

    Answer for Q 15 on page 82

16. Which of the following conditions is NOT an ectopic condition?
    (a) Fordyce's granules
    (b) Latent bone cyst
    (c) White spongy nevus
    (d) Lingual thyroid nodule

    Answer for Q 16 on page 83

17. One of the following conditions is caused by somatic mutation:
    (a) Treacher Collins syndrome
    (b) Crouzon syndrome
    (c) Albright's syndrome
    (d) Pierre Robin syndrome

    Answer for Q 17 on page 83

18. One the following conditions is hereditary:
    (a) Leukoedema
    (b) Ankyloglossia
    (c) Witkop's disease
    (d) Congenital syphilis

    Answer for Q 18 on page 83

19. Which term refers to a defect present at birth?
    (a) Inherited defect
    (b) Acquired defect
    (c) Congenital defect
    (d) Developmental defect

    Answer for Q 19 on page 83

20. Regarding cleft lip and palate, one of the following statements is **correct**:
    (a) They are example of multi-factorial inheritance
    (b) Cleft upper lip is always associated with cleft palate
    (c) Cleft palate is always associated with cleft upper lip
    (d) None of the above

    Answer for Q 20 on page 83

21. Which of the following developmental defects is considered as ectopic condition?
    (a) Torus palatinus
    (b) Lingual thyroid nodule
    (c) Congenital lip pit
    (d) Ankyloglossia

    Answer for Q 21 on page 83

22. The classic triad of Pierre Robin syndrome includes mandibular hypoplasia, cleft palate and:
    (a) microglossia
    (b) macroglossia
    (c) ankyloglossia
    (d) glossoptosis

    Answer for Q 22 on page 83

23. One of the following conditions is due to failure of migration of neural crest cells:
    (a) Melkersson-Rosenthal syndrome
    (b) Crouzon's syndrome
    (c) Treacher Collins syndrome
    (d) Albright's syndrome

    Answer for Q 23 on page 83

24. Fordyce's Spots are due to:
    (a) improper fusion of the embryonic processes
    (b) presence of sweat glands in the oral mucosa
    (c) improper maturation of the oral epithelium
    (d) presence of sebaceous glands in the oral mucosa

    Answer for Q 24 on page 83
25. Fissured tongue is one of the clinical feature associated with:
    (a) Gardener's syndrome
    (b) Crouzon's syndrome
    (c) Pierre Robin's syndrome
    (d) Down's syndrome –

    Answer for Q 25 on page 83
26. One of the following hereditary conditions is transmitted as autosomal recessive disorder:
    (a) Xeroderma pigmentosa
    (b) Cleidocranial dysplasia
    (c) Dentinogenesis imperfecta
    (d) Peutz-Jegher's syndrome

    Answer for Q 26 on page 83
27. Basket weave appearance is a common histological feature of:
    (a) Fordyce's granules
    (b) Chelitis granulomatosa
    (c) White spongy nevus
    (d) Chelitis glandularis

    Answer for Q 27 on page 83
28. One of the following disorders is considered as precancerous condition:
    (a) White spongy nevus
    (b) Fibromatosis gingivae
    (c) Chelitis glandularis
    (d) Lingual thyroid nodule

    Answer for Q 28 on page 83

29. One of the following conditions is associated with circum-oral melanin pigmentation:
    (a) Melanotic neuroectodermal tumor
    (b) Pigmented nevus
    (c) Xeroderma pigmentosa
    (d) Peutz-Jegher syndrome –

    Answer for Q 29 on page 83

30. One the following conditions is non-developmental condition:
    (a) Leukoedema
    (b) Black tongue
    (c) Witkop's disease
    (d) Congenital syphilis

    Answer for Q 30 on page 84

31. Delayed ossification of sutures and fontanelles is a common feature of:
    (a) Cleidocranial dysplasia
    (b) Cherubism
    (c) Facial fibrous dysplasia
    (d) Paget's disease of bone

    Answer for Q 31 on page 84

32. The improper posterior point of fusion of tuberculum impar and the two lateral lingual swellings (tubercles) shows the absence of:
    (a) Filiform papilla
    (b) Circumvallate papilla
    (c) Fungiform papilla
    (d) Foramen cecum

    Answer for Q 32 on page 84

33. Loss of tongue papillae occurs in:
    (a) Black hairy tongue
    (b) Lingual thyroid nodule
    (c) Median rhomboid glossitis
    (d) Tongue hypermobility

    Answer for Q 33 on page 84

34. All of the following are characteristic features of chromosomal abnormalities **except**:
    (a) Follow Medellin pattern of inheritance
    (b) May be structural or numerical
    (c) May involve autosomes or sex chromosomes
    (d) May involve deletion or duplication

    Answer for Q 34 on page 84

35. One of the following conditions is an example of multifactorial inheritance:
    (a) Crouzon syndrome
    (b) cleft lip and palate
    (c) ectodermal dysplasia
    (d) mongolism

    Answer for Q 35 on page 84

36. Langhan's giant cell is a histologic feature of:
    (a) Cheilitis glandularis
    (b) Cheilitis granulomatosa
    (c) Dyskeratosis congenita
    (d) Xeroderma pigmentosa

    Answer for Q 36 on page 84

37. Hereditary hemorrhagic telangiectasia is also known as:
    (a) Rendu-Osler Weber syndrome
    (b) Sturge-Weber syndrome
    (c) Plummer-Vinson syndrome
    (d) All of the above

    Answer for Q 37 on page 84

38. Decreased osteoclastic activity is a feature of:
    (a) Achondroplasia
    (b) Cleidocranial dysplasia
    (c) Crouzon syndrome
    (d) Osteopetrosis

    Answer for Q 38 on page 84

39. Macrognathia is associated with following conditions **except**:
    (a) Acromegaly
    (b) Fibrous dysplasia
    (c) Paget's disease
    (d) Pierre-Robin syndrome

    Answer for Q 39 on page 84

40. Geographic tongue is characterized by:
    (a) Atrophy of fungiform and persistence of filiform papilla
    (b) Atrophy of foliate and persistence of circumvallate papilla
    (c) Atrophy of foliate and persistence of filiform papilla
    (d) Atrophy of filiform and persistence of fungiform papilla

    Answer for Q 40 on page 84

41. Downs syndrome results usually from:
    (a) Chromosomal inversion
    (b) Dysjunction during meiosis
    (c) Non-dysjunction during mitosis
    (d) Non-dysjunction during meiosis

    Answer for Q 41 on page 84

42. Atrophy of the pharyngeal and gastric mucosa, spoon nails and predisposition to carcinoma in post-menopausal women are features of:
    (a) Pernicious anemia
    (b) Iron deficiency anemia
    (c) Plummer-Vinson syndrome
    (d) Sturge-Weber syndrome

    Answer for Q 42 on page 84

43. Development of the central face begin around:
    (a) 4th week
    (b) 6–7 week
    (c) 12 weeks
    (d) 18 weeks

    Answer for Q 43 on page 84

44. Condylar hyperplasia in the right side will result:
    (a) Mandibular shift the right side
    (b) Mandibular shift to the left side
    (c) Hemifacial hypertrophy
    (d) Will not have any effect on the jaw

    Answer for Q 44 on page 84

45. "Coup de sabre" is a description term to[1]:
    (a) Line of demarcation separate atrophic area of the face from normal area
    (b) Line of demarcation separate hypertrophy of the face from normal area
    (c) Abnormal enlarged area of the nose
    (d) Deviated mouth

    Answer for Q 45 on page 84

46. Macroglossia could be associated with one of the following conditions:
    (a) Pierre Robin syndrome
    (b) Apert syndrome
    (c) Down's syndrome
    (d) Acher syndrome

    Answer for Q 46 on page 85

47. The main difference between Apert and Crouzon syndromes is:
    (a) Head shape
    (b) Cleft in the palate
    (c) Fused fingers
    (d) Premature suture closure

    Answer for Q 47 on page 85

48. Mandibulofacial dysostosis is associated with the following cleft:
    (a) Oblique facial cleft
    (b) Lateral facial cleft
    (c) Median cleft of the upper lip
    (d) Median maxillary anterior alveolar clefts

    Answer for Q 48 on page 85

[1] From French en coup de sabre (literally "by/in a strike of the sword"), so-called because of its resemblance to the scar of a sabre wound.

49. Van der Woude syndrome has all of the following **Except**:
    - (a) Cleft lip
    - (b) Paramedian pit
    - (c) Cleft palate
    - (d) Tongue tie

    Answer for Q 49 on page 85

50. Complex hemihyperplasia is called when:
    - (a) One whole side of the body is affected
    - (b) Both side of the body are affected
    - (c) Single limb is affected with complication
    - (d) Single limb is affected without complication

    Answer for Q 50 on page 85

51. Metastatic tumor that results in radiopaque mass in the jaw is:
    - (a) Renal cancer
    - (b) Lung cancer
    - (c) Prostate cancer
    - (d) Thyroid cancer

    Answer for Q 51 on page 85

52. Fordyce spots are due to:
    - (a) Improper fusion of embryonic processes
    - (b) Presence of sweat glands in oral mucosa
    - (c) Improper maturation of oral epithelium
    - (d) Presence of sebaceous glands in oral mucosa

    Answer for Q 52 on page 85

53. Typical features of Asher Syndrome consist of blepharochalasis, thyroid enlargement and
    - (a) Mandibular dysostosis
    - (b) Cleft lip
    - (c) Cleft palate
    - (d) Double lip

    Answer for Q 53 on page 85

54. White lesions of the oral mucosa are characteristic of the following **except**:

(a) Leukodema

(b) Morsicatio buccarum

(c) Acanthosis

(d) Median rhomboid glossitis

Answer for Q 54 on page 85

55. Failure of the tuberculum impar to retract prior to fusion of lateral lingual swellings results in:

(a) Bifid tongue

(b) Scrotal tongue

(c) Median rhomboid glossitis

(d) Lingual thyroid nodule

Answer for Q 55 on page 85

56. Transverse facial cleft is due to failure of fusion of:

(a) Mandibular and maxillary processes

(b) Maxillary and lateral nasal processes

(c) Median nasal process and lateral nasal process

(d) None of the above

Answer for Q 56 on page 85

57. Crouzon syndrome is also called as:

(a) Mandibulofacial dysostosis

(b) Craniofacial dysostosis

(c) Osteopetrosis

(d) Osteitis deformans

Answer for Q 57 on page 85

58. Which is associated with defect in DNA repair:

(a) Xeroderma pigmentosum

(b) Albinism

(c) Icthyosis

(d) Sickle cell anemia

Answer for Q 58 on page 85

59. Which vitamin deficiency is the commonest cause of craniofacial anomalies?
   (a) Folk acid
   (b) Pantothenic acid
   (c) Ascorbic acid
   (d) Retinoic acid

   Answer for Q 59 on page 85

60. The most common congenital craniofacial anomalies seen at birth is:
   (a) Cleft lip and or palate
   (b) Oligodontia
   (c) Hemifacial microsomia
   (d) Hemangioma

   Answer for Q 60 on page 85

61. A mild form of cleft lip is:
   (a) Paramedian lip
   (b) Lip pits
   (c) Double lip
   (d) Notching of lip

   Answer for Q 61 on page 85

62. Premature closure of cranial sutures in an infant result in:
   (a) Cleft lip and/or palate
   (b) Craniosynostosis
   (c) Pierre Robin syndrome
   (d) Hemifacial microsomia

   Answer for Q 62 on page 85

63. Synostosis is a feature of all the following **except**:
   (a) Craniosynostosis
   (b) Apert syndrome
   (c) Romberg syndrome (Parry Romberg Syndrome)[2]
   (d) Treacher Collins syndrome

   Answer for Q 63 on page 86

[2] Parry Romberg syndrome (PRS) or progressive hemifacial atrophy is a progressive idiopathic disorder, presenting in early childhood.

64. The genetic constitution of an individual is his/her:
    (a) Phenotype
    (b) Heritability
    (c) Genotype
    (d) None of the above

Answer for Q 64 on page 86

65. If both the copies of gene in a chromosome are identical the individual is described as:
    (a) Heterozygous
    (b) Homozygous
    (c) Alleles
    (d) Pleiotrophic

Answer for Q 65 on page 86

66. If a trait or a disease manifests itself when the affected person carries only one copy of gene responsible along with one normal allele in somatic chromosome, the mode of inheritance is:
    (a) Dominant
    (b) X linked
    (c) Recessive
    (d) None of the above

Answer for Q 66 on page 86

67. Agents that cause birth defects when present in fetal environment are known as:
    (a) Mutants
    (b) Carcinogens
    (c) Toxins
    (d) Teratogens

Answer for Q 67 on page 86

68. Agnathia (Otocephaly) is a lethal anomaly characterized by mode of inheritance:
    (a) Autosomal recessive
    (b) Autosomal dominant
    (c) X linked recessive
    (d) X linked dominant

Answer for Q 68 on page 86

69. Micrognathia of maxilla frequently occurs due to deficiency of:
   (a) Lateral nasal swelling
   (b) Premaxillary area
   (c) Zygomatic process
   (d) Frontal process

   Answer for Q 69 on page 86

70. True mandibular micrognathia is characterized by all features **except**:
   (a) Severe retrusion of chin
   (b) Steep mandibular angle
   (c) Prominent maxilla
   (d) Deficient chin

   Answer for Q 70 on page 86

71. Excessive condylar growth may predispose to:
   (a) Mandibular retrognathism
   (b) Maxillary retrognathism
   (c) Maxillary prognathism
   (d) Mandibular prognathism

   Answer for Q 71 on page 86

72. The pathology in facial hemihypertrophy is:
   (a) Hypoplasia
   (b) Hypotrophy
   (c) Hyperplasia
   (d) Hypertrophy

   Answer for Q 72 on page 86

73. The affected side dentition in facial hemihypertrophy reveals:
   (a) Increased size of teeth
   (b) Increased rate of development
   (c) Premature eruption
   (d) All of the above

   Answer for Q 73 on page 86

74. The "coup de sabre" near midline of face separates between normal tissue and affected tissue in:
    (a) Hemifacial hyperplasia
    (b) Hemifacial atrophy
    (c) Scleroderma
    (d) None of the above

    Answer for Q 74 on page 86

75. Van der Woude syndrome, an orofacial anomaly, is characterized by[3]:
    (a) Occurs due to abnormal fusion of palate and lips at 30-50 days post-conception.
    (b) Deletion in lq32
    (c) Cleft lip or palate with distinctive lower lip pits
    (d) All of the above

    Answer for Q 75 on page 86

76. Failure in the fusion of the median nasal and maxillary process leads to the formation of:
    (a) Cleft lip
    (b) Cleft uvula
    (c) Cleft palate
    (d) Lip pits

    Answer for Q 76 on page 86

77. Cleft of the secondary palate is:
    (a) Median
    (b) Lateral
    (c) Always with cleft lip
    (d) Not isolated

    Answer for Q 77 on page 86

78. The cause of clefting of lip/palate is:
    (a) Polygenic
    (b) Multifactorial
    (c) Syndromic
    (d) All of the above

    Answer for Q 78 on page 86

---

[3] From French en coup de sabre (literally "by/in a strike of the sword"), so-called because of its resemblance to the scar of a sabre wound.

79. The line of cleft lip always starts at:
   (a) Midline
   (b) Commisure of lip
   (c) Medial to commisure
   (d) Lateral part of lip to philtrum

   Answer for Q 79 on page 87

80. A soft well circumscribed, sessile nodule occurring bilaterally, located lingually to mandibular cuspid is:
   (a) Mandibular tori
   (b) Median mandibular cyst
   (c) Lateral periodontal cyst
   (d) Retrocuspid papilla

Answer for Q 80 on page 87

81. Failure of fusion of lateral lingual swelling results in:
   (a) Cleft palate
   (b) Cleft lip
   (c) Cleft tongue
   (d) Orofacial cleft

   Answer for Q 81 on page 87

82. 46. The incomplete clefting of tongue is manifested as:
   (a) Scrotal tongue
   (b) Cleft tongue
   (c) Bifid tongue
   (d) Deep groove

   Answer for Q 82 on page 87

83. The current accepted etiology of fissured tongue is:
   (a) Candidal infection
   (b) Improper fusion of later al lingual swelling
   (c) Polygenic
   (d) Nutritional deficiency

   Answer for Q 83 on page 87

84. The improper posterior point of fusion of tuberculum impar and lingual tubercles shows the absence of:

    (a) Filiform papilla

    (b) Circumvallate papilla

    (c) Fungiform papilla

    (d) Foramen cecum

    Answer for Q 84 on page 87

85. When an erythematous patch occurs in the posterior middle area of the tongue at the area of foramen caecum, the lesion is better described as:

    (a) Posterior midline atrophic candidiasis

    (b) Kissing lesion

    (c) Angular chelitis

    (d) Median rhomboid glossitis

    Answer for Q 85 on page 87

86. Benign migratory glossitis is related to:

    (a) Geographical tongue

    (b) Psoriasis

    (c) Candidal infection

    (d) Lichen planus

    Answer for Q 86 on page 87

87. Decreased desquamation of filiform papillae on dorsal surface of tongue leads to:

    (a) Benign migratory glossitis

    (b) Papillitis

    (c) Hairy tongue

    (d) Anemia

    Answer for Q 87 on page 87

88. The lingual thyroid nodule arises from the remnants of tissue that does not involutes after its:

    (a) Anterior ascent

    (b) Medial descent

    (c) Downward descent

    (d) Lateral migration

    Answer for Q 88 on page 87

89. A radiolucency ovoid in shape located between the inferior alveolar canal and inferior border of mandible is probably the:
   (a) Stafne bone cyst
   (b) Hemorrhagic bone cyst
   (c) Dentigerous cyst
   (d) Pleomorphic adenoma

   Answer for Q 89 on page 87

90. Microdontia involving only single teeth is most often associated with:
   (a) Mandibular central incisor
   (b) Maxillary lateral incisor
   (c) Maxillary second premolar
   (d) Mandibular second premolar

   Answer for Q 90 on page 87

91. Which one of the following is considered as a precancerous condition?
   (a) Leukodema
   (b) Lingual thyroid nodule
   (c) Geographic tongue
   (d) Xeroderma pigmentosa

   Answer for Q 91 on page 87

92. Regarding cleft lip and palate, one of the following statements is **correct**:
   (a) They are example of multifactorial inheritance
   (b) Cleft upper lip is always associated with cleft palate
   (c) Cleft palate is always associated with cleft upper lip
   (d) None of the above

   Answer for Q 92 on page 87

93. Fissured tongue is one clinical feature associated with:
   (a) Gardener's syndrome
   (b) Crouzon's syndrome
   (c) Pierre Robin's syndrome
   (d) Down's syndrome

   Answer for Q 93 on page 87

94. One of the following hereditary conditions is transmitted as autosomal recessive disorder:

(a) Xeroderma pigmentosa

(b) Cleidocranial dysplasia

(c) Dentinogenesis imperfecta

(d) Peutz-Jeghers syndrome

Answer for Q 94 on page 87

95. Basket weave appearance is a common histological feature of:

(a) Fordyce's granules

(b) Chelitis granulomatosa

(c) White spongy nevus

(d) Chelitis glandularis

Answer for Q 95 on page 87

96. One of the following disorders is considered as precancerous condition:

(a) White spongy nevus

(b) Fibromatosis gingivae

(c) Chelitis glandularis

(d) Lingual thyroid nodule

Answer for Q 96 on page 88

97. One of the following conditions is associated with circum-oral melanin pigmentation:

(a) Melanotic neuroectodermal tumor

(b) Pigmented nevus

(c) Xeroderma pigmentosa

(d) Peutz-Jeghers syndrome

Answer for Q 97 on page 88

98. One the following conditions is non-developmental:

(a) Leukoedema

(b) Black tongue

(c) Witkop's disease

(d) Congenital syphilis

Answer for Q 98 on page 88

99. Chelitis granulomatosa may be a manifestation of one of the following
   (a) Cherubism
   (b) Melkersson-Rosenthal syndrome
   (c) Syphilis
   (d) Peutz–Jeghers syndrome

   Answer for Q 99 on page 88

100. Orofacial granulomatosis includes:
   (a) Cheilitis granulomatosa
   (b) Melkersson Rosenthal syndrome
   (c) Sarcoidosis
   (d) Oral lesions of Crohn's disease
   (e) All of the above

   Answer for Q 100 on page 88

101. Focal dermal hypoplasia syndrome is characterized by:
   (a) Enamel hypoplasia
   (b) Increased thickness of cementum
   (c) Absence of cellular cementum
   (d) Early eruption of teeth

   Answer for Q 101 on page 88

102. One of the following is **not** characterized by fissured tongue:
   (a) Melkersson–Rosenthal syndrome
   (b) Down syndrome
   (c) Cowden's syndrome
   (d) Hereditary ectodermal dysplasia

   Answer for Q 102 on page 88

103. One or more of the following is true regarding gingival fibromatosis (fibromatosis gingivae; elephantiasis gingivae):
   (a) Autosomal dominant
   (b) Autosomal recessive
   (c) Incomplete penetrance
   (d) Variable expressivity
   (e) All of the above

   Answer for Q 103 on page 88

3.2 Answers with Comments:

1. The correct answer is **C** – White spongy nevus is not an ectopic conditions. The ectopic condition is defined as presence of normal tissue in an abnormal anatomical site.

   Back to Q 1 on page 61

2. The correct answer is **A** – No explanation is available for this answer.

   Back to Q 2 on page 61

3. The correct answer is **B** – Torus palatinus is an excessive formation of normal bone in normal site and thus is not considered as an ectopic lesion.

   Back to Q 3 on page 61

4. The correct answer is **C** – The surface of median rhomboidal glossitis is devoid of filiform papillae.

   Back to Q 4 on page 62

5. The correct answer is **D** – No explanation is available for this answer.

   Back to Q 5 on page 62

6. The correct answer is **D** – No explanation is available for this answer.

   Back to Q 6 on page 62

7. The correct answer is **C** – No explanation is available for this answer.

   Back to Q 7 on page 62

8. The correct answer is **D** – No explanation is available for this answer.

   Back to Q 8 on page 62

9. The correct answer is **B** – No explanation is available for this answer.

   Back to Q 9 on page 62

10. The correct answer is **A** – No explanation is available for this answer.

    Back to Q 10 on page 63

11. The correct answer is **D** – No explanation is available for this answer.

    Back to Q 11 on page 63

12. The correct answer is **D** – No explanation is available for this answer.

    Back to Q 12 on page 63

13. The correct answer is **B** – No explanation is available for this answer.

    Back to Q 13 on page 63

14. The correct answer is **C** – No explanation is available for this answer.

    Back to Q 14 on page 64

15. The correct answer is **B** – No explanation is available for this answer.

Back to Q 15 on page 64

16. The correct answer is **C** – No explanation is available for this answer.

Back to Q 16 on page 64

17. The correct answer is **C** – No explanation is available for this answer.

Back to Q 17 on page 64

18. The correct answer is **C** – No explanation is available for this answer.

Back to Q 18 on page 64

19. The correct answer is **C** – No explanation is available for this answer.

Back to Q 19 on page 64

20. The correct answer is **A** – No explanation is available for this answer.

Back to Q 20 on page 65

21. The correct answer is **B** – No explanation is available for this answer.

Back to Q 21 on page 65

22. The correct answer is **D** – No explanation is available for this answer.

Back to Q 22 on page 65

23. The correct answer is **C** – No explanation is available for this answer.

Back to Q 23 on page 65

24. The correct answer is **D** – No explanation is available for this answer.

Back to Q 24 on page 65

25. The correct answer is **D** – Fissured tongue is a condition frequently seen in the general population and it is characterized by grooves that vary in depth and are noted along the dorsal and lateral aspects of the tongue. Although a definitive etiology is unknown, a polygenic mode of inheritance is suspected because the condition is seen clustering in families who are affected. Patients are usually asymptomatic, and the condition is initially noted on routine intraoral examination as an incidental finding. The condition is relatively common, with an estimated prevalence of 6.8%–11% [4].

Back to Q 25 on page 66

26. The correct answer is **A** – No explanation is available for this answer.

Back to Q 26 on page 66

27. The correct answer is **C** – No explanation is available for this answer.

Back to Q 27 on page 66

28. The correct answer is **C** – No explanation is available for this answer.

Back to Q 28 on page 66

29. The correct answer is **D** – No explanation is available for this answer.

Back to Q 29 on page 66

30. The correct answer is **B** – No explanation is available for this answer.

Back to Q 30 on page 75

31. The correct answer is **A** – No explanation is available for this answer.

Back to Q 31 on page 67

32. The correct answer is **A** – No explanation is available for this answer.

Back to Q 32 on page 67

33. The correct answer is **C** – No explanation is available for this answer.

Back to Q 33 on page 67

34. The correct answer is **A** – No explanation is available for this answer.

Back to Q 34 on page 67

35. The correct answer is **B** – No explanation is available for this answer.

Back to Q 35 on page 68

36. The correct answer is **B** – No explanation is available for this answer.

Back to Q 36 on page 68

37. The correct answer is **A** – No explanation is available for this answer.

Back to Q 37 on page 68

38. The correct answer is **D** – No explanation is available for this answer.

Back to Q 38 on page 68

39. The correct answer is **D** – No explanation is available for this answer.

Back to Q 39 on page 68

40. The correct answer is **D** – No explanation is available for this answer.

Back to Q 40 on page 69

41. The correct answer is **D** – No explanation is available for this answer.

Back to Q 41 on page 69

42. The correct answer is **C** – No explanation is available for this answer.

Back to Q 42 on page 69

43. The correct answer is **A** – No explanation is available for this answer.

Back to Q 43 on page 69

44. The correct answer is **B** – No explanation is available for this answer.

Back to Q 44 on page 69

45. The correct answer is **A** – No explanation is available for this answer.

Back to Q 45 on page 70

46. The correct answer is **C** – No explanation is available for this answer.

Back to Q 46 on page 70

47. The correct answer is **B** – No explanation is available for this answer.

Back to Q 47 on page 70

48. The correct answer is **C** – No explanation is available for this answer.

Back to Q 48 on page 70

49. The correct answer is **D** – No explanation is available for this answer.

Back to Q 49 on page 70

50. The correct answer is **A** – No explanation is available for this answer.

Back to Q 50 on page 71

51. The correct answer is **C** – No explanation is available for this answer.

Back to Q 51 on page 71

52. The correct answer is **D** – No explanation is available for this answer.

Back to Q 52 on page 71

53. The correct answer is **D** – No explanation is available for this answer.

Back to Q 53 on page 71

54. The correct answer is **D** – No explanation is available for this answer.

Back to Q 54 on page 71

55. The correct answer is **C** – No explanation is available for this answer.

Back to Q 55 on page 72

56. The correct answer is **A** – No explanation is available for this answer.

Back to Q 56 on page 72

57. The correct answer is **B** – No explanation is available for this answer.

Back to Q 57 on page 72

58. The correct answer is **A** – No explanation is available for this answer.

Back to Q 58 on page 72

59. The correct answer is **A** – No explanation is available for this answer.

Back to Q 59 on page 72

60. The correct answer is **A** – No explanation is available for this answer.

Back to Q 60 on page 73

61. The correct answer is **D** – No explanation is available for this answer.

Back to Q 61 on page ??

62. The correct answer is **B** – No explanation is available for this answer.

Back to Q 62 on page 73

63. The correct answer is **D** – No explanation is available for this answer.

Back to Q 63 on page 73

64. The correct answer is **C** – No explanation is available for this answer.

Back to Q 64 on page 73

65. The correct answer is **B** – No explanation is available for this answer.

Back to Q 65 on page 74

66. The correct answer is **A** – No explanation is available for this answer.

Back to Q 66 on page 74

67. The correct answer is **D** – No explanation is available for this answer.

Back to Q 67 on page 74

68. The correct answer is **B** – No explanation is available for this answer.

Back to Q 68 on page 74

69. The correct answer is **B** – No explanation is available for this answer.

Back to Q 69 on page 74

70. The correct answer is **C** – No explanation is available for this answer.

Back to Q 70 on page 75

71. The correct answer is **D** – No explanation is available for this answer.

Back to Q 71 on page 75

72. The correct answer is **A** – No explanation is available for this answer.

Back to Q 72 on page 75

73. The correct answer is **A** – No explanation is available for this answer.

Back to Q 73 on page 75

74. The correct answer is **C** – No explanation is available for this answer.

Back to Q 74 on page ??

75. The correct answer is **C** – No explanation is available for this answer.

Back to Q 75 on page 76

76. The correct answer is **A** – No explanation is available for this answer.

Back to Q 76 on page 76

77. The correct answer is **A** – No explanation is available for this answer.

Back to Q 77 on page 76

78. The correct answer is **D** – No explanation is available for this answer.

Back to Q 78 on page 76

79. The correct answer is **D** – No explanation is available for this answer.

Back to Q 79 on page 76

80. The correct answer is **D** – No explanation is available for this answer.

Back to Q 80 on page 77

81. The correct answer is **C** – No explanation is available for this answer.

Back to Q 81 on page 77

82. The correct answer is **D** – No explanation is available for this answer.

Back to Q 82 on page 77

83. The correct answer is **C** – No explanation is available for this answer.

Back to Q 83 on page 77

84. The correct answer is **A** – No explanation is available for this answer.

Back to Q 84 on page 77

85. The correct answer is **D** – No explanation is available for this answer.

Back to Q 85 on page 78

86. The correct answer is **A** – No explanation is available for this answer.

Back to Q 86 on page 78

87. The correct answer is **C** – No explanation is available for this answer.

Back to Q 87 on page 78

88. The correct answer is **C** – No explanation is available for this answer.

Back to Q 88 on page 78

89. The correct answer is **A** – No explanation is available for this answer.

Back to Q 89 on page 78

90. The correct answer is **B** – No explanation is available for this answer.

Back to Q 90 on page 79

91. The correct answer is **D** – No explanation is available for this answer.

Back to Q 91 on page 79

92. The correct answer is **A** – No explanation is available for this answer.

Back to Q 92 on page 79

93. The correct answer is **D** – No explanation is available for this answer.

Back to Q 93 on page 79

94. The correct answer is **A** – No explanation is available for this answer.

Back to Q 94 on page 79

95. The correct answer is **C** – No explanation is available for this answer.

Back to Q 95 on page 80

96. The correct answer is **C** – No explanation is available for this answer.

Back to Q 96 on page 80

97. The correct answer is **D** – No explanation is available for this answer.

Back to Q 97 on page 80

98. The correct answer is **B** – No explanation is available for this answer.

Back to Q 98 on page 80

99. The correct answer is **B** – No explanation is available for this answer.

Back to Q 99 on page 80

100. The correct answer is **E** – No explanation is available for this answer.

Back to Q 100 on page 81

101. The correct answer is **A** – No explanation is available for this answer.

Back to Q 101 on page 81

102. The correct answer is **D** – Fissured tongue is seen in Melkersson–Rosenthal syndrome, Down syndrome and Cowden's syndrome.

Back to Q 102 on page 81

103. The correct answer is **E** – All the items are true regarding gingival fibromatosis.

Back to Q 103 on page 81

CHAPTER 4
DENTAL CARIES

Dental caries is a progressive, mostly irreversible bacterial damage affecting hard tooth structure exposed to oral environment.

4.1 MCQs Questions

Choose **one or more** of the most appropriate answers. Some questions may have **more than one** correct answer. You have to choose all the correct answers as best as you can.

1. The most common transmission of *S. mutans* occurs mainly through:
   (a) saliva
   (b) skin
   (c) mother to child
   (d) blood transfusion
   Answer for Q 1 on page 103
2. Which of the following statement is **incorrect** about dental caries?
   (a) Caries prevalence increases when populations become exposed to sucrose-rich diets
   (b) Intrinsic sugars are more damaging than extrinsic sugars
   (c) Sucrose is the most cariogenic sugar
   (d) Frequency of sugar intake is of more importance than total amount consumed
   Answer for Q 2 on page 103
3. Which of the following zone is an area of active remineralization:
   (a) surface zone
   (b) body of the lesion
   (c) dark zone
   (d) translucent zone
   Answer for Q 3 on page 103

4. A substance used as a non-cariogenic substitute for sugar is:
   (a) Fructose
   (b) Glucose
   (c) Lactose
   (d) Maltose
   (e) Sorbitol

   Answer for Q 4 on page 103

5. Mottled enamel is produced by:
   (a) Syphilis
   (b) Febrile diseases
   (c) Fluorine
   (d) Acids
   (e) Tuberculosis

   Answer for Q 5 on page 103

6. The structures of enamel that are more resistant to the actions of acids are:
   (a) Enamel cuticles
   (b) Enamel lamellae
   (c) Enamel rods
   (d) Interprismatic substance of enamel
   (e) Ameloblast

   Answer for Q 6 on page 103

7. In an early carious lesion, the first structure to show evidence of destruction is the:
   (a) Enamel prism
   (b) Cuticle
   (c) Interprismatic substance
   (d) Enamel lamellae
   (e) Dead tracts

   Answer for Q 7 on page 103

8. Which one of the following main constituents of saliva acts as a buffering agent?
   (a) Enzymes
   (b) Immunoglobulins
   (c) Inorganic ions
   (d) Leukocytes

   Answer for Q 8 on page 103

9. The most common cause for tooth loss in adults is:
   (a) Dental caries
   (b) Chronic periodontitis
   (c) Trauma
   (d) Neoplasm

   Answer for Q 9 on page 103

10. Which of the following is cariogenic / caries promoting?
   (a) Selenium
   (b) Vanadium
   (c) Strontium
   (d) Molybdenum

   Answer for Q 10 on page 103

11. Widely accepted theory of dental caries:
   (a) Proteolytic theory
   (b) Proteolytic chelation theory
   (c) Acidogenic theory
   (d) Autoimmune theory

   Answer for Q 11 on page 103

12. Early invading bacteria in carious lesions are called:
   (a) Microcosm
   (b) Pioneer bacteria
   (c) Advancing bacteria
   (d) Anaerobic bacteria

   Answer for Q 12 on page 103

13. Bacteria free zone of dentinal caries is:
   (a) Zone of decomposed dentin
   (b) Zone of bacterial invasion
   (c) Zone of decalcification
   (d) Zone of dentinal sclerosis

   Answer for Q 13 on page 103

14. Pioneer bacteria in dental caries are in:
    (a) Enamel
    (b) Dentin
    (c) Pulp
    (d) Cementum

    Answer for Q 14 on page 103

15. Linear enamel caries lesions in deciduous teeth predominate in: (See image, source: [5])
    (a) Maxillary anterior teeth
    (b) Maxillary posterior teeth
    (c) Mandibular posterior teeth
    (d) Mandibular anterior teeth

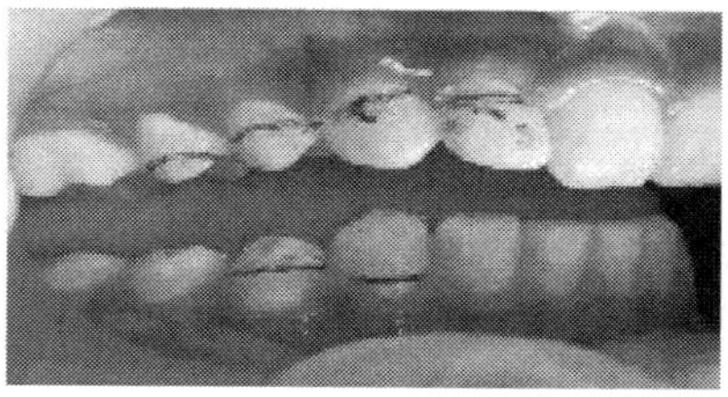

16. From the list of oral microorganisms, which is primarily responsible for the initiation of dental caries?
    (a) *Mutans streptococci*
    (b) *Bifidobacteria*
    (c) *Lactobacilli*
    (d) *Porphyromonas gingivalis*

    Answer for Q 16 on page 104

17. Oral bacterial synthesis extracellular glucans (dextran and mutan) from which host dietary component?
    (a) Glucose
    (b) Alpha limit dextrins
    (c) Sucrose
    (d) Polysaccharides

    Answer for Q 17 on page 104

18. A deficiency of which vitamin has been associated with enamel defects and increased risk of dental caries?
    (a) Vitamin A
    (b) Folic acid
    (c) Vitamin C
    (d) Vitamin D

    Answer for Q 18 on page 104

19. The best available evidence for an association between amount of sugars and risk of dental caries comes from which type of study design:
    (a) Randomized controlled
    (b) Non-randomized controlled
    (c) Cross sectional observational
    (d) Cohort

    Answer for Q 19 on page 104

20. Chemico-parasitic theory of dental caries is proposed by:
    (a) G.V. Black
    (b) Miller
    (c) Gottlieb
    (d) Schwartz

    Answer for Q 20 on page 104

21. Which of the following organisms is found in deep carious lesions rather than in incipient lesions?
    (a) Streptococci
    (b) Lactobacilli
    (c) Veillonella
    (d) Bacteroides

    Answer for Q 21 on page 104

22. Pioneer bacteria in dental caries are in:
    (a) Enamel
    (b) Dentin
    (c) Pulp
    (d) Cementum

    Answer for Q 22 on page 104

23. The most pronounced effect on the oral microflora of a reduction in rate of salivary flow is a:
    (a) Significant increase in number of oral bacteria
    (b) Shift towards more acidogenic microflora
    (c) Significant decrease in number of oral bacteria
    (d) shift towards more aerobic microflora

    Answer for Q 23 on page 104

24. Ammonia causes:
    (a) increase in plaque formation
    (b) increase in calculus formation
    (c) decrease in plaque formation
    (d) precipitation of salivary proteins

    Answer for Q 24 on page 104

25. Cavity formation in a tooth, due to dental caries is due to:
    (a) Destructive potential of Streptococcus mutans
    (b) Destructive potential of Lactobacillus acidophilus
    (c) Lateral spread of caries along DEJ and weakening of the outer covering enamel
    (d) Mastectomy force and unrelated to the extent of carious process

    Answer for Q 25 on page 105

26. Animals maintained in a germ-free environment did not develop caries fed on a high carbohydrate diet is given by:
    (a) Gottlieb
    (b) Miller
    (c) Snyder
    (d) Orland

    Answer for Q 26 on page 105

27. Which of the following factors in the Stephan's curve is related to the caries incidence and sugar intake?
    (a) Physical form of sugar
    (b) Frequency of sugar intake
    (c) pH of plaque
    (d) Quantity of sugar intake

    Answer for Q 27 on page 105

28. Initiation of caries by Streptococcus mutans is by the production of the:
    (a) Dextranase and soluble dextran
    (b) Insoluble dextran and glycosyl transferase
    (c) Soluble dextran and glycosyl transferase
    (d) None of the above

    Answer for Q 28 on page 105

29. The attachment of Actinomyces species to the tooth surface is facilitated by:
    (a) Fimbriae
    (b) Cilia
    (c) Flagella
    (d) Pseudopodia

    Answer for Q 29 on page 105

30. Caries associated with pre-eruptive enamel hypoplasia:
    (a) Secondary caries
    (b) Chronic caries
    (c) Occult caries
    (d) Incipient caries

    Answer for Q 30 on page 105

31. Bacteria free zone of dentinal caries is:
    (a) Zone of decomposed dentin
    (b) Zone of bacterial invasion
    (c) Zone of decalcification
    (d) Zone of dentinal sclerosis

    Answer for Q 31 on page 105

32. The legend of worms, endogenous theories, chemical theories and parasitic theory are early theories explaining:
    (a) Dental caries
    (b) Gingivitis
    (c) Periodontitis
    (d) Osteomyelitis

    Answer for Q 32 on page 105

33. Lactobacilli are numerous in carious lesions because they:
    (a) Are the main causative agent
    (b) Can produce insoluble extracellular polysaccharides
    (c) Can attach to smooth enamel surfaces
    (d) Are secondary invaders and powerful acidogenic

    Answer for Q 33 on page 105

34. Starch is considered to be less cariogenic than monosaccharides and disaccharides because it:
    (a) Does not diffuse through plaque
    (b) is rapidly hydrolyzed in the mouth
    (c) enhances remineralization
    (d) raises the pH in the oral cavity

    Answer for Q 34 on page 105

35. The extra cellular polysaccharides synthesized by cariogenic streptococci in the presence of excess sucrose are best described as:
    (a) Mucopolysaccharide
    (b) Dextran-like glucan
    (c) Glycogen like glucan
    (d) Amylopectin

    Answer for Q 35 on page 105

36. Organism involved in smooth surface caries is: 1. Streptococcus mutans; 2. Actinomyces viscosus; 3. Lactobacillus; 4. Campylobacter:
    (a) only 1
    (b) only 2
    (c) 1 and 3
    (d) All of the above

    Answer for Q 36 on page 105

37. In patient with reduced salivary flow the carious incidence is:
    (a) more than the patient with normal salivary flow
    (b) less than the patient with normal salivary flow
    (c) unaffected
    (d) none of the above

    Answer for Q 37 on page 105

38. Which of the following is a cariostatic element?
   (a) Fluoride
   (b) Strontium
   (c) Vanadium
   (d) Molybdenum

   Answer for Q 38 on page 105

39. The number of dentinal zones in dentinal caries is:
   (a) one
   (b) two
   (c) four
   (d) five

   Answer for Q 39 on page 105

40. Dental caries is associated with:
   (a) *Streptococcus Agalactiae*
   (b) *Streptococcus Mutans*
   (c) *Streptococcus Bovis*
   (d) *Streptococcus Anginosus*

   Answer for Q 40 on page 106

41. Widely accepted theory of dental caries is:
   (a) Proteolytic theory
   (b) Proteolytic chelation theory
   (c) Acidogenic theory
   (d) Autoimmune theory

   Answer for Q 41 on page 106

42. The correct order of microscopic zones of dentinal caries starting from the DEJ is:
   (a) Zone of sclerosis, decalcification zone, bacterial invasion
   (b) Bacterial invasion, decalcification zone, zone of sclerosis
   (c) Zone of sclerosis, bacterial invasion, decalcification zone
   (d) Decalcification zone, Zone of sclerosis, bacterial invasion

   Answer for Q 42 on page 106

43. Streptococcus mutans is involved in dental caries initiation. Other bacteria also involved is:

    (a) *S. Sarcinus*

    (b) *S. Macae*

    (c) *S. Sanguis*

    (d) *S. Salivarius*

    Answer for Q 43 on page 106

44. The dietary carbohydrate most likely involved in etiology of dental caries is:

    (a) Glucose

    (b) Sucrose

    (c) Dextran

    (d) Polysaccharides

    Answer for Q 44 on page 106

45. Bacteria responsible for initiation of caries is:

    (a) *Actinomyces*

    (b) *Streptococcus mutans*

    (c) *Lactobacillus*

    (d) *Streptococcus viridans*

    Answer for Q 45 on page 106

46. What is the pH at which initiation of caries begins?

    (a) 4.3-4.5

    (b) 5.2-5.5

    (c) 4.9-5.1

    (d) 3.5-4.5

    Answer for Q 46 on page 106

47. Oral foci of Miller's are seen in:

    (a) Dental caries

    (b) Lichen planus

    (c) Herpes simplex

    (d) Syphilis

    Answer for Q 47 on page 106

48. In the earliest stages of carious lesion, there is loss of:
   (a) Enamel cuticle
   (b) Interprismatic substance
   (c) Organic matrix
   (d) Enamel lamellae

   Answer for Q 48 on page 106

49. Smooth surface caries is characterized by spread of caries in enamel and dentin as cones. These alignment in enamel and dentin is:
   (a) Base to base
   (b) Apex to base
   (c) Apex to apex
   (d) None of the above

   Answer for Q 49 on page 106

50. Least cariogenic among these:
   (a) Raw starch
   (b) Cooked starch
   (c) Sucrose
   (d) Fructose

   Answer for Q 50 on page 106

51. Which tooth in the permanent dentition is the most susceptible to dental caries?
   (a) Maxillary first premolar
   (b) Maxillary second molar
   (c) Mandibular first molar
   (d) Mandibular second molar

   Answer for Q 51 on page 106

52. Turbid dentin in carious tooth is all **except**:
   (a) Zone of bacterial invasion
   (b) Zone which cannot be remineralized
   (c) Zone in which collagen is irreversibly denatured
   (d) Zone that need not be removed before restoration

   Answer for Q 52 on page 107

53. Primary destruction in process of dental caries is characterized by:
   (a) Demineralization of organic substances
   (b) Both processes occur simultaneously
   (c) Destruction of organic substances
   (d) None of the above

   Answer for Q 53 on page 107

54. Microorganisms found in the dentinal tubules, before the clinical evidence of dental caries are termed:
   (a) Primary bacteria
   (b) Acidogenic bacteria
   (c) Pioneer bacteria
   (d) Proteolytic bacteria

   Answer for Q 54 on page 107

55. Famous Vipeholm study was conducted to:
   (a) Find out role of sticky and non-sticky form of sugars
   (b) Find out the role of water fluoridation on dental caries
   (c) Find out role of xylitol on dental caries
   (d) All of the above

   Answer for Q 55 on page 107

56. Dead tracts appear:
   (a) Black in transmitted light
   (b) White in transmitted light
   (c) Black in reflected light
   (d) Same in both transmitted and reflected light

   Answer for Q 56 on page 107

57. Primary dentin has:
   (a) fewer tubules than secondary dentin
   (b) same number of tubules as secondary dentin
   (c) more number of tubules than secondary dentin
   (d) none of the above

   Answer for Q 57 on page 107

58. In carious process, the pioneer bacteria are present in:
   (a) enamel lamellae
   (b) enamel tufts
   (c) dentinal tubules
   (d) peritubular dentin

   Answer for Q 58 on page 107

59. Which of the following mechanisms is responsible for formation of liquifaction foci?
   (a) focal coalescence and breakdown of enamel lamellae
   (b) focal coalescence and breakdown of enamel tufts
   (c) generalized breakdown of dentinal tubules
   (d) focal coalescence and breakdown of dentinal tubules

   Answer for Q 59 on page 107

60. In pit and fissure caries of occlusal surface, apex of the cone-shaped carious lesion is present towards:
   (a) dentino-enamel junction
   (b) occlusal surface of tooth
   (c) buccal surface of tooth
   (d) lingual surface of tooth

   Answer for Q 60 on page 108

61. Primary destruction in process of dental caries is characterized by:
   (a) Demineralization of inorganic substance
   (b) Destruction of organic substance
   (c) Both processes occur simultaneously
   (d) None of the above

   Answer for Q 61 on page 108

62. Primitive raw foods influence on dental caries:
   (a) Increase the incidence of dental caries
   (b) Decrease the incidence of dental caries
   (c) No influence on dental caries
   (d) Similar effect as modern diet

   Answer for Q 62 on page 108

63. Transverse clefts found in dentin cares are:

    (a) Similar to enamel tufts in caries enamel

    (b) Liquefaction foci occurring along one of the lateral branches of a dentinal tubules

    (c) Acids collected at the amelodentinal junction

    (d) Developmental malformations during matrix apposition of dentin

    Answer for Q 63 on page 108

64. Aciduric bacteria:

    (a) Can survive in an alkaline media

    (b) Can produce acids by fermenting carbohydrates

    (c) Can survive in an acidic media

    (d) Can produce proteolytic enzymes

    Answer for Q 64 on page 108

65. *Mutans streptococci* the major pathogens of dental caries because:

    (a) They are highly acidogenic

    (b) They are highly aciduric

    (c) Can produce water-insoluble extracellular polysaccharides (glucans)

    (d) All of the above

    Answer for Q 65 on page 108

66. Oral bacteria synthesize extracellular glucans (dextran and mutan) from which host dietary component?

    (a) Glucose

    (b) Alpha limit dextrins

    (c) Sucrose

    (d) Polysaccharides

    Answer for Q 66 on page 108

67. ♣ Some of the following may be true regarding the Vipeholm experiments:

    (a) Were a series of experiments held in a hospital for the intellectually disabled

    (b) Are considered to have violated the principles of medical ethics

    (c) Showed that fluoride application could enhance caries resistance

    (d) Showed that frequency of intake the most important factor in cariogenicity of carbohydrates

    Answer for Q 67 on page 108

4.2 Answers with Comments:

1. The correct answer is **C** – No explanation is available for this answer.

   Back to Q 1 on page 89

2. The correct answer is **B** – Intrinsic sugars which are the results of body metabolism are not amenable to be digested by oral cariogenic bacteria.

   Back to Q 2 on page 89

3. The correct answer is **A** – No explanation is available for this answer.

   Back to Q 3 on page 89

4. The correct answer is **E** – Sorbitol cannot be metabolized by cariogenic bacteria.

   Back to Q 4 on page 90

5. The correct answer is **C** – No explanation is available for this answer.

   Back to Q 5 on page 90

6. The correct answer is **A** – No explanation is available for this answer.

   Back to Q 6 on page 90

7. The correct answer is **C** – No explanation is available for this answer.

   Back to Q 7 on page 90

8. The correct answer is **C** – No explanation is available for this answer.

   Back to Q 8 on page 90

9. The correct answer is **A** – No explanation is available for this answer.

   Back to Q 9 on page 91

10. The correct answer is **A** – Cariostatic elements: F, P; Mildly cariostatic Mo, V, Cu, Sr, B, Li, Au; Doubtful: Be, Co, Mn, Sn, Zn, Br, I; Caries inert: Ba, Al, Ni, Fe, Pd, Ti; Caries promoting: Se, Mg, Cd, Pt, Pb, Si.

    Back to Q 10 on page 91

11. The correct answer is **C** – Acidogenic theory was proposed by miller. According to this, initial decalcification of enamel and dentin is followed by dissolution of softened residue.

    Back to Q 11 on page 91

12. The correct answer is **B** – Pioneer bacteria or primary bacteria are streptococcus *mutans, lactobacillus* and *Actinomyces* species

    Back to Q 12 on page 91

13. The correct answer is **D** – Zone of dentinal sclerosis is a defective mechanism of pulp-dentin complex to guard against invading bacteria and its products such as acids.

    Back to Q 13 on page 91

14. The correct answer is **B** – Pioneer bacteria begin to invade dentin during their journey to the pulp.

Back to Q 14 on page 92

15. The correct answer is **A** – Linear enamel caries (odontoclasia) is seen to occur in the region of the neonatal line of the maxillary anterior teeth in children. The line, which represent a metabolic defect such as hypocalcemia or trauma of birth, may predispose to caries, leading to gross destruction of the labial surface of the teeth.

Back to Q 15 on page 92

16. The correct answer is **A** – *Streptococcus mutans* is capable for production of acids and dextran. The later is the material responsible for good adhesion to the tooth surfaces. Other organisms although capable of production of acids, yet they cannot produce such dextran. Mutans Streptococci initiate the dental caries process and other bacteria such as *Lactobacilli* become involved at a later state when the plaque pH is lower. *Porphyromonas gingivalis* is a bacterium that causes gingival inflammation. *Bifidobacteria* can metabolize dietary sugars to acids and contribute to dental caries, but these bacteria are not responsible for initiating caries.

Back to Q 16 on page 92

17. The correct answer is **C** – Plaque glucans are synthesized from dietary sucrose by glucosyletransferase.

Back to Q 17 on page 92

18. The correct answer is **D** – Vitamin D: A deficiency is a risk factor for enamel hypocalcification and this increases risk of caries. Although there are limitations with some studies a systematic review has suggested that vitamin D supplementation may decrease risk of dental caries.

Back to Q 18 on page 93

19. The correct answer is **D** – In the absence of any randomized controlled trials investigating sugars and dental caries the best available data come from cohort studies. Cross sectional observational studies provide weaker data as they only measure sugars and caries at one point in time and do not provide evidence on the association between sugars and development of dental caries over time.

Back to Q 19 on page 93

20. The correct answer is **B** – No explanation is available for this answer.

Back to Q 20 on page 93

21. The correct answer is **B** – No explanation is available for this answer.

Back to Q 21 on page 93

22. The correct answer is **B** – No explanation is available for this answer.

Back to Q 22 on page 93

23. The correct answer is **B** – No explanation is available for this answer.

Back to Q 23 on page 94

24. The correct answer is **C** – No explanation is available for this answer.

    Back to Q 24 on page 94

25. The correct answer is **C** – No explanation is available for this answer.

    Back to Q 25 on page 94

26. The correct answer is **D** – Orland et. al., (1954) showed that rats fed a diet which is normally cariogenic failed to develop dental decay in the absence of bacteria. This observation was confirmed and extended by Fitzgerald and Keyes (1960). It was Keyes (1960), however, who showed that caries is an infectious and transmissible disease in the hamster.

    Back to Q 26 on page 94

27. The correct answer is **C** – No explanation is available for this answer.

    Back to Q 27 on page 94

28. The correct answer is **B** – No explanation is available for this answer.

    Back to Q 28 on page 95

29. The correct answer is **A** – No explanation is available for this answer.

    Back to Q 29 on page 95

30. The correct answer is **C** – No explanation is available for this answer.

    Back to Q 30 on page 95

31. The correct answer is **D** – No explanation is available for this answer.

    Back to Q 31 on page 95

32. The correct answer is **A** – No explanation is available for this answer.

    Back to Q 32 on page 95

33. The correct answer is **D** – No explanation is available for this answer.

    Back to Q 33 on page 96

34. The correct answer is **A** – No explanation is available for this answer.

    Back to Q 34 on page 96

35. The correct answer is **B** – No explanation is available for this answer.

    Back to Q 35 on page 96

36. The correct answer is **A** – No explanation is available for this answer.

    Back to Q 36 on page 96

37. The correct answer is **A** – No explanation is available for this answer.

    Back to Q 37 on page 96

38. The correct answer is **A** – No explanation is available for this answer.

    Back to Q 38 on page 97

39. The correct answer is **D** – No explanation is available for this answer.

    Back to Q 39 on page 97

40. The correct answer is **B** – No explanation is available for this answer.

    Back to Q 40 on page 97

41. The correct answer is **C** – No explanation is available for this answer.

    Back to Q 41 on page 97

42. The correct answer is **B** – No explanation is available for this answer.

    Back to Q 42 on page 97

43. The correct answer is **C** – *S. Sanguis* plays the second most important role after *S. Mutans.*

    Back to Q 43 on page 98

44. The correct answer is **B** – Sucrose can provide bacteria with dextrans and levans. Both are required in the initiation of caries process as the former act as a binding agent and the latter acts as a store of carbohydrates readily consumed by the bacteria after the dietary carbohydrates are washed away.

    Back to Q 44 on page 98

45. The correct answer is **B** – *Streptococcus mutans* is an acidogenic bacteria, in addition it can produce dextran and levan which are sticky polymers that can attach the dental plaque firmly to the tooth surface.

    Back to Q 45 on page 98

46. The correct answer is **B** – The pH of 5.2–5.5 is termed the critical pH at which enamel minerals begin to dissolve.

    Back to Q 46 on page 98

47. The correct answer is **A** – In present medical consensus, a focal infection is a localized infection, often asymptomatic, that causes disease elsewhere in the body. As dental caries is a chronic latent infectious disease, it was considered as a focus of infection.

    Back to Q 47 on page 98

48. The correct answer is **B** – The interprismatic substance is less calcified than the enamel rods and so it is more vulnerable for acid attack. The enamel cuticle is lost very early after tooth eruption.

    Back to Q 48 on page 99

49. The correct answer is **B** – This is because acids of caries follow the direction of enamel rods and dentinal tubules.

    Back to Q 49 on page 99

50. The correct answer is **A** – Raw starch cannot ferment easily in the oral cavity and is of large molecular weight that prevent its penetration into the dental plaque.

    Back to Q 50 on page 99

51. The correct answer is **C** – Mandibular first molar erupts at an early stage of childhood and hence in more susceptible to the sugary diet which is consumed in abundance during childhood period.

Back to Q 51 on page 99

52. The correct answer is **D** – Turbid dentin is the zone of bacterial invasion. Widening and distortion of the dentinal tubules which are filled with bacteria. There is very little mineral present and the collagen in this zone is irreversibly denatured. The dentin in this zone will not self-repair.

Back to Q 52 on page 99

53. The correct answer is **A** – No explanation is available for this answer.

Back to Q 53 on page 100

54. The correct answer is **B** – No explanation is available for this answer.

Back to Q 54 on page 100

55. The correct answer is **A** – No explanation is available for this answer.

Back to Q 55 on page 100

56. The correct answer is **A** – No explanation is available for this answer.

Back to Q 56 on page 100

57. The correct answer is **B** – No explanation is available for this answer.

Back to Q 57 on page 100

58. The correct answer is **B** – No explanation is available for this answer.

Back to Q 58 on page 101

59. The correct answer is **D** – No explanation is available for this answer.

Back to Q 59 on page 101

60. The correct answer is **C** – No explanation is available for this answer.

    Back to Q 60 on page 101

61. The correct answer is **A** – No explanation is available for this answer.

    Back to Q 61 on page 101

62. The correct answer is **B** – No explanation is available for this answer.

    Back to Q 62 on page 101

63. The correct answer is **B** – No explanation is available for this answer.

    Back to Q 63 on page 102

64. The correct answer is **C** – Aciduric bacteria are the bacterial which can tolerate an acidic medium.

    Back to Q 64 on page 102

65. The correct answer is **D** – Much research has identified mutans streptococci (MS) as the major pathogens of dental caries. This is because, first, MS are frequently isolated from cavitated caries lesions; second, MS induce caries formation in animals fed a sucrose-rich diet; third, MS are highly acidogenic and aciduric; and fourth, MS are able to produce surface antigens I/II and water-insoluble glucan, which promote bacterial adhesion to the tooth surface and to other bacteria.

    Back to Q 65 on page 102

66. The correct answer is **C** – Plaque glucans are synthesized from dietary sucrose by glucosyltransferase.

    Back to Q 66 on page 102

67. The correct answer is **ABD** – The Vipeholm trials, which took place between 1945 and 1955, involved feeding excessive quantities of sweets to patients at the Vipeholm Hospital for the Intellectually Handicapped in Lund, Sweden, in order to test the effect of carbohydrates on dental caries. Today, nevertheless, it is believed that they violated medical ethic's fundamental rules. The experiment led to the conclusion that frequency of intake, followed by stickiness of carbohydrates were the most important factors in the cariogenicity of carbohydrates.

    Back to Q 67 on page 102

Chapter 5
Diseases of Pulp and Periapical Tissues

The pulp is a small tissue with a big issue which is usually attributed to the characteristic anatomy and histology of the dental pulp.

5.1 MCQs Questions

Choose **one or more** of the most appropriate answers. Some questions may have **more than one** correct answer. You have to choose all the correct answers as best as you can.

1. The most common complication of periapical granuloma is:
   (a) Fracture of the mandible
   (b) Pulp necrosis
   (c) Cyst formation
   (d) Malignancy
   Answer for Q 1 on page 117
2. Pulp polyp (chronic hyperplastic pulpitis) usually affects:
   (a) Upper third molar
   (b) First permanent molar
   (c) Upper deciduous canine
   (d) Lower permanent canine
   Answer for Q 2 on page 117
3. Focal reversible pulpitis is a reversible condition because it is characterized by presence of micro-abscesses in the pulp tissue
   (a) Both statements are incorrect
   (b) The second statement is only correct
   (c) Both statements are correct
   (d) The first statement is only correct

Answer for Q 3 on page 117

4. The most common location of chronic hyperplastic pulpitis is:
   (a) Permanent upper incisors
   (b) Deciduous upper incisors
   (c) deciduous or succedaneous molars
   (d) Permanent premolar

Answer for Q 4 on page 117

5. Which of the following statement is incorrect about pulpitis?
   (a) Carbohydrates is the most important etiological factor
   (b) dental caries is the commonest cause
   (c) bacteria can also reach the pulp by other local routes
   (d) trauma to the dentin and/or pulp may cause pulpitis and/or reactionary changes in the pulpo-dentinal

Answer for Q 5 on page 117

6. Most cases of pulpitis are caused by
   (a) injudicious cavity preparation
   (b) chemical irritation from sterilizing agent
   (c) bacterial invasion from bloodstream
   (d) bacterial invasion from carious lesion

Answer for Q 6 on page 118

7. The most common route by which infection may reach the pulp is through:
   (a) The blood streams
   (b) Traumatic injuries
   (c) Dental caries
   (d) Erosion
   (e) Periosteum

Answer for Q 7 on page 118

8. Acute inflammation would attract:
   (a) Monocytes
   (b) Plasma cells
   (c) Neutrophils
   (d) Eosinophils

Answer for Q 8 on page 118

9. The rationale for treatment of periapical granuloma is:
   (a) Pathological fracture
   (b) Cyst formation
   (c) Malignancy
   (d) Face disfigurement

   Answer for Q 9 on page 118

10. The most common complication of periapical granuloma is:
   (a) Fracture of the mandible
   (b) Cyst formation
   (c) Malignancy
   (d) Pulp necrosis

   Answer for Q 10 on page 118

11. Aerodontalgia is:
   (a) Pain resulting from hot application on the tooth
   (b) Pain resulting from percussion test
   (c) Pain felt in persons flying at high altitudes
   (d) Pain resulting from presence of two dissimilar metals in the oral cavity

   Answer for Q 11 on page 118

12. One of the following components is responsible for converting periapical granuloma into a cyst:
   (a) Cholesterol clefts
   (b) Epithelial rests of Malassez
   (c) Macrophages
   (d) Cholesterol crystals

   Answer for Q 12 on page 118

13. Sensitivity of a tooth to percussion test is a prominent feature of:
   (a) Periapical abscess
   (b) Pulp abscess
   (c) Cementicles
   (d) Acute suppurative pulpitis

   Answer for Q 13 on page 118

14. Focal reversible pulpitis is a reversible condition because it is characterized by presence of micro-abscesses in the pulp tissue
    (a) The second statement is only correct
    (b) The first statement is only correct
    (c) Both statements are correct
    (d) Both statements are incorrect

    Answer for Q 14 on page 118

15. The epithelium that might cover pulp polyp originates from:
    (a) Within pulp tissue
    (b) Saliva
    (c) Endothelium of pulpal blood vessels
    (d) Blood born

    Answer for Q 15 on page 118

16. Pulp polyp (chronic hyperplastic pulpitis) usually affects:
    (a) Lower permanent canine
    (b) Upper third molar
    (c) First permanent molar
    (d) Upper deciduous canine

    Answer for Q 16 on page 118

17. The most common cause of pulpitis is:
    (a) Trauma to a tooth
    (b) Blood born infection
    (c) Dental caries
    (d) Iatrogenic causes

    Answer for Q 17 on page 118

18. Pain originating from within dental pulp can be localized by the patient because, pulp tissue is mesenchymal in origin:
    (a) Both statements are correct and related
    (b) The first statement is only correct
    (c) The second statement is only correct
    (d) Both statements are correct but not related

    Answer for Q 18 on page 118

19. The best line of treatment for periapical granuloma is the use of antibiotics, because granuloma is an infectious process resulting from ingress of bacteria into the periapical region:
    (a) Both statements are correct but not related
    (b) Both statements are correct and related
    (c) The second statement is only correct
    (d) The first statement is only correct

    Answer for Q 19 on page 118

20. The predominant cell in acute pulpitis is:
    (a) Lymphocyte
    (b) Plasma cell
    (c) Polymorph nuclear leukocyte
    (d) Multinucleated giant cell

    Answer for Q 20 on page 118

21. In pulp hyperemia, the tooth is sensitive to:
    (a) Cold application
    (b) Hot application
    (c) Thermal changes particularly cold application
    (d) Percussion

    Answer for Q 21 on page 118

22. In irreversible pulpitis the pain normally
    (a) Is exacerbated by biting down on the affected tooth
    (b) Is poorly localized
    (c) Is of short, less than 10 minutes, duration
    (d) Does not respond to simple analgesics such as paracetamol

    Answer for Q 22 on page 118

23. All of the following are characteristics of dental pulp **except**:
    (a) Absence of collateral circulation
    (b) Constricted apical foramen
    (c) Presence of of proprioceptors
    (d) Dental pulp shows an unlimited power for healing

    Answer for Q 23 on page 119

24. Aerodontalgia is the tooth ache in cases of persons flying at high altitude due to:
    (a) Fall of atmospheric pressure
    (b) Increased atmospheric pressure
    (c) Decreased blood supply of the pulp
    (d) Dissolution of blood gases

    Answer for Q 24 on page 119

25. In reversible pulpitis, the pain is:
    (a) Persistent
    (b) Momentary
    (c) Spontaneous
    (d) Could be elicited by percussion

    Answer for Q 25 on page 119

26. In acute pulpitis, the pain is:
    (a) Persistent
    (b) Momentary
    (c) Cannot be spontaneous
    (d) Could be elicited by percussion

    Answer for Q 26 on page 119

27. The main clinical feature of pulp stones is:
    (a) Severe pain
    (b) Discomfort
    (c) Sensitivity to percussion
    (d) None of the above

    Answer for Q 27 on page 119

28. Acute pulpitis is treated only by removal of the irritating cause, because dental pulp shows an extensive power for healing:
    (a) The second statement is only correct
    (b) Both statements are incorrect
    (c) The first statement is only correct
    (d) Both statements are correct and related

    Answer for Q 28 on page 119

29. In chronic pulpitis, pain is usually described as:
    (a) Sharp lancinating spontaneous
    (b) Dull aching, intermittent being non-localizable by the patient
    (c) Dull aching, intermittent being well-localizable by the patient
    (d) Intermittent sharp shooting

    Answer for Q 29 on page 119

30. All of the following is true for acute apical periodontitis **except**:
    (a) Can results from extension of infection from pulp tissue
    (b) Histologically shows foam cells. cholesterol clefts and multinucleated giant cells
    (c) May result from acute exacerbation of periapical granuloma
    (d) Severe throbbing pain

    Answer for Q 30 on page 119

31. Russell bodies are usually found in:
    (a) Pulp stones
    (b) Acute apical periodontitis
    (c) Acute periapical abscess
    (d) Periapical granuloma

    Answer for Q 31 on page 119

32. The most important difference between pulp polyp and gingival polyp is:
    (a) Gingival polyp is always inflamed while pulp polyp is not
    (b) Gingival polyp is sensitive to manipulation while pulp polyp is not
    (c) Gingival polyp is always related to carious tooth with large cavity
    (d) Gingival polyp appears radiographically as a radiopaque mass

    Answer for Q 32 on page 119

33. Chronic pulpitis is usually characterized by:
    (a) Dull aching pain
    (b) Severe throbbing pain
    (c) Not pain at all
    (d) Pain elicited by percussion

    Answer for Q 33 on page 119

34. Which of the following statements is false?

    (a) A periapical granuloma can develop into a periapical cyst.

    (b) An apical periodontitis always causes radiographic periapical changes.

    (c) A periapical granuloma is a circumscribed area of chronically inflamed tissue.

    (d) A periapical granuloma may contain epithelial rests.

    Answer for Q 34 on page 119

35. Intensity of pain increased when patient lies down, is a characteristic feature of:

    (a) focal reversible pulpitis

    (b) chronic pulpitis

    (c) acute pulpitis

    (d) chronic hyperplastic pulpitis

    Answer for Q 35 on page 119

36. In contrast to acute pulpitis, in chronic pulpitis threshold for stimulation by electric pulp tester is:

    (a) increased

    (b) unaffected

    (c) decreased

    (d) may increase or decrease

    Answer for Q 36 on page 119

37. A granuloma, cyst and an abscess may be accurately distinguished by:

    (a) pulp vitality test

    (b) radiographic examination

    (c) percussion

    (d) histologic examination

    Answer for Q 37 on page 119

38. Acute exacerbation of a chronic periapical inflammatory lesion might lead to the development of

    (a) Phoenix abscess

    (b) Radicular cyst

    (c) Periapical granuloma

    (d) Chronic periodontitis

    Answer for Q 38 on page 119

39. Barodontalgia is:
    (a) Pain felt in the teeth due to difference in barometric pressure
    (b) Pain resulting from cold application on the tooth
    (c) Pain resulting from percussion test
    (d) Pain resulting from electric pulp tester

    Answer for Q 39 on page 120

40. What is meant by iatrogenic pulpitis?
    (a) Pain felt when persons are flying at high altitude
    (b) Pulpitis caused by errors made by dentists
    (c) Pulpitis caused by excessive occlusal forces
    (d) Any pulpitis caused by infection

    Answer for Q 40 on page 120

41. Pain of reversible pulpitis:
    (a) Persists for several hours after removal of the stimulus
    (b) Can be spontaneous and unpredictable
    (c) Disappears instantly after removal of the stimulus
    (d) Cannot be elicited by electric pulp tester

    Answer for Q 41 on page 120

5.2 Answers with Comments:

1. The correct answer is **C** – The epithelial rests of Malassez found in granuloma can undergo inflammatory proliferation and hence converting the granuloma into a cyst.

   Back to Q 1 on page 109

2. The correct answer is **B** – Remember the requisites for the formation of chronic hyperplastic pulpitis.

   Back to Q 2 on page 109

3. The correct answer is **D** – No explanation is available for this answer.

   Back to Q 3 on page 109

4. The correct answer is **C** – No explanation is available for this answer.

   Back to Q 4 on page 110

5. The correct answer is **A** – No explanation is available for this answer.

   Back to Q 5 on page 110

6. The correct answer is **D** – No explanation is available for this answer.

   Back to Q 6 on page 110

7. The correct answer is **C** – No explanation is available for this answer.

   Back to Q 7 on page 110

8. The correct answer is **C** – No explanation is available for this answer.

   Back to Q 8 on page 110

9. The correct answer is **B** – No explanation is available for this answer.

   Back to Q 9 on page 111

10. The correct answer is **B** – No explanation is available for this answer.

    Back to Q 10 on page 111

11. The correct answer is **C** – No explanation is available for this answer.

    Back to Q 11 on page 111

12. The correct answer is **B** – No explanation is available for this answer.

    Back to Q 12 on page 111

13. The correct answer is **A** – No explanation is available for this answer.

    Back to Q 13 on page 111

14. The correct answer is **B** – No explanation is available for this answer.

    Back to Q 14 on page 112

15. The correct answer is **B** – No explanation is available for this answer.

    Back to Q 15 on page 112

16. The correct answer is **C** – No explanation is available for this answer.

    Back to Q 16 on page 112

17. The correct answer is **C** – No explanation is available for this answer.

    Back to Q 17 on page 112

18. The correct answer is **C** – No explanation is available for this answer.

    Back to Q 18 on page 112

19. The correct answer is **C** – No explanation is available for this answer.

    Back to Q 19 on page 113

20. The correct answer is **C** – No explanation is available for this answer.

    Back to Q 20 on page 113

21. The correct answer is **C** – No explanation is available for this answer.

    Back to Q 21 on page 113

22. The correct answer is **B** – No explanation is available for this answer.

Back to Q 22 on page 113

23. The correct answer is **C** – No explanation is available for this answer.

Back to Q 23 on page 113

24. The correct answer is **A** – No explanation is available for this answer.

Back to Q 24 on page 114

25. The correct answer is **B** – No explanation is available for this answer.

Back to Q 25 on page 114

26. The correct answer is **A** – No explanation is available for this answer.

Back to Q 26 on page 114

27. The correct answer is **D** – No explanation is available for this answer.

Back to Q 27 on page 114

28. The correct answer is **B** – No explanation is available for this answer.

Back to Q 28 on page 114

29. The correct answer is **B** – No explanation is available for this answer.

Back to Q 29 on page 115

30. The correct answer is **B** – No explanation is available for this answer.

Back to Q 30 on page 115

31. The correct answer is **D** – Russel bodies are scattered eosinophilic globules of gamma globulin found at the aggregates of plasma cells.

Back to Q 31 on page 115

32. The correct answer is **B** – The so called pulp polyp does not contain nerve endings so it is insensitive to manipulation.

Back to Q 32 on page 115

33. The correct answer is **A** – No explanation is available for this answer.

Back to Q 33 on page 115

34. The correct answer is **B** – No explanation is available for this answer.

Back to Q 34 on page 116

35. The correct answer is **B** – No explanation is available for this answer.

Back to Q 35 on page 116

36. The correct answer is **A** – No explanation is available for this answer.

Back to Q 36 on page 116

37. The correct answer is **D** – No explanation is available for this answer.

Back to Q 37 on page 116

38. The correct answer is **A** – No explanation is available for this answer.

    Back to Q 38 on page 116

39. The correct answer is **A** – No explanation is available for this answer.

    Back to Q 39 on page 117

40. The correct answer is **B** – No explanation is available for this answer.

    Back to Q 40 on page 117

41. The correct answer is **C** – Pain of reversible pulpitis cannot be spontaneous, disappears immediately after removal of the stimulus and poorly localized by the patient.

    Back to Q 41 on page 117

CHAPTER 6
CYSTS & CYST-LIKE LESIONS

Cysts, cyst-like, and cystic tumors are common pathologies of the jaws and soft tissues surrounding the jaws. They usually appear as painless swellings that could be mistaken for tumors; however, they are not neoplastic in nature.

6.1 MCQs Questions

Choose **one or more** of the most appropriate answers. Some questions may have **more than one** correct answer. You have to choose all the correct answers as best as you can.

1. Which of the following cyst arises from glands of Serres ((Serres pearls)?
    (a) Odontogenic keratocyst
    (b) Dentigerous cysts
    (c) Radicular cysts
    (d) Paradental cyst
    Answer for Q 1 on page 135
2. A constant feature associated with radicular cyst is
    (a) Impacted tooth
    (b) Missing tooth
    (c) None vital tooth
    (d) Anomalous tooth
    Answer for Q 2 on page 135
3. High recurrence rate of keratocysts is due to all factors **except:**
    (a) satellite cysts
    (b) difficulty of surgical removal
    (c) focal areas of active growth of the cyst wall
    (d) cystic contents have a low soluble protein level

Answer for Q 3 on page 135

4. Cyst resembling the bunch of grapes is
   (a) Gingival cyst
   (b) developmental lateral periodontal cyst (botyroid cyst)
   (c) dentigerous cyst
   (d) OKC

Answer for Q 4 on page 136

5. Which of the following lesion resembles frog's belly?
   (a) ranula
   (b) Retention mucocele
   (c) extravasation mucocele
   (d) dermoid cyst

Answer for Q 5 on page 136

6. Which one of the following is most commonly a midline lesion?
   (a) Epidermoid cyst
   (b) Branchial cleft cyst
   (c) Nasolabial cyst
   (d) Dermoid cyst

Answer for Q 6 on page 136

7. Which of the following is a **true** statement about thyroglossal duct cysts?
   (a) They occur in the lateral neck, just anterior to the sternocleidomastoid muscle
   (b) They are associated with high incidence of malignant transformation
   (c) They are pseudocysts
   (d) They may be associated with thyroid follicles

Answer for Q 7 on page 136

8. The most frequent odontogenic developmental cyst is the:
   (a) dentigerous cyst
   (b) gingival cyst of adult
   (c) lateral periodontal cyst
   (d) glandular odontogenic cyst

Answer for Q 8 on page 136

9. The most common frequent site of lateral periodontal cyst is the:
   (a) Anterior mandible
   (b) Canine-premolar area of mandible
   (c) Anterior maxilla
   (d) Posterior maxilla

   Answer for Q 9 on page 136

10. Nasolabial cysts are:
    (a) Three times more common in men
    (b) Usually, bilateral
    (c) Radiolucent
    (d) Occasionally lined by apocrine and ciliated columnar epithelial cells

    Answer for Q 10 on page 136

11. What is the most common developmental non-odontogenic cyst in head and neck?
    (a) Nasolabial cysts
    (b) Nasopalatine duct cyst
    (c) Branchial cleft cyst
    (d) Oral lymphoepithelial cyst

    Answer for Q 11 on page 136

12. Which of the following radiographic descriptions is considered characteristic for traumatic bone cyst?
    (a) "Sun-ray" appearance
    (b) "Scalloping between roots" appearance
    (c) "Cotton-wool" appearance
    (d) "Onion-skin" appearance

    Answer for Q 12 on page 136

13. Nevoid basal cell carcinoma syndrome is characterized by basal cell carcinomas, calcified falx cerebri and multiple:
    (a) Osteomas
    (b) Odontomas
    (c) Odontogenic keratocysts
    (d) Mucosal neuromas

    Answer for Q 13 on page 136

14. A well-defined radiolucency near the angle of the mandible and below the inferior alveolar canal on a radiograph is most likely a:
    (a) Dentigerous cyst
    (b) Traumatic bone cyst
    (c) Stafne bone defect
    (d) Cervical lymphoepithelial cyst

    Answer for Q 14 on page 136

15. Epstein pearls (palatal cysts of newborn) are:
    (a) Same as enamel pearls
    (b) Imperfection in the tooth bud
    (c) Seen in vitamin D deficiency
    (d) Small keratin cysts of newborn infant

    Answer for Q 15 on page 137

16. A pear-shaped radiolucency causing displacement of the roots of vital maxillary lateral and cuspid teeth is characteristics of:
    (a) Globulomaxillary cyst
    (b) Apical periodontal cyst
    (c) Primordial cyst
    (d) Nasoalveolar cyst
    (e) Lateral Periodontal Cyst

    Answer for Q 16 on page 137

17. Lesion that characteristically occurs on the alveolar ridges of infants is:
    (a) Congenital lymphangioma
    (b) Fordyce granules
    (c) Bohn's nodules
    (d) White sponge nevus
    (e) Retrocuspid papilla

    Answer for Q 17 on page 137

18. A cyst occurring under the tongue, caused by obstruction of a salivary gland duct, is called a:
    (a) Follicular cyst
    (b) Dentigerous cyst
    (c) Ranula
    (d) Dermoid cyst
    (e) Epidermoid cyst

    Answer for Q 18 on page 137

19. All the following developmental cysts of the jaws present as radiolucent lesions **except**:
    (a) Median palatal cyst
    (b) Nasopalatine duct cyst
    (c) Nasoalveolar
    (d) Globulomaxillary cyst
    (e) Epidermoid cyst

    Answer for Q 19 on page 137

20. Which of the following is **not** an advantage of marsupialization?
    (a) Exposure of very little bone
    (b) Preservation of vital structure
    (c) Rapid healing
    (d) Conserve surgical sutures

    Answer for Q 20 on page 137

21. Needle aspiration of a central bone lesion is useful to:
    (a) Rule out a vascular lesion
    (b) Determine thickness of buccal plate
    (c) Determine the position of the furcation
    (d) Feel root surfaces

    Answer for Q 21 on page 137

22. The aspirate from a keratocyst will have:
    (a) A low soluble protein content
    (b) A high soluble protein content
    (c) Cholesterol crystal
    (d) Inflammatory cells

    Answer for Q 22 on page 137

23. An empty cavity in the mandible with no lining is most likely to be:

    (a) Aneurysmal bone cyst

    (b) Idiopathic bone cavity

    (c) Dentigerous cyst

    (d) Keratocyst

    Answer for Q 23 on page 137

24. A 14-year-old boy has delayed eruption of the second molar. Radiography shows a dentigerous cyst surrounding the crown of the tooth. The treatment of choice is:

    (a) Extraction of the molar

    (b) Aspiration of the cyst

    (c) Observe

    (d) Expose the crown and keep it exposed

    Answer for Q 24 on page 137

25. Expected surgical procedure most frequently indicated for odontogenic cysts is:

    (a) Incision and drainage

    (b) Sclerosing solution

    (c) Marsupialization

    (d) Enucleation

    Answer for Q 25 on page 137

26. The cyst is deroofed and the surrounding periosteum is sutured to the margins of the cyst wall in:

    (a) Decortication

    (b) Marsupialization

    (c) Saucerization

    (d) Enucleation

    Answer for Q 26 on page 137

27. Best treatment of the large cyst:

    (a) Enucleation

    (b) Marsupialization

    (c) Marsupialization followed by Enucleation

    (d) Enucleation followed by Marsupialization

    Answer for Q 27 on page 137

28. Protein content of less than 4 mg/ml is seen in:
    (a) Dentigerous cyst
    (b) Periapical abscess
    (c) Keratocyst
    (d) Periodontal cyst

    Answer for Q 28 on page 137

29. Marsupialization is the procedure done in:
    (a) large cyst
    (b) periodontal cyst
    (c) Aneurysmal bone cyst
    (d) Stafne cyst

    Answer for Q 29 on page 137

30. Apical cyst having a direct connection with apical foramen have been termed as:
    (a) Residual
    (b) Bay cyst[1]
    (c) Paradental
    (d) Collateral

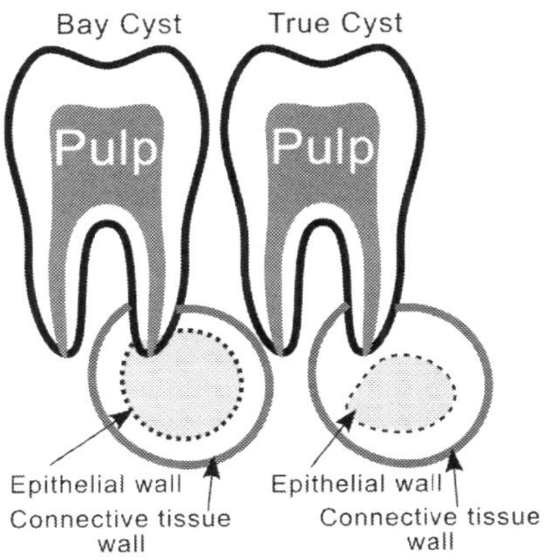

Answer for Q 30 on page 138

[1] It has been suggested that radicular cysts can be divided into two main categories, bay cysts and true cysts. Bay cysts can be described as open bags where the cyst lumen is continuous with the necrotic root canal. True cysts, on the other hand, are structurally independent lesions inside the body of the periapical lesion (apical periodontitis) without continuity with the root canal. Diagnosis between bay cyst and true cyst would require serial histological sectioning which may be too complex for routine procedures. However, a distinction of bay cysts from true cysts offers a possible explanation why some cysts apparently respond to conservative endodontic therapy (bay cysts) while others do not (true cysts). It also may explain the occurrence of residual cysts found after extraction of the tooth with true cysts. See associated picture.

31. Carnoy's[2] solution is used in the treatment of:
    (a) Odontogenic keratocyst
    (b) Ameloblastoma
    (c) Dentigerous cyst
    (d) Mucocele

    Answer for Q 31 on page 138

32. Maintaining continuity of jaw: Which of the following substances is filled in the bone cavity after enucleation of a cyst:
    (a) Hydroxyapatite
    (b) Autogenous cortical bone chips
    (c) Autogenous medullary bone chips
    (d) Allogenic bone chips

    Answer for Q 32 on page 138

33. A cyst can be differentiated from granuloma by:
    (a) Radiopaque dyes
    (b) Polyacrylamide gel electrophoresis
    (c) Biopsy
    (d) All of the above

    Answer for Q 33 on page 138

34. A cyst can be differentiated from tumor by:
    (a) Radiography
    (b) CT scan
    (c) Aspiration biopsy
    (d) Percussion

    Answer for Q 34 on page 138

35. Chemical cauterization in odontogenic keratocyst is done by:
    (a) Hydrogen peroxide
    (b) Carnoy's solution
    (c) Superoxide solution
    (d) Betadine

    Answer for Q 35 on page 138

[2] Carnoy's solution is a fixative and caustic composed of 60% ethanol, 30% chloroform and 10% glacial acetic acid, 1 gram of ferric chloride.

36. Multiple bilateral dentigerous cysts are seen in?
    (a) Down's syndrome
    (b) Maroteaux-lamy syndrome (Mucopolysaccharidosis Type VI (MPS-VI))
    (c) Teacher collins syndrome
    (d) Gorlin Goltz syndrome

    Answer for Q 36 on page 138

37. The most aggressive and destructive cyst is:
    (a) Periapical cyst
    (b) Odontogenic keratocyst
    (c) Globulomaxillary cyst
    (d) Nasopalatine cyst

    Answer for Q 37 on page 138

38. The most common odontogenic cyst is:
    (a) Primordial cyst
    (b) Dentigerous cyst
    (c) Radicular cyst
    (d) Mucocele

    Answer for Q 38 on page 138

39. Dentigerous cyst is associated with the following
    (a) Impacted 3rd molar
    (b) Impacted supernumerary tooth
    (c) Odontome
    (d) All of the above

    Answer for Q 39 on page 138

40. After entering a radiolucent lesion in a 30 years old man, a hollow cavity without epithelial lining was seen, the most probable diagnosis is:
    (a) Aneurysmal bone cyst
    (b) Static bone cavity
    (c) Hemorrhagic bone cyst
    (d) Ameloblastoma

    Answer for Q 40 on page 138

41. Dentigerous cyst is suspected if the follicular space is more than:

    (a) 2–3 mm

    (b) 3–4 mm

    (c) 1–2 mm

    (d) >5 mm

    Answer for Q 41 on page 138

42. All of the following lesions may be classified as odontogenic tumors **except**:

    (a) Acanthomatous ameloblastoma

    (b) Branchial cleft cyst

    (c) Odontogenic myxoma

    (d) Simple ameloblastoma

    Answer for Q 42 on page 138

43. Bifid ribs, Multiple radiolucent lesions of the jaws, multiple basal cell nevi and falx cerebri calcification are found in:

    (a) Basal cell nevus syndrome

    (b) Sturge weber syndrome

    (c) Horner syndrome

    (d) Hereditary internal polyposis

    Answer for Q 43 on page 138

44. Botryoid odontogenic cyst is a variant of:

    (a) Lateral periodontal cyst

    (b) Apical periodontal cyst

    (c) Gingival cysts of the newborn

    (d) Gingival cysts of adult

    Answer for Q 44 on page 139

45. Eruption cyst:

    (a) Transforms into dentigerous cyst

    (b) Will not regresses after eruption of the tooth

    (c) Is found in the place of the missing tooth

    (d) Is a type of dentigerous teeth

    Answer for Q 45 on page 139

46. Which of the following shows the presence of cholesterol crystals?
    (a) Keratocyst
    (b) Periodontal cyst
    (c) Aneurysmal cyst
    (d) Hemorrhagic cyst

    Answer for Q 46 on page 139

47. Basal layer in primordial cyst is arranged in the form of:
    (a) Tennis racket
    (b) Picket fence
    (c) Linear
    (d) Irregular

    Answer for Q 47 on page 139

48. One of them is not a true cyst:
    (a) Hemorrhagic cyst
    (b) Medial palatal
    (c) Globulomaxillary
    (d) Nasolabial

    Answer for Q 48 on page 139

49. Dentigerous cyst is likely to cause which neoplasia?
    (a) Ameloblastoma
    (b) Osteogenic sarcoma
    (c) Squamous cell carcinoma
    (d) Osteoclastoma

    Answer for Q 4 on page 139

50. Odontogenic Keratocyst has the following feature:
    (a) Occurs due to infection periapically
    (b) is developmental in origin
    (c) Can be treated by aspiration
    (d) Has low recurrence rate

    Answer for Q 50 on page 139

51. Primordial cyst develops:
    (a) In place of missing teeth
    (b) In teeth in which crown development is completed
    (c) In periapical region
    (d) In mandibular body

    Answer for Q 51 on page 139

52. The most ideal explanation for recurrence of odontogenic keratocyst is:
    (a) Increased mitotic activity of the epithelial lining
    (b) Friability of the epithelial lining
    (c) Presence of satellite cysts or daughter cysts
    (d) Continued proliferation of rests of dental lamina

    Answer for Q 52 on page 139

53. The cyst with highest recurrence rate is:
    (a) Keratocyst
    (b) Periapical cyst
    (c) Nasoalveolar cyst
    (d) Globulomaxillary cyst

    Answer for Q 53 on page 139

54. A multilocular cyst of the jaw is most likely:
    (a) Dental cyst
    (b) Dentigerous cyst
    (c) Keratocyst
    (d) Simple bone cyst

    Answer for Q 54 on page 139

55. keratocyst has all of the following features **except**:
    (a) It is more common in mandible
    (b) May be filled with thin straw-colored fluid
    (c) Low recurrence rate
    (d) Expansion of bone clinically seen

    Answer for Q 55 on page 139

56. Each of the following cyst is associated with an impacted tooth **except**:
    (a) Dentigerous cyst
    (b) Calcifying epithelial odontogenic cyst
    (c) Keratocyst
    (d) Primordial cyst

    Answer for Q 56 on page 139

57. Which of the following is wrong about keratocyst?
    (a) has low recurrence rate
    (b) has low protein content
    (c) high recurrence rate
    (d) B and C

    Answer for Q 57 on page 139

58. Which histopathological type of odontogenic keratocyst is commoner, more invasive and has a greater tendency for recurrence?
    (a) Orthokeratinized
    (b) Parakeratinized
    (c) Non keratinized
    (d) Dyskeratinized

    Answer for Q 58 on page 139

59. Multiple odontogenic keratocyst are associated with:
    (a) Gardner's syndrome
    (b) Gorlin-Goltz Syndrome
    (c) Goldenhar Syndrome[3]
    (d) Grinspan syndrome[4]

    Answer for Q 59 on page 139

60. All of the following is true about primordial cyst **except**:
    (a) Can occur in place of a missing tooth
    (b) The term "Primordial cyst" is considered an outdated term and should be avoided
    (c) Most "primordial cysts" are actually Keratocyst odontogenic tumors (KOT's)
    (d) Most commonly arise in the area of mandibular third molars.

    Answer for Q 60 on page 140

---

[3] A rare congenital disease characterized by incomplete development of the ear, nose, soft palate, lip and mandible on usually one side of the body.

[4] A syndromic complex which comprises a triad of hypertension, diabetes, and oral lichen planus.

61. A 35-year-old female came to the clinic for a routine dental checkup. Tooth number 35 has a big defective restoration. The tooth negatively responded to the vitality test. The X-ray showed a well-defined radiolucency associate with the apex of tooth number 35. The patient reported that the tooth was endodontically treated 6 months prior this visit. After taking a biopsy, the microscopic examination revealed connective tissue wall lined by stratified squamous epithelium. What is the diagnosis of this case?

    (a) Periapical abscess

    (b) Periapical granuloma

    (c) Periapical cyst

    (d) Residual cyst

    Answer for Q 61 on page 140

62. The most common source of epithelium that forms a periapical cyst is:

    (a) Epithelial rest of Malassez

    (b) The superficial epithelium

    (c) Epithelial rests of Serres

    (d) Dental lamina

    Answer for Q 62 on page 140

63. Which of the following is TRUE statement about thyroglossal duct cysts?

    (a) They occur in the lateral neck, just anterior to the sternocleidomastoid muscle.

    (b) They are associated with high incidence of malignant transformation

    (c) They are pseudocysts

    (d) They may be associated with thyroid follicles.

    Answer for Q 63 on page 140

64. Nasolabial cysts are:

    (a) Three times more common in men

    (b) Usually, bilateral

    (c) Radiolucent

    (d) Occasionally lined by apocrine and ciliated columnar epithelial cells

    Answer for Q 64 on page 140

65. Which of the following is a synonym for traumatic bone cyst?
    (a) Solitary bone cyst
    (b) Static bone cyst
    (c) Stafne bone defect
    (d) Aneurysmal bone cyst

    Answer for Q 65 on page 140

66. A patient having routine dental radiographs was found to have a radiolucent lesion near the angle of the mandible. Given the classic characteristic radiographic features, the patient was diagnosed as a Stafne defect and that no treatment was need. If a pathology specimen was obtained, what would be expected microscopically?
    (a) Cystic lesion lined by columnar basal cells in a palisading arrangement with vacuolated cytoplasm and nuclei polarized away from basement membrane
    (b) Normal appearing salivary gland tissue
    (c) Squamous epithelium with a wavy "corrugated" surface and basal cell layer with palisading
    (d) A and C
    (e) None of the above

    Answer for Q 66 on page 140

6.2 Answers with Comments:

1. The correct answer is **A**:
    (a) Derived from epithelial residues of the tooth-forming organ
    (b) The main cyst types derived from each residue are:
        - dental lamina rests/glands of Serres – odontogenic keratocyst
        - reduced enamel epithelium – dentigerous cysts and paradental cyst
        - rests of Malassez – radicular cysts

    Back to Q 1 on page 121

2. The correct answer is **C** – Apical, residual, or lateral are sub-types of apical cysts, the apical is commonest type. All are associated with non-vital tooth. apical radiolucency indistinguishable from a periapical granuloma. May be symptomless. Enlargement of cyst leads to bone expansion.

    Back to Q 2 on page 121

3. The correct answer is **D**:
   (a) Tendency to recur related to difficulty of surgical removal
   (b) Thin, easily ruptured wall
   (c) Projections into cancellous spaces easily torn
   (d) Satellite cysts in capsule
   (e) Cyst enlargement involves - focal areas of active growth of the cyst wall - extension of proliferating areas along cancellous spaces - production of bone resorbing factors

   Back to Q 3 on page 121
4. The correct answer is **B** – Occasionally, developmental lateral periodontal cysts are multilocular and may be described by the adjective “botryoid” because of their resemblance to a bunch of grapes (botryoid odontogenic cyst).

   Back to Q 4 on page 122
5. The correct answer is **A** – Ranula is a clinical term used to describe a swelling of the floor of the mouth which is said to resemble a frog’s belly. Histologically, most ranulae are mucous extravasation cysts. Occasionally, a ranula may extend through the mylohyoid muscle and present in the submandibular area or neck, referred to clinically as a plunging ranula.

   Back to Q 5 on page 122
6. The correct answer is **D** – No explanation is available for this answer.

   Back to Q 6 on page 122
7. The correct answer is **D** – No explanation is available for this answer.

   Back to Q 7 on page 122
8. The correct answer is **A** – No explanation is available for this answer.

   Back to Q 8 on page 122
9. The correct answer is **C** – No explanation is available for this answer.

   Back to Q 9 on page 123
10. The correct answer is **D** – No explanation is available for this answer.

    Back to Q 10 on page 123
11. The correct answer is **C** – No explanation is available for this answer.

    Back to Q 11 on page 123
12. The correct answer is **B** – No explanation is available for this answer.

    Back to Q 12 on page 123
13. The correct answer is **C** – No explanation is available for this answer.

    Back to Q 13 on page 123

14. The correct answer is **C** – No explanation is available for this answer.

Back to Q 14 on page 124

15. The correct answer is **D** – No explanation is available for this answer.

Back to Q 15 on page 124

16. The correct answer is **A** – No explanation is available for this answer.

Back to Q 16 on page 124

17. The correct answer is **C** – No explanation is available for this answer.

Back to Q 17 on page 124

18. The correct answer is **C** – No explanation is available for this answer.

Back to Q 18 on page 125

19. The correct answer is **C** – No explanation is available for this answer.

Back to Q 19 on page 125

20. The correct answer is **C** – Marsupialization preserves vital tissues, however, one of its drawbacks is the slow healing process.

Back to Q 20 on page 125

21. The correct answer is **A** – No explanation is available for this answer.

Back to Q 21 on page 125

22. The correct answer is **A** – No explanation is available for this answer.

Back to Q 22 on page 125

23. The correct answer is **B** – Idiopathic bone cavity (*traumatic bone cyst, solitary bone cyst*) is not a true cyst but an empty cavity in the bone.

Back to Q 23 on page 126

24. The correct answer is **D** – By exposure of the crown, the tooth will continue to erupt and the cyst usually vanishes.

Back to Q 24 on page 126

25. The correct answer is **D** – No explanation is available for this answer.

Back to Q 25 on page 126

26. The correct answer is **B** – No explanation is available for this answer.

Back to Q 26 on page 126

27. The correct answer is **C** – No explanation is available for this answer.

Back to Q 27 on page 126

28. The correct answer is **C** – No explanation is available for this answer.

Back to Q 28 on page 127

29. The correct answer is **A** – No explanation is available for this answer.

    Back to Q 29 on page 127

30. The correct answer is **B** – No explanation is available for this answer.

    Back to Q 30 on page 127

31. The correct answer is **A** – No explanation is available for this answer.

    Back to Q 31 on page 128

32. The correct answer is **C** – No explanation is available for this answer.

    Back to Q 32 on page 128

33. The correct answer is **D** – No explanation is available for this answer.

    Back to Q 33 on page 128

34. The correct answer is **C** – Aspiration biopsy yields a fluid while tumors are solid with no aspirating fluids.

    Back to Q 34 on page 128

35. The correct answer is **B** – No explanation is available for this answer.

    Back to Q 35 on page 128

36. The correct answer is **B** – Bilateral and multiple dentigerous cysts have been reported in Basal cell nevus syndrome, Mucopolysaccharidosis, Cleidocranial dysplasia and after prolonged concurrent use of cyclosporine A and calcium channel blockers. Multiple dentigerous cysts have also been reported with Klippel Feil Syndrome.

    Back to Q 36 on page 129

37. The correct answer is **B** – No explanation is available for this answer.

    Back to Q 37 on page 129

38. The correct answer is **C** – No explanation is available for this answer.

    Back to Q 38 on page 129

39. The correct answer is **D** – No explanation is available for this answer.

    Back to Q 39 on page 129

40. The correct answer is **C** – No explanation is available for this answer.

    Back to Q 40 on page 129

41. The correct answer is **D** – No explanation is available for this answer.

    Back to Q 41 on page 130

42. The correct answer is **B** – No explanation is available for this answer.

    Back to Q 42 on page 130

43. The correct answer is **A** – No explanation is available for this answer.

Back to Q 43 on page 130

44. The correct answer is **A** – No explanation is available for this answer.

Back to Q 44 on page 130

45. The correct answer is **D** – No explanation is available for this answer.

Back to Q 45 on page 130

46. The correct answer is **A** – No explanation is available for this answer.

Back to Q 46 on page 131

47. The correct answer is **B** – No explanation is available for this answer.

Back to Q 47 on page 131

48. The correct answer is **A** – No explanation is available for this answer.

Back to Q 48 on page 131

49. The correct answer is **A** – No explanation is available for this answer.

Back to Q 49 on page 131

50. The correct answer is **B** – No explanation is available for this answer.

Back to Q 50 on page 131

51. The correct answer is **A** – No explanation is available for this answer.

Back to Q 51 on page 132

52. The correct answer is **C** – No explanation is available for this answer.

Back to Q 52 on page 132

53. The correct answer is **A** – No explanation is available for this answer.

Back to Q 53 on page 132

54. The correct answer is **C** – No explanation is available for this answer.

Back to Q 54 on page 132

55. The correct answer is **C** – No explanation is available for this answer.

Back to Q 55 on page 132

56. The correct answer is **D** – No explanation is available for this answer.

Back to Q 56 on page 133

57. The correct answer is **A** – No explanation is available for this answer.

Back to Q 57 on page 133

58. The correct answer is **B** – No explanation is available for this answer.

Back to Q 58 on page 133

59. The correct answer is **B** – No explanation is available for this answer.

Back to Q 59 on page 133

60. The correct answer is **B** – No explanation is available for this answer.

    Back to Q 60 on page 133

61. The correct answer is **C** – No explanation is available for this answer.

    Back to Q 61 on page 134

62. The correct answer is **A** – No explanation is available for this answer.

    Back to Q 62 on page 134

63. The correct answer is **D** – No explanation is available for this answer.

    Back to Q 63 on page 134

64. The correct answer is **D** – No explanation is available for this answer.

    Back to Q 64 on page 134

65. The correct answer is **A** – No explanation is available for this answer.

    Back to Q 65 on page 135

66. The correct answer is **B** – No explanation is available for this answer.

    Back to Q 66 on page 135

CHAPTER 7
PHYSICAL, CHEMICAL & IDIOPATHIC PATHOLOGY OF TEETH

Pathological changes in the dental tissues that include a variety of alterations, which are neither inflammatory nor developmental, have been traditionally described in older literature as "***regressive alterations of teeth***". Some of these lesions may be associated with the general aging process, while others arise because of injury to the dental tissues or other obscure causes.

7.1 MCQs Questions

Choose **one or more** of the most appropriate answers. Some questions may have **more than one** correct answer. You have to choose all the correct answers as best as you can.

1. Teeth loss due to tooth-to-tooth contact is called:

   (a) Erosion

   (b) Abrasion

   (c) Attrition

   (d) Abfraction

   Answer for Q 1 on page 144

2. Erosion is:

   (a) Loss of tooth structure due to tooth-to-tooth contact

   (b) Loss of tooth structure due to tooth to abrasive particles contact

   (c) Loss of tooth structure due chemical exposure

   (d) Loss of tooth structure due to flexion of the tooth

   Answer for Q 2 on page 144

3. Pathological attrition may result from:
   (a) Excessive intake of acid beverages
   (b) Faulty tooth brushing
   (c) Abnormal occlusion
   (d) Habits of pipe smoking

   Answer for Q 3 on page 144

4. Chronic alcoholics may present with the features of:
   (a) Erosion
   (b) Resorption
   (c) Abrasion
   (d) Attrition

   Answer for Q 4 on page 144

5. It is advised that a patient avoids excessive consumption of which one of the following in order to reduce the occurrence of enamel erosion?
   (a) Ascorbic acid
   (b) Citric acid
   (c) Lactic acid
   (d) Phosphoric acid

   Answer for Q 5 on page 145

6. The chemical disintegration of enamel is referred to as:
   (a) Abrasion
   (b) Attrition
   (c) Erosion
   (d) Hypoplasia
   (e) Pitting

   Answer for Q 6 on page 145

7. The cells responsible for root resorption are:
   (a) Fibroblasts
   (b) Cementoblasts
   (c) Osteoblasts
   (d) Osteoclasts
   (e) Odontoblast

   Answer for Q 7 on page 145

8. Erosion is most frequently found on:
   (a) Lingual surfaces
   (b) Proximal surfaces
   (c) Facial surfaces
   (d) Incisal or occlusal surfaces

   Answer for Q 8 on page 145

9. Generalized hypercementosis characteristically seen in:
   (a) fibrous dysplasia
   (b) Hyperparathyroidism
   (c) Paget's disease
   (d) cherubism

   Answer for Q 9 on page 145

10. With age, the alteration in size of pulp chamber is a direct result of:
    (a) deposition of primary dentin
    (b) pulp fibrosis
    (c) deposition of secondary dentin
    (d) metaplasia

    Answer for Q 10 on page 145

11. Internal resorption is usually seen in a tooth with:
    (a) Aerodontalgia (barodontalgia)
    (b) Chronic trauma
    (c) Galvanic shock
    (d) Pulp stones

    Answer for Q 11 on page 145

12. Eburnated[1] dentin is seen in:
    (a) Recurrent caries
    (b) Acute caries
    (c) Nursing caries
    (d) Arrested caries

    Answer for Q 12 on page 145

---

[1]A condition observed in arrested dental caries wherein decalcified dentin is burnished and takes on a polished, often brown-stained appearance.

13. Bacterial chemical loss of tooth structure is called:
    (a) erosion
    (b) attrition
    (c) abrasion
    (d) caries

    Answer for Q 13 on the next page

14. Pink tooth of Mummery is a term given to:
    (a) External root resorption at the apex
    (b) Internal root resorption of the pulp chamber
    (c) Abfraction of the tooth
    (d) Pink external stain of the tooth

    Answer for Q 14 on the facing page

15. Abfraction is:
    (a) Similar to attrition but results from chemicals
    (b) Loss of tooth surface at the cervical areas of teeth
    (c) Caused by excessive use of mouth washes
    (d) Induced by forceful tooth brushing

    Answer for Q 15 on the next page

7.2 Answers with Comments:

1. The correct answer is **C** – Pathological attrition may result from:
    (a) Abnormal occlusion - either developmental or following extractions;
    (b) Bruxism and habits such as tobacco and betel chewing;
    (c) Abnormal tooth structure, for example amelogenesis imperfecta, dentinogenesis imperfecta.

    Back to Q 1 on page 141

2. The correct answer is **C** – No explanation is available for this answer.

    Back to Q 2 on page 141

3. The correct answer is **C** – No explanation is available for this answer.

    Back to Q 3 on page 142

4. The correct answer is **A** – A similar pattern of erosion may also be seen in other patients with gastroesophageal reflux, and chronic alcoholics, where gastric reflux is probably associated with chronic gastritis.

Back to Q 4 on page 142

5. The correct answer is **B** – Citric acid is the most commonly used acidifier in beverages.

Back to Q 5 on page 142

6. The correct answer is **C** – Is the pathologic loss (dissolution) of tooth substance by chemicals, usually non-bacterial acids.

Back to Q 6 on page 142

7. The correct answer is **D** – No explanation is available for this answer.

Back to Q 7 on page 142

8. The correct answer is **B** – No explanation is available for this answer.

Back to Q 8 on page 143

9. The correct answer is **C** – Hypercementosis may be one of the complications of Paget's disease of bone in the form of generalized hypercementosis.

Back to Q 9 on page 143

10. The correct answer is **C** – The overall pulp cavity may become smaller by the addition of secondary or tertiary dentin that cause pulp recession.

Back to Q 10 on page 143

11. The correct answer is **B** – No explanation is available for this answer.

Back to Q 11 on page 143

12. The correct answer is **D** – No explanation is available for this answer.

Back to Q 12 on page 143

13. The correct answer is **D** – Bacterial chemicals of caries are organic acids which can dissolve the inorganic elements of tooth structures.

Back to Q 13 on the facing page

14. The correct answer is **B** – No explanation is available for this answer.

Back to Q 14 on the preceding page

15. The correct answer is **B** – No explanation is available for this answer.

Back to Q 15 on the facing page

CHAPTER 8
SPREAD OF DENTAL INFECTION

Odontogenic Infections are one of the most common causes of sever infectious swellings in the head and neck region. It can spread from the original site to remote areas resulting in serious and sometimes fatal consequences.

8.1 MCQs Questions

Choose **one or more** of the most appropriate answers. Some questions may have **more than one** correct answer. You have to choose all the correct answers as best as you can.

1. The spread of infection through the fascial planes of the soft tissue is known as:
   (a) Osteomyelitis
   (b) Cellulitis
   (c) Periapical abscess
   (d) Dry socket
   Answer for Q 1 on page 157
2. Trismus associated with infection of lateral pharyngeal space is related to irritation of the:
   (a) Buccinator
   (b) Masseter
   (c) Lateral pterygoid
   (d) Medial pterygoid
   Answer for Q 2 on page 157
3. Death in Ludwig's angina occurs due to:
   (a) Sepsis
   (b) Respiratory obstruction
   (c) Cavernous sinus thrombosis
   (d) Carotid blow-out

Answer for Q 3 on page 157

4. The roof of pterygomandibular space is formed by:
   (a) Temporalis muscle
   (b) Medial pterygoid muscle
   (c) Cranial base
   (d) lateral pterygoid

Answer for Q 4 on page 157

5. Retropharyngeal space infection is mainly due to spread of:
   (a) Cervical tuberculosis
   (b) Meningoencephalitis
   (c) Mumps
   (d) Odontogenic infections

Answer for Q 5 on page 157

6. The distinguishing feature of masticatory space infection is:
   (a) Pain
   (b) Dysphagia
   (c) Trismus
   (d) Swelling

Answer for Q 6 on page 157

7. The greatest barrier to infection is:
   (a) Connective tissue
   (b) Epithelium
   (c) Muscle
   (d) Fascia

Answer for Q 7 on page 157

8. A mandibular dental infection which exits the buccal cortical plate above the muscle attachment will cause abscess of:
   (a) Buccal space
   (b) Masseter space
   (c) Vestibular sulcus
   (d) Masticatory space

Answer for Q 8 on page 157

9. Which of the following is not a primary mandibular space?
   (a) Buccal
   (b) Sublingual
   (c) Submandibular
   (d) Pterygomandibular

   Answer for Q 9 on page 157

10. Odontogenic infections are most commonly caused by:
    (a) Mixed bacteria
    (b) Anaerobic bacteria
    (c) Aerobic bacteria
    (d) Streptococci

    Answer for Q 10 on page 157

11. The infection from a lower third molar pericoronal area spreads mostly to the following space"
    (a) Submandibular
    (b) Submental space
    (c) Pterygomandibular space
    (d) Buccal space

    Answer for Q 11 on page 157

12. The facial space that is divided by styloid process into an anterior and posterior compartment is:
    (a) Pterygomandibular
    (b) Lateral pharyngeal
    (c) Retropharyngeal
    (d) Infratemporal

    Answer for Q 12 on page 158

13. The most definite clinical sign indicating odontogenic infection in to the masticatory space is:
    (a) trismus
    (b) xerostomia
    (c) difficulty in swallowing
    (d) swelling in submental area

    Answer for Q 13 on page 158

14. Which of the following does not suggest post operative infection?
    (a) Increase in temperature
    (b) Swelling
    (c) Pain
    (d) Pitting edema

    Answer for Q 14 on page 158

15. Ludwig's angina is characterized by:
    (a) Raised tongue
    (b) Elevation of ear lobe
    (c) Trismus
    (d) Unilateral swelling

    Answer for Q 15 on page 158

16. In a 19-year-old patient with a swelling over the left angle of the mandible, temperature of 39 degrees centigrade and negative history of trauma, one should suspect:
    (a) spontaneous fracture of the mandible
    (b) pericoronal infection
    (c) Mumps
    (d) Sjogren's syndrome

    Answer for Q 16 on page 158

17. The most dangerous type of spread of infection from apical abscess is to:
    (a) Infratemporal fossa
    (b) Pterygoid
    (c) Parapharyngeal space
    (d) Submandibular space

    Answer for Q 17 on page 158

18. Cavernous sinus thrombosis following infection of anterior maxillary teeth most often from infection along:
    (a) Facial artery
    (b) Angular artery
    (c) Ophthalmic vein
    (d) Pterygoid plexus

    Answer for Q 18 on page 158

19. Infection of masticatory space is usually associated with:
    (a) tonsillar abscess
    (b) mandibular molar
    (c) lateral pharyngeal space
    (d) Parotid space infection

    Answer for Q 19 on page 158

20. A diagnosis of cavernous sinus thrombosis is made on the basis of: i) known site of infection ii) septicemia iii) venous obstruction in retina, conjunctiva, or eyelid iv) Paresis of third, fourth, and sixth nerves v) Abscess formation of neighboring soft tissues vi) Nuchal rigidity.
    (a) 1,2,3,4,5
    (b) 3,4,5
    (c) 1,2,5,6
    (d) All of the above correct

    Answer for Q 20 on page 158

21. Lateral pharyngeal space is **not** connected directly to:
    (a) Buccal space
    (b) Sublingual space
    (c) Submandibular space
    (d) Retropharyngeal space

    Answer for Q 21 on page 158

22. In any dental abscess, what is the fate of the infection?
    (a) Usually spreads along the path of least resistance
    (b) Always perforate to the lingual cortical palate
    (c) The maxillary lateral incisors drain to the buccal cortical plate
    (d) The mandibular molars drain the temporal space

    Answer for Q 22 on page 158

23. A periapical abscess of a mandibular second molar space spreads most commonly to the:
    (a) Submandibular space
    (b) Temporal space
    (c) Sublingual space
    (d) Infratemporal space

    Answer for Q 23 on page 158

24. Palatal abscess most commonly results from infection of:
    (a) Maxillary centrals
    (b) Maxillary laterals
    (c) Maxillary canine
    (d) Maxillary premolars

Answer for Q 24 on page 158

25. Infection from maxillary first molar drains into:
    (a) Submandibular space
    (b) Infratemporal space
    (c) Buccal space
    (d) Infraorbital space

Answer for Q 25 on page 158

26. After incision and drainage of an abscess, the infectious process has failed to regress in spite of the patient being on high doses of an antibiotic. It would be wise to:
    (a) Insert a large drain
    (b) Repeat culture and sensitivity tests
    (c) Debride and irrigate the area with a fibrinolytic agent
    (d) Begin the parenteral administration of proteolytic enzymes to augment the antibiotics

Answer for Q 26 on page 158

27. Which of the following is **not** present in pterygomandibular space?
    (a) Auriculotemporal nerve
    (b) Lingual nerve
    (c) Mandibular nerve
    (d) Mylohyoid nerve

Answer for Q 27 on page 158

28. The incision for drainage in Ludwig's angina extends:
    (a) up to neck
    (b) to the angle of mandible
    (c) floor of mouth
    (d) all of the above

Answer for Q 28 on page 158

29. Boundaries of the pterygomandibular space includes all of the following **except**:
    (a) Lateral pterygoid muscle
    (b) Parotid gland
    (c) Masseter muscle
    (d) Buccinator muscle

    Answer for Q 29 on page 159

30. After extraction of upper central incisor, patient develops opthalmoplegia, meningitis and lateral rectus paralysis. The diagnosis is:
    (a) Cavernous sinus thrombosis
    (b) Not related
    (c) Cellulitis
    (d) Ludwig's angina

    Answer for Q 30 on page 159

31. Pericoronitis is seen in relation to:
    (a) Impacted third molars only
    (b) Around incompletely erupted crown
    (c) Completely erupted crowns only
    (d) None of the above

    Answer for Q 31 on page 159

32. Subperiosteal abscess, penetrating deep is seen after extraction of:
    (a) Maxillary third molar
    (b) Mandibular third molar
    (c) Maxillary first molar
    (d) Mandibular first molar

    Answer for Q 32 on page 159

33. In infection involving the submandibular space when extra oral incision and drainage are necessary, which of the following structures should be divided?
    (a) Skin only
    (b) Skin, superficial fascia only
    (c) Skin, superficial fascia, platysma and masseter muscle
    (d) Skin, superficial fascia, platysma, masseter and deep cervical fascia

    Answer for Q 33 on page 159

34. In pericoronal abscess related to distoangular impacted lower third molars, the infection may spread to:
    (a) Submasseteric space
    (b) Sublingual space
    (c) Submental space
    (d) Buccal space

    Answer for Q 34 on page 159

35. Masticatory space infection usually occurs from:
    (a) Infections of the last two lower molar
    (b) Non aseptic technique in local anesthesia
    (c) External or internal trauma to the mandibular angle region
    (d) All of the above

    Answer for Q 35 on page 159

36. Dumb bell-shaped swelling is characteristic of which type of odontogenic space infections?
    (a) Submandibular space infection
    (b) Buccal space infection
    (c) Submasseteric space infection
    (d) Temporal space infection

    Answer for Q 36 on page 159

37. All of the following are present in pterygomandibular space **except**:
    (a) Nerve to mylohyoid
    (b) Chorda tympani
    (c) Long buccal nerve
    (d) Nerve to pterygoid

    Answer for Q 37 on page 159

38. Cavernous sinus thrombosis can occur due to spread of odontogenic infection via:
    (a) Tissue Spaces
    (b) Lymphatic route
    (c) Hematogenous route
    (d) All of the above

    Answer for Q 38 on page 159

39. Standard airway for Ludwig's angina:
    (a) Tracheostomy
    (b) Cricothyrotomy
    (c) Nasal intubation
    (d) Oral intubation

    Answer for Q 39 on page 159

40. Which of the following is a secondary site of spread of odontogenic infection involving pterygomandibular space?
    (a) Infratemporal space
    (b) Canine space
    (c) Buccal space
    (d) Sublingual space

    Answer for Q 40 on page 159

41. "Hot potato"[1] voice is characteristically seen in:
    (a) Pterygomandibular space infection
    (b) Retropharyngeal space infection
    (c) Pre-tracheal space infection
    (d) Lateral pharyngeal space infection

    Answer for Q 41 on page 159

42. Ludwig's angina is usually caused by:
    (a) Streptococci and various mixed anaerobes
    (b) Anaerobic infection by Prevotella and Fusobacterium
    (c) Paramyxovirus
    (d) Candida species

    Answer for Q 42 on page 159

43. The most common serious complication which can occur following surgery in maxillary incisor region:
    (a) Iritis
    (b) Cellulitis
    (c) Periapical abscess
    (d) Cavernous sinus thrombosis

    Answer for Q 43 on page 159

[1] Severe sore throat leading to the phenomenon of "hot potato voice". The term "hot potato voice" is used for a defect of resonance in which the speech has a muffled quality, similar to a person speaking with a hot potato in the mouth. Seen also in peritonsillar abscess.

44. There is a fluctuant swelling with respect to maxillary lateral incisor, in the last 48 hours. The swelling is hot and palpable, rebound on pressure. The treatment of choice is:

   (a) Incision and drainage

   (b) Antibiotic coverage

   (c) Antibiotics of heat only

   (d) Aspiration

   Answer for Q 44 on page 159

45. In oral and maxillofacial surgery, "danger space" is known as:

   (a) carotid sheath

   (b) Posterior to carotid sheath in posterior triangle of neck

   (c) posterior to transverse process of vertebrae

   (d) space between alar and prevertebral fascia

   Answer for Q 45 on page 160

46. **Untrue** regarding Ludwig's angina:

   (a) Involves submandibular, sublingual, and submental space

   (b) Involves bilateral mandibular spaces and lymphadenopathy

   (c) Bilateral submandibular, sublingual and submental spaces along with salivary gland enlargements

   (d) None of the above

   Answer for Q 46 on page 160

47. Sublingual space is divided from submandibular space by:

   (a) Fibers of mylohyoid

   (b) Submandibular gland

   (c) Body of mandible

   (d) Geniohyoid

   Answer for Q 47 on page 160

48. Penrose[2] drain is:

   (a) a simple rubber tube which opens at one end

   (b) simple rubber tube which opens at both ends

   (c) Modified corrugated rubber drain

   (d) Modified Foley's catheter

   Answer for Q 48 on page 160

[2] A Penrose drain is a soft, flat, flexible tube made of latex. It lets blood and other fluids move out of the area of your surgery. This keeps fluid from collecting under your incision (surgical cut) and causing infection.

49. A patient comes to the emergency with Ludwig's angina. Which of the following is done first?
    (a) Incision and drainage
    (b) Antibiotic and IV fluid infusion
    (c) Fiberoptic nasotracheal intubation/tracheostomy under local anesthesia
    (d) Tracheostomy under general anesthesia

    Answer for Q 49 on page 160

8.2 Answers with Comments:

1. The correct answer is **B** – An infection which is spread along the fascial planes is termed cellulitis, while localized infection with formation of pus is termed abscess.

   Back to Q 1 on page 147
2. The correct answer is **D** – No explanation is available for this answer.

   Back to Q 2 on page 147
3. The correct answer is **B** – The most common and dangerous complications of Ludwig's angina is suffocation due to obstruction of the airway.

   Back to Q 3 on page 147
4. The correct answer is **D** – No explanation is available for this answer.

   Back to Q 4 on page 148
5. The correct answer is **D** – No explanation is available for this answer.

   Back to Q 5 on page 148
6. The correct answer is **C** – No explanation is available for this answer.

   Back to Q 6 on page 148
7. The correct answer is **D** – Fascia is the most tough tissue among the mentioned tissues.

   Back to Q 7 on page 148
8. The correct answer is **C** – No explanation is available for this answer.

   Back to Q 8 on page 148
9. The correct answer is **D** – No explanation is available for this answer.

   Back to Q 9 on page 149
10. The correct answer is **A** – Due to the nature of oral flora, almost all dental infections are mixed.

    Back to Q 10 on page 149
11. The correct answer is **C** – No explanation is available for this answer.

    Back to Q 11 on page 149

12. The correct answer is **B** – No explanation is available for this answer.

    Back to Q 12 on page 149

13. The correct answer is **A** – No explanation is available for this answer.

    Back to Q 13 on page 149

14. The correct answer is **D** – No explanation is available for this answer.

    Back to Q 14 on page 150

15. The correct answer is **A** – No explanation is available for this answer.

    Back to Q 15 on page 150

16. The correct answer is **B** – No explanation is available for this answer.

    Back to Q 16 on page 150

17. The correct answer is **C** – No explanation is available for this answer.

    Back to Q 17 on page 150

18. The correct answer is **C** – No explanation is available for this answer.

    Back to Q 18 on page 150

19. The correct answer is **B** – No explanation is available for this answer.

    Back to Q 19 on page 151

20. The correct answer is **D** – No explanation is available for this answer.

    Back to Q 20 on page 151

21. The correct answer is **A** – No explanation is available for this answer.

    Back to Q 21 on page 151

22. The correct answer is **A** – No explanation is available for this answer.

    Back to Q 22 on page 151

23. The correct answer is **A** – No explanation is available for this answer.

    Back to Q 23 on page 151

24. The correct answer is **B** – No explanation is available for this answer.

    Back to Q 24 on page 152

25. The correct answer is **C** – No explanation is available for this answer.

    Back to Q 25 on page 152

26. The correct answer is **B** – No explanation is available for this answer.

    Back to Q 26 on page 152

27. The correct answer is **A** – No explanation is available for this answer.

    Back to Q 27 on page 152

28. The correct answer is **C** – No explanation is available for this answer.

Back to Q 28 on page 152

29. The correct answer is **C** – No explanation is available for this answer.

Back to Q 29 on page 153

30. The correct answer is **A** – No explanation is available for this answer.

Back to Q 30 on page 153

31. The correct answer is **B** – Pericoronitis is usually associated with partially erupted crowns.

Back to Q 31 on page 153

32. The correct answer is **B** – No explanation is available for this answer.

Back to Q 32 on page 153

33. The correct answer is **D** – No explanation is available for this answer.

Back to Q 33 on page 153

34. The correct answer is **A** – No explanation is available for this answer.

Back to Q 34 on page 154

35. The correct answer is **D** – No explanation is available for this answer.

Back to Q 35 on page 154

36. The correct answer is **D** – No explanation is available for this answer.

Back to Q 36 on page 154

37. The correct answer is **C** – No explanation is available for this answer.

Back to Q 37 on page 154

38. The correct answer is **C** – No explanation is available for this answer.

Back to Q 38 on page 154

39. The correct answer is **B** – No explanation is available for this answer.

Back to Q 39 on page 155

40. The correct answer is **A** – No explanation is available for this answer.

Back to Q 40 on page 155

41. The correct answer is **D** – No explanation is available for this answer.

Back to Q 41 on page 155

42. The correct answer is **A** – No explanation is available for this answer.

Back to Q 42 on page 155

43. The correct answer is **D** – No explanation is available for this answer.

Back to Q 43 on page 155

44. The correct answer is **A** – No explanation is available for this answer.

Back to Q 44 on page 156

45. The correct answer is **D** – No explanation is available for this answer.

    Back to Q 45 on page 156

46. The correct answer is **C** – No explanation is available for this answer.

    Back to Q 46 on page 156

47. The correct answer is **A** – No explanation is available for this answer.

    Back to Q 47 on page 156

48. The correct answer is **B** – No explanation is available for this answer.

    Back to Q 48 on page 156

49. The correct answer is **C** – No explanation is available for this answer.

    Back to Q 49 on page 157

Chapter 9
Oral Tumors and Tumor-Like Lesions – Preamble

In this chapter, the students should be acquainted with different terms used to describe tumors, neoplasms, hyperplastic growths and reactive lesions.

9.1 MCQs Questions

Choose **one or more** of the most appropriate answers. Some questions may have **more than one** correct answer. You have to choose all the correct answers as best as you can.

1. Any tumor consists of:
   (a) Neoplastic cells
   (b) Stroma with blood supply
   (c) Matrix
   (d) All of the above

   Answer for Q 1 on page 174

2. One of the following gives the tumor its characteristic behavior?
   (a) Matrix
   (b) Stroma cells
   (c) Neoplastic cells
   (d) None of the above

   Answer for Q 2 on page 174

3. Differentiation of tumors is:
   (a) The degree of similarity of the tumor cells to their mother cell (i.e. the cell of origin)
   (b) The ability of the tumor to send distant metastasis
   (c) The ability of the tumor to form a capsule
   (d) None of the above

   Answer for Q 3 on page 174

4. Incidence of most common malignant tumors in women is:
   (a) Breast
   (b) Lung
   (c) Cervix
   (d) Ovary

   Answer for Q 4 on page 174

5. Carcinogens induce tumors, they are:
   (a) Chemicals
   (b) Radiation
   (c) Viruses
   (d) All of the above

   Answer for Q 5 on page 174

6. Oncogenic viruses in human are:
   (a) HPV
   (b) EBV
   (c) Hepatitis-B virus
   (d) All of the above

   Answer for Q 6 on page 174

7. Most tumors are:
   (a) Biclonal in origin
   (b) Monoclonal in origin
   (c) Polyclonal in origin
   (d) None of the above

   Answer for Q 7 on page 174

8. The wasting syndrome associated in cancer is
   (a) Achalasia
   (b) Cachexia
   (c) Atelexis
   (d) Cacoguesia

   Answer for Q 8 on page 174

9. Malignant neoplasms show all the following features **except**:
   (a) Disorganized cell structure
   (b) Encapsulation
   (c) Invasion of blood vessels
   (d) Rapid, erratic growth

   Answer for Q 9 on page 174

10. The term metaplasia refers to:
    (a) Irregular, atypical proliferative changes in epithelial or mesenchymal cells
    (b) Loss of cell substance producing shrinkage of the cells
    (c) Replacement of one type of adult cell by another type of adult cell
    (d) Increase in the size of the cells

    Answer for Q 10 on page 174

11. Exfoliative cytology is mostly indicated in:
    (a) Heavily keratinized lesions of oral cavity
    (b) Pre-cancerous lesions of oral cavity
    (c) Cigarette smokers
    (d) Mass screening of cervical cancer

    Answer for Q 11 on page 174

12. Gardner syndrome is characterized by jaw osteomas, epidermoid cyst **and:**
    (a) Intestinal polyp
    (b) Elevated alkaline phosphatase
    (c) Basal cell carcinomas
    (d) Mucosal neuromas

    Answer for Q 12 on page 174

13. Change in structure and functions of a tissue is called:
    (a) Dysplasia
    (b) Metaplasia
    (c) Anaplasia
    (d) Aplasia

    Answer for Q 13 on page 174

14. The most definite and dangerous feature of a malignant tumor is:
    (a) Hemorrhage
    (b) Increased mitoses
    (c) Metastasis
    (d) Necrosis

    Answer for Q 14 on page 174

15. The increase in size of individual cells is referred as:
    (a) Hypertrophy
    (b) Hyperplasia
    (c) Hypodontia
    (d) Differentiation

    Answer for Q 15 on page 175

16. Increased proliferation of cells is called:
    (a) Hypertrophy
    (b) Atrophy
    (c) Hyperplasia
    (d) Metaplasia

    Answer for Q 16 on page 175

17. Malignant tumor of skeletal muscle is:
    (a) Rhabdomyoma
    (b) Rhabdomyosarcoma
    (c) Leiomyoma
    (d) Leiomyosarcoma

    Answer for Q 17 on page 175

18. Epstein Barr virus is associated with
    (a) Nasopharyngeal carcinoma
    (b) Burkitt's lymphoma
    (c) Infectious mononucleosis
    (d) All of the above

    Answer for Q 18 on page 175

19. Immune response to tumor is mediated by
    (a) Cytotoxic T - lymphocytes
    (b) Natural killer cells
    (c) Humoral mechanism
    (d) All of the above

    Answer for Q 19 on page 175

20. Pap smear is used to detect dysplasia, carcinoma in situ and invasive carcinoma of uterine cervix. This is based on the principle of:
    (a) Neoplastic cells are cohesive
    (b) Neoplastic cells are non-cohesive
    (c) Hyper chromatic and pleomorphism of tumor cells
    (d) All of the above

    Answer for Q 20 on page 175

21. Tumor which shows origin from more than one germ layers is known as:
    (a) Teratoma
    (b) Pleomorphic tumors
    (c) Choristoma
    (d) Hamartoma

    Answer for Q 21 on page 175

22. Malignant tumor of epithelial origin is:
    (a) Carcinoma
    (b) Sarcomas
    (c) Papilloma
    (d) All of the above

    Answer for Q 22 on page 175

23. In dysplasia mitotic figures are seen in:
    (a) In basal layers of epithelium
    (b) In surface layers only
    (c) From basal layer to surface
    (d) None of the above

    Answer for Q 23 on page 175

24. Nuclear cytoplasmic ratio in malignant cells is:
    (a) 1 : 6
    (b) 1 : 5
    (c) 1 : 1
    (d) 6 : 4

    Answer for Q 24 on page 175

25. The **reversible** change including the replacement of one type of adult cells with the other type is called:
    (a) Hyperplasia
    (b) Metaplasia
    (c) Dysplasia
    (d) Neoplasia

    Answer for Q 25 on page 175

26. The disordered **reversible** cellular changes such as pleomorphism, nuclear hyperchromatin are seen in:
    (a) Hyperplasia
    (b) Metaplasia
    (c) Dysplasia
    (d) Neoplasia

    Answer for Q 26 on page 175

27. When the cells in malignancy resemble their undifferentiated primitive cells, they are said to be:
    (a) Anaplastic
    (b) Dysplastic
    (c) Hyperplastic
    (d) Metaplasia

    Answer for Q 27 on page 175

28. Which of the following is not a feature of neoplasia?
    (a) Hyperkeratosis
    (b) Anaplasia
    (c) Abnormal mitosis
    (d) Pleomorphism

    Answer for Q 28 on page 175

29. Lack of differentiation of cells is known as:
    (a) Anaplasia
    (b) Metaplasia
    (c) Dysplasia
    (d) Hypertrophy

    Answer for Q 29 on page 176

30. The most common type of epithelial metaplastic changes seen in bronchial mucosa of cigarette smokers is:
    (a) Cuboidal cells to columnar cells
    (b) Squamous cells to cuboid cells
    (c) Cuboidal to stratified squamous cells
    (d) Columnar to cuboidal cells

    Answer for Q 30 on page 176

31. There is increase in the size of heart following myocardial infarction or long-standing hypertension. This is an example of:
    (a) Hyperplasia
    (b) Hypertrophy
    (c) Metaplasia
    (d) Hyperplastic

    Answer for Q 31 on page 176

32. The increase in the size of uterus during pregnancy is an example of:
    (a) Hyperplasia
    (b) Hypertrophy
    (c) Both of the above
    (d) None of the above

    Answer for Q 32 on page 176

33. Which of the following are correctly matched?
    (a) Increase in size of breast during puberty - Physiological hyperplasia
    (b) Increase in size of cardiac muscle and skeletal muscle - Hypertrophy
    (c) Increase in the size of left kidney following removal of right kidney - Compensatory hyperplasia
    (d) All of the above

    Answer for Q 33 on page 176

34. Which of the following constituents of tobacco are carcinogens?

    (a) Nitrosamine, N-nitrosonornicotine (NNN), nicotine

    (b) Polycyclic aromatic hydrocarbons, benzopyrene, phenol

    (c) Benzopyrene, Carbon mono oxide, formaldehyde

    (d) Nicotine, benzopyrene, phenol

    Answer for Q 34 on page 176

35. A simple bacterial test for mutagenic carcinogens is:

    (a) Ames test

    (b) Redox test

    (c) Bacteriophage

    (d) Gene splicing

    Answer for Q 35 on page 176

36. All the following methods are used to detect mutations **except**:

    (a) Single stranded conformational polymorphism

    (b) Denaturating gradient gel electrophoresis

    (c) Gel electrophoresis

    (d) Northern blot analysis

    Answer for Q 36 on page 176

37. Presence of dermoid cyst in ovary is an example of:

    (a) Choristoma

    (b) Hamartoma

    (c) Neoplasia

    (d) Teratoma

    Answer for Q 37 on page 176

38. A benign tumor of smooth muscle such as myometrium of uterus is called:

    (a) Leiomyoma

    (b) Rhabdomyoma

    (c) Leiomyosarcoma

    (d) Rhabdomyosarcoma

    Answer for Q 38 on page 176

39. Neoplasia of blood vessel is called:
    (a) Angioma
    (b) Hematoma
    (c) Lymphosarcoma
    (d) Papilloma

    Answer for Q 39 on page 176

40. Compared to normal cellular growth, cell growth in benign neoplasm is:
    (a) 10 times greater than normal cell growth
    (b) Never exceeds normal cell growth
    (c) Very rapid
    (d) Is very less than normal cell growth

    Answer for Q 40 on page 176

41. Which of the following is a feature of malignant neoplasm?
    (a) Encapsulation
    (b) Metastasis
    (c) Hypertrophy
    (d) Metaplasia

    Answer for Q 41 on page 176

42. One of the following is among the genes that is responsible for carcinogenesis:
    (a) SRY genes
    (b) Tabby genes
    (c) Oncogenes
    (d) COL1A1 genes

    Answer for Q 42 on page 176

43. The most characteristic feature of a neoplasm as opposed to inflammatory hyperplasia is:
    (a) Abnormal mitosis
    (b) Size of the lesion
    (c) Progressive growth after removal of causative stimuli
    (d) Tendency to grow rapidly

    Answer for Q 43 on page 176

44. The tumor that is highly radiosensitive but not radiocurable is:
    (a) Squamous cell carcinoma
    (b) Malignant lymphoma
    (c) Ewing's sarcoma
    (d) Osteoblastoma

    Answer for Q 44 on page 176

45. Which of the following is most radiosensitive neoplasm of oral cavity?
    (a) Squamous cell carcinoma
    (b) Basal cell carcinoma
    (c) Fibroma
    (d) Osteogenic sarcoma

    Answer for Q 45 on page 177

46. Tumor which shows poor differentiation with immature anaplastic cells and increased mitosis are generally:
    (a) Radioresistant
    (b) Radiosensitive
    (c) Radiostable
    (d) Radiorefractive

    Answer for Q 46 on page 177

47. A benign tumor developing from glands is called:
    (a) Adenoma
    (b) Fibroma
    (c) Lipoma
    (d) Nevus

    Answer for Q 47 on page 177

48. The loss of weight associated in cancer is called:
    (a) Achalasia
    (b) Cachexia
    (c) Atelexis
    (d) Cacogeusia

    Answer for Q 48 on page 177

49. Immune response to tumor is mediated by:
    (a) Cytotoxic T lymphocytes
    (b) Natural killer cells
    (c) Humoral mechanism
    (d) All of the above

    Answer for Q 49 on page 177

50. Most potent stimulators of naive T cells are:
    (a) Follicular dendritic cells
    (b) Mature dendritic cells
    (c) Mast cells
    (d) B lymphocytes

    Answer for Q 50 on page 177

51. Immunohistochemistry is mainly employed for which of the following processes?
    (a) To localize the cell of origin of tumor
    (b) To distinguish benign and malignant lesions
    (c) To distinguish neoplastic from non-neoplastic proliferation
    (d) To detect autoantibodies in the serum

    Answer for Q 51 on page 177

52. PAP smear is used to detect dysplasia, carcinoma in situ and invasive carcinoma of uterine cervix. This is based on the principle of:
    (a) Neoplastic cells are cohesive
    (b) Neoplastic cells are non-cohesive
    (c) Hyperchromatic and pleomorphism of tumor cells
    (d) All of the above

    Answer for Q 52 on page 177

53. Exfoliative cytology is indicated in:
    (a) Heavily keratinized lesions of oral cavity
    (b) Precancerous lesions of oral cavity
    (c) Cigarette smokers
    (d) Mass screening of cervical cancer

    Answer for Q 53 on page 177

54. Prostate specific antigen is used as:
    (a) Tumor marker
    (b) Proto-oncogene
    (c) Oncogene
    (d) Bacterial antigen

    Answer for Q 54 on page 177

55. Old male demonstrates urinary retention and difficulty in voiding his bladder, otherwise he is healthy without cachexia. He may be suffering most likely from:
    (a) Prostate malignant neoplasm
    (b) Benign nodular prostatic hyperplasia
    (c) Malignant neoplasm of bladder
    (d) Neoplasm of testicles

    Answer for Q 55 on page 177

56. The basic effect of radiation on living tissue is:
    (a) Denaturation
    (b) Precipitation
    (c) Ionization
    (d) All of the above

    Answer for Q 56 on page 177

57. Least sensitive phase of a cell cycle to radiation is:
    (a) S phase
    (b) G1 phase
    (c) G2 phase
    (d) M phase

    Answer for Q 57 on page 177

58. Which of the following is most radiosensitive?
    (a) Spermatogonium[1]
    (b) Endothelium
    (c) Smooth muscle
    (d) Alimentary canal lining

    Answer for Q 58 on page 177

[1] A cell produced at an early stage in the formation of spermatozoa, formed in the wall of a seminiferous tubule and giving rise by mitosis to spermatocytes.

59. The least radiosensitive cell is:
    (a) Endothelium
    (b) Alimentary canal mucosal cells
    (c) Lining smooth muscle cells
    (d) Osteocyte

    Answer for Q 59 on page 177

60. Most radiosensitive among the following is:
    (a) Lymphocytes
    (b) Endothelial cells
    (c) Nerve cells
    (d) Muscle cell

    Answer for Q 60 on page 177

61. The radiosensitivity of a tissue is dependent on:
    (a) Type of cells and their mitotic rate
    (b) Size of cells and their cytoplasmic content
    (c) Amount of RNA in the cytoplasm
    (d) All of the above

    Answer for Q 61 on page 178

62. Which of the following adult cells have no ability to proliferate?
    (a) Neurons of CNS, skeletal and cardiac muscle cells
    (b) Smooth muscle cells, fibroblasts, vascular endothelium and bone and cartilage cells
    (c) Hematopoietic cells of bone marrow and cells of lymph nodes and spleen
    (d) Surface epithelial cells, lining mucosa of alimentary, respiratory and urinary tracts

    Answer for Q 62 on page 178

63. Which of the following cells have no capacity for regeneration?
    (a) Neurons
    (b) Smooth muscle cells
    (c) Hematopoietic cells of bone marrow
    (d) Parenchyma of liver

    Answer for Q 63 on page 178

9.2 Answers with Comments:

1. The correct answer is **D** – Tumors consist of neoplastic cells and stroma. The matrix also is sometimes a term given to the stroma.

   Back to Q 1 on page 161

2. The correct answer is **C** – Neoplastic cells give the tumor its characteristics and behavior.

   Back to Q 2 on page 161

3. The correct answer is **A** – Differentiation in pathology is the degree of similarity of the tumor cells to their mother cell (cell of origin).

   Back to Q 3 on page 161

4. The correct answer is **A** – Breast cancer is the most common malignancy in females while lung cancer is the most common malignancy in males.

   Back to Q 4 on page 162

5. The correct answer is **D** – The principle carcinogenic agents are chemicals, radiation and viruses.

   Back to Q 5 on page 162

6. The correct answer is **D** – No explanation is available for this answer.

   Back to Q 6 on page 162

7. The correct answer is **B** – Most tumors start as monoclonal and some my end by being polyclonal in nature.

   Back to Q 7 on page 162

8. The correct answer is **B** – No explanation is available for this answer.

   Back to Q 8 on page 162

9. The correct answer is **B** – Encapsulation is a feature of benign tumors.

   Back to Q 9 on page 163

10. The correct answer is **C** – No explanation is available for this answer.

    Back to Q 10 on page 163

11. The correct answer is **D** – No explanation is available for this answer.

    Back to Q 11 on page 163

12. The correct answer is **A** – No explanation is available for this answer.

    Back to Q 12 on page 163

13. The correct answer is **B** – No explanation is available for this answer.

    Back to Q 13 on page 163

14. The correct answer is **C** – Metastasis is the most dangerous feature of malignant tumors as it will result in formation of secondary tumors in remote tissues and organs. This can lead to loss of function of vital organs.

    Back to Q 14 on page 164

15. The correct answer is **A** – No explanation is available for this answer.

    Back to Q 15 on page 164

16. The correct answer is **C** – No explanation is available for this answer.

    Back to Q 16 on page 164

17. The correct answer is **B** – No explanation is available for this answer.

    Back to Q 17 on page 164

18. The correct answer is **D** – Evidences indicate that Epstein Barr virus is responsible in the 3 types of mentioned tumors.

    Back to Q 18 on page 164

19. The correct answer is **D** – No explanation is available for this answer.

    Back to Q 19 on page 165

20. The correct answer is **B** – Loss of cohesiveness is a prominent feature of neoplastic cells.

    Back to Q 20 on page 165

21. The correct answer is **A** – No explanation is available for this answer.

    Back to Q 20 on page 165

22. The correct answer is **A** – No explanation is available for this answer.

    Back to Q 22 on page 165

23. The correct answer is **C** – The basal cell layer is the germinal layer of epithelium and hence they are more liable for the occurrence of mitotic figures.

    Back to Q 23 on page 165

24. The correct answer is **C** – No explanation is available for this answer.

    Back to Q 24 on page 166

25. The correct answer is **B** – No explanation is available for this answer.

    Back to Q 25 on page 166

26. The correct answer is **C** – Many cases of epithelial dysplasia can regress and/or reverse back to normal upon removal of the predisposing factors.

    Back to Q 26 on page 166

27. The correct answer is **A** – No explanation is available for this answer.

    Back to Q 27 on page 166

28. The correct answer is **A** – Hyperkeratosis can occur in non-neoplatic lesions such as chronic mechanical irritation.

    Back to Q 28 on page 166

29. The correct answer is **A** – No explanation is available for this answer.

    Back to Q 29 on page 167

30. The correct answer is **C** – No explanation is available for this answer.

    Back to Q 30 on page 167

31. The correct answer is **B** – No explanation is available for this answer.

    Back to Q 31 on page 167

32. The correct answer is **C** – No explanation is available for this answer.

    Back to Q 32 on page 167

33. The correct answer is **D** – No explanation is available for this answer.

    Back to Q 33 on page 167

34. The correct answer is **A** – No explanation is available for this answer.

    Back to Q 34 on page 168

35. The correct answer is **A** – No explanation is available for this answer.

    Back to Q 35 on page 168

36. The correct answer is **D** – No explanation is available for this answer.

    Back to Q 36 on page 168

37. The correct answer is **D** – No explanation is available for this answer.

    Back to Q 37 on page 168

38. The correct answer is **A** – No explanation is available for this answer.

    Back to Q 38 on page 168

39. The correct answer is **A** – No explanation is available for this answer.

    Back to Q 39 on page 169

40. The correct answer is **B** – No explanation is available for this answer.

    Back to Q 40 on page 169

41. The correct answer is **B** – No explanation is available for this answer.

    Back to Q 41 on page 169

42. The correct answer is **C** – No explanation is available for this answer.

    Back to Q 42 on page 169

43. The correct answer is **C** – No explanation is available for this answer.

    Back to Q 43 on page 169

44. The correct answer is **B** – No explanation is available for this answer.

Back to Q 44 on page 170

45. The correct answer is **A** – No explanation is available for this answer.

Back to Q 45 on page 170

46. The correct answer is **B** – No explanation is available for this answer.

Back to Q 46 on page 170

47. The correct answer is **A** – No explanation is available for this answer.

Back to Q 47 on page 170

48. The correct answer is **B** – No explanation is available for this answer.

Back to Q 48 on page 170

49. The correct answer is **D** – No explanation is available for this answer.

Back to Q 49 on page 171

50. The correct answer is **B** – No explanation is available for this answer.

Back to Q 50 on page 171

51. The correct answer is **A** – No explanation is available for this answer.

Back to Q 51 on page 171

52. The correct answer is **B** – No explanation is available for this answer.

Back to Q 52 on page 171

53. The correct answer is **D** – No explanation is available for this answer.

Back to Q 53 on page 171

54. The correct answer is **A** – No explanation is available for this answer.

Back to Q 54 on page 172

55. The correct answer is **B** – No explanation is available for this answer.

Back to Q 55 on page 172

56. The correct answer is **C** – No explanation is available for this answer.

Back to Q 56 on page 172

57. The correct answer is **A** – No explanation is available for this answer.

Back to Q 57 on page 172

58. The correct answer is **A** – No explanation is available for this answer.

Back to Q 58 on page 172

59. The correct answer is **D** – No explanation is available for this answer.

Back to Q 59 on page 173

60. The correct answer is **A** – No explanation is available for this answer.

Back to Q 60 on page 173

61. The correct answer is **A** – No explanation is available for this answer.

Back to Q 61 on page 173

62. The correct answer is **A** – No explanation is available for this answer.

Back to Q 62 on page 173

63. The correct answer is **A** – No explanation is available for this answer.

Back to Q 63 on page 173

CHAPTER 10

BENIGN NON-ODONTOGENIC TUMORS AND TUMOR-LIKE LESIONS

In this chapter true oral neoplasms as well as the traditionally described tumor (although most of them are not true neoplastic) are to be discussed.

10.1 MCQs Questions

Choose **one or more** of the most appropriate answers. Some questions may have **more than one** correct answer. You have to choose all the correct answers as best as you can.

1. The most common benign tumor occurring in the oral cavity is the:
   (a) Papilloma
   (b) Adenoma
   (c) Fibroma
   (d) Hemangioma
   (e) Lipoma
   Answer for Q 1 on page 182
2. Features of familial multiple neurofibroma with café-au-lait spots of the skin are typical of:
   (a) Von Recklinghausen's disease of skin
   (b) Peget's disease of skin
   (c) Hereditary ectodermal dysplasia
   (d) Familial fibrous dysplasia
   (e) Papillon-Lefevre Syndrome
   Answer for Q 2 on page 182

3. A 5 cm suspicious looking lesion of oral mucosa should be:
   - (a) Incised and sent for biopsy
   - (b) Excised and sent for biopsy
   - (c) Irradiated
   - (d) Offered palliative treatment

   Answer for Q 3 on page 182

4. Biopsy specimens removed for examinations are immediately placed in:
   - (a) 10% ethanol
   - (b) 10% formalin
   - (c) Hydrogen peroxide
   - (d) 1% formalin

   Answer for Q 4 on page 182

5. Pigmented cellular nevi are considered as:
   - (a) Ectopic lesion
   - (b) Hamartomatous lesion
   - (c) Neoplastic lesion
   - (d) None of the above

   Answer for Q 5 on page 182

6. Crater shaped lesion with central keratin plug and downwards growth of the epithelium are histological features of:
   - (a) Squamous cell carcinoma
   - (b) Verrucous carcinoma
   - (c) Multifocal epithelial hyperplasia
   - (d) Keratoacanthoma

   Answer for Q 6 on page 183

7. Pale hypopigmented border is a clinical manifestation of:
   - (a) Blue nevus
   - (b) Spitz nevus
   - (c) Halo nevus
   - (d) Malignant melanoma

   Answer for Q 7 on page 183

8. Verruca vulgaris is a viral-induced epithelial hyperplasia caused by:
   (a) Human papilloma virus
   (b) Epstein-Barr virus
   (c) Cytomegalovirus
   (d) Herpes simplex virus

   Answer for Q 8 on page 183

9. Nevus cells are
   (a) Altered melanocytes
   (b) Cells containing excessive melanin pigment
   (c) Melanocytes which are functionally more active
   (d) Large melanocytes

   Answer for Q 9 on page 183

10. Most frequently stimulating factor in the occurrence of pyogenic granuloma is:
   (a) Pregnancy
   (b) Large carious lesions
   (c) Local irritant
   (d) Puberty

   Answer for Q 10 on page 183

11. A person on diet will not lose fat from:
   (a) Buccal pad of fat
   (b) Adipose layer of dermis
   (c) Abdomen
   (d) Lipoma

   Answer for Q 11 on page 183

12. Which of the following tumors may undergo spontaneous regression?
   (a) Basal cell carcinoma
   (b) Verrucous carcinoma
   (c) Keratoacanthoma
   (d) Granular cell myoblastoma

   Answer for Q 12 on page 183

13. Verruca vulgaris is a viral-induced lesion caused by:
    (a) Paramyxovirus
    (b) Human papilloma virus
    (c) Epstein-Barr virus
    (d) Cytomegalovirus

    Answer for Q 13 on the next page
14. A 20-year-old female attended the dental clinic complaining of a small, flat, blue lesion on the palate. Histological examination revealed collections of spindle shaped cells located deep in the connective tissue. The most probable diagnosis is:
    (a) Spitz nevus
    (b) Halo nevus
    (c) Blue nevus
    (d) Malignant melanoma

    Answer for Q 14 on the facing page
15. Which of the following is TRUE statement about lymphangioma?
    (a) Most common on or in the lower extremities
    (b) Cavernous lymphangioma may be termed a cystic hygroma
    (c) Cystic hygroma is more common in posterior triangle of lateral neck
    (d) The most common location of oral lympahngiomas is floor of the mouth.

    Answer for Q 15 on the next page

10.2 Answers with Comments:

1. The correct answer is **C** – No explanation is available for this answer.

   Back to Q 1 on page 179
2. The correct answer is **A** – No explanation is available for this answer.

   Back to Q 2 on page 179
3. The correct answer is **A** – No explanation is available for this answer.

   Back to Q 3 on page 180
4. The correct answer is **B** – No explanation is available for this answer.

   Back to Q 4 on page 180
5. The correct answer is **B** – No explanation is available for this answer.

   Back to Q 5 on page 180

6. The correct answer is **D** – No explanation is available for this answer.

   Back to Q 6 on page 180

7. The correct answer is **C** – No explanation is available for this answer.

   Back to Q 7 on page 180

8. The correct answer is **A** – No explanation is available for this answer.

   Back to Q 8 on page 181

9. The correct answer is **A** – No explanation is available for this answer.

   Back to Q 9 on page 181

10. The correct answer is **C** – No explanation is available for this answer.

    Back to Q 10 on page 181

11. The correct answer is **D** – No explanation is available for this answer.

    Back to Q 11 on page 181

12. The correct answer is **C** – No explanation is available for this answer.

    Back to Q 12 on page 181

13. The correct answer is **B** – No explanation is available for this answer.

    Back to Q 13 on the facing page

14. The correct answer is **C** – No explanation is available for this answer.

    Back to Q 14 on the preceding page

15. The correct answer is **B** – No explanation is available for this answer.

    Back to Q 15 on the facing page

Chapter 11
Potentially Malignant Disorders of the Oral Cavity

A premalignant lesion (or potentially malignant lesion) is an altered tissue in which cancer is more likely to occur and is characterized by presence of epithelial dysplasia.

Recent research showed that, while there is statistical evidence that some of these lesions can progress into cancer, nevertheless the probability of such progress is still small. Thus, rather than precancerous lesion, a term that more accurately reflects current understanding is preferred: *potentially malignant disorder* [6]

11.1 MCQs Questions

Choose **one or more** of the most appropriate answers. Some questions may have **more than one** correct answer. You have to choose all the correct answers as best as you can.

1. An increased thickness of the spinous cell layer is termed
   (a) Acanthosis
   (b) Hyperparakeratosis
   (c) Hyperorthokeratosis
   (d) Hypertrophy
   Answer for Q 1 on page 191
2. Oral submucous fibrosis:
   (a) Typically produces thickening of the buccal mucosa and soft palate with loss of elasticity, resulting in limited mouth opening and difficulty in swallowing
   (b) Is a hereditary disorder
   (c) Is a part of a syndrome known as Peutz–Jeghers syndrome
   (d) Results in excessive salivation
   Answer for Q 2 on page 191

3. Oral submucous fibrosis:
   - (a) Is caused by chewing betel nuts
   - (b) Is a hereditary disorder
   - (c) Is a part of a syndrome known as Gardener's syndrome (adenomatous polyposis coli)
   - (d) Results in decreased salivation

   Answer for Q 3 on page 191
4. Oral submucous fibrosis:
   - (a) Is a part of a syndrome known as multiple neurofibromatosis (Von-Recklinghausen's disease of skin)
   - (b) Is a hereditary disorder
   - (c) Has oral epithelium that usually shows atrophy
   - (d) Results from vitamin C deficiency

   Answer for Q 4 on page 191
5. Oral submucous fibrosis:
   - (a) Results from vitamin C deficiency and is a form of scurvy
   - (b) Is a hereditary disorder
   - (c) Has oral epithelium that shows papillary projections which is finger-like
   - (d) Results in the presence of a fine fibrillary collagen layer in the lamina propria

   Answer for Q 5 on page 191
6. Oral submucous fibrosis:
   - (a) Typically produces thickening of the buccal mucosa, resulting in limited mouth opening and difficulty in swallowing
   - (b) Is caused by chewing betel nuts or areca nuts
   - (c) Has a hereditary background
   - (d) All of the above

   Answer for Q 6 on page 191
7. Oral submucous fibrosis:
   - (a) Has oral epithelium that usually shows atrophy
   - (b) Results in the presence of hyalinization in the lamina propria
   - (c) May be related to Iron and Vitamin B12 deficiency
   - (d) All of the above

   Answer for Q 7 on page 191

8. Histopathological features of oral epithelial dysplasia:
   (a) Interobserver agreement of oral epithelial dysplasia grade amongst specialist pathologists is excellent
   (b) Includes acanthosis and hyperkeratosis
   (c) Indicate carcinoma in situ when the dysplasia involves the entire thickness of the epithelium
   (d) Mild dysplasia will progress through moderate to severe dysplasia

   Answer for Q 8 on page 191

9. Oral submucous fibrosis appears clinically as:
   (a) Leukoplakia
   (b) Erythoplakia
   (c) Pale mucosa with erythematous or leukoplakia-like patches
   (d) Verrucous surface

   Answer for Q 9 on page 191

10. Histopathological features of oral epithelial dysplasia:
    (a) Interobserver agreement of oral epithelial dysplasia grade amongst specialist pathologists is excellent
    (b) Includes acanthosis and hyperkeratosis
    (c) Mild dysplasia should progress through moderate to severe dysplasia
    (d) Dysplastic oral epithelium may be found in non-smokers and non-drinkers

    Answer for Q 10 on page 191

11. A 37-year-old woman presents for routine dental examination. Diffuse, red, velvety lesions are present on the buccal mucosa and retromolar areas in a bilateral distribution. The patient smokes 30 cigarettes per day and drink alcohol. Biopsy showed a drop-shaped rete pegs and marked cellular atypia involving the whole thickness of the epithelium. What is the most probable diagnosis?
    (a) Lichen planus
    (b) Carcinoma in situ
    (c) Erythema multiforme
    (d) Benign Mucous Membrane Pemphigoid

    Answer for Q 11 on page 191

12. Difficulty in opening the mouth or even complete trismus is a late complication of:
    (a) Erythroplakia
    (b) Malignant melanoma
    (c) Oral submucous fibrosis
    (d) Actinic cheilitis

    Answer for Q 12 on page 191

13. One of the following is a feature of epithelial dysplasia:
    (a) Acanthosis
    (b) Hyperkeratosis
    (c) Hyperchromatism
    (d) Hyperplasia

    Answer for Q 13 on page 191

14. Dysplasia involving the entire thickness of the epithelium top to bottom change. is referred to as:
    (a) Mild dysplasia
    (b) Moderate dysplasia
    (c) Severe dysplasia
    (d) Carcinoma in situ

    Answer for Q 14 on page 191

15. Hairy leukoplakia is a variant of leukoplakia characterized by:
    (a) Caused by human papilloma virus
    (b) Common on the floor of mouth
    (c) Develop in immunocompromised patients
    (d) Presence of hair in the lesion

    Answer for Q 15 on page 192

16. Which of the following is not a precancerous condition?
    (a) Senile keratosis
    (b) Seborrhic keratosis
    (c) Erythroplakia
    (d) Leukoplakia

    Answer for Q 16 on page 192

17. The most common potentially malignant state of oral mucosa is:
    (a) Leukoplakia
    (b) Erythroplakia
    (c) Hairy leukoplakia
    (d) Oral submucous fibrosis

    Answer for Q 17 on page 192

18. An abnormal epithelium that histopathologically lacks keratin production, atrophic in some foci and normal in other areas is referred as:
    (a) Leukoplakia
    (b) Erythroplakia
    (c) Speckled leukoplakia
    (d) Leukodema

    Answer for Q 18 on page 192

19. Severe burning sensation, red patch and loss of elasticity of oral mucosa are clinical features of:
    (a) Erythroplakia
    (b) Leukoplakia
    (c) Oral submucous fibrosis
    (d) Oral squamous cell carcinoma

    Answer for Q 19 on page 192

20. The following are critical features of epithelial dysplasia **except**:
    (a) Nuclear hypochromatism
    (b) Abnormal mitosis
    (c) Hyperkeratosis
    (d) Altered nuclear-cytoplasmic ratio

    Answer for Q 20 on page 192

21. Altered nuclear-cytoplasmic ratio in epithelial dysplasia is indicative of:
    (a) Abnormal DNA production
    (b) Abnormal RNA production
    (c) Increased DNA synthesis
    (d) Decreased RNA synthesis

    Answer for Q 21 on page 192

22. A patient reported with an asymptomatic white patch on buccal mucosa which cannot be rubbed off. The patch was present for the last 3 months. Patient is a heavy cigarette smoker. Most probable diagnosis of the lesion is:
    (a) Candidiasis
    (b) Frictional keratosis
    (c) Leukoplakia
    (d) White spongy nevus

    Answer for Q 22 on page 192

23. Which of the following is caused by areca nut?
    (a) Oral squamous carcinoma
    (b) Oral submucous fibrosis
    (c) Leukoplakia
    (d) Smokeless tobacco keratosis

    Answer for Q 23 on page 192

24. "A white patch or plaque that cannot be characterized clinically or pathologically as any other disease" Which of the following represent the previous statement?
    (a) Erythroleukoplakia
    (b) Erythroplakia
    (c) Leukoplakia
    (d) Actinic cheilitis

    Answer for Q 24 on page 192

25. One of the following is a cytological feature of epithelial dysplasia:
    (a) Hyperkeratosis
    (b) Acanthosis
    (c) Loss of polarity
    (d) Hyperplasia

    Answer for Q 25 on page 192

26. Nuclear beading due to extensive HHV 4 replication is evident in:
    (a) Candidiasis
    (b) Kaposi sarcoma
    (c) Oral hairy leukoplakia
    (d) Oral squamous cell carcinoma

    Answer for Q 26 on page 192

11.2 Answers with Comments:

1. The correct answer is **A** – No explanation is available for this answer.

   Back to Q 1 on page 185

2. The correct answer is **A** – Excessive fibrosis with fibrous bands are often visible in the buccal mucosa and the affected areas appear pale and thickened on microscopic and clinical examination.

   Back to Q 2 on page 185

3. The correct answer is **A** – Results from betel nut, areca nut and paan chewing.

   Back to Q 3 on page 186

4. The correct answer is **C** – At the later stages, decreased vascularity results in atrophy of the epithelium which can be reduced to only a few cell layers in thickness.

   Back to Q 4 on page 186

5. The correct answer is **D** – Submucous fibrosis is characterized by deposition of fine collagen fibers beneath the oral epithelium. The papillary lamina propria is reduced and the abnormal collagen fibers tend to be orientated parallel to the surface of the mucosa.

   Back to Q 5 on page 186

6. The correct answer is **D** – No explanation is available for this answer.

   Back to Q 6 on page 186

7. The correct answer is **D** – No explanation is available for this answer.

   Back to Q 7 on page 186

8. The correct answer is **C** – No explanation is available for this answer.

   Back to Q 8 on page 187

9. The correct answer is **C** – No explanation is available for this answer.

   Back to Q 9 on page 187

10. The correct answer is **D** – No explanation is available for this answer.

    Back to Q 10 on page 187

11. The correct answer is **B** – No explanation is available for this answer.

    Back to Q 11 on page 187

12. The correct answer is **C** – No explanation is available for this answer.

    Back to Q 12 on page 188

13. The correct answer is **C** – No explanation is available for this answer.

    Back to Q 13 on page 188

14. The correct answer is **D** – No explanation is available for this answer.

Back to Q 14 on page 188

15. The correct answer is **C** – No explanation is available for this answer.

Back to Q 15 on page 188

16. The correct answer is **B** – No explanation is available for this answer.

Back to Q 16 on page 188

17. The correct answer is **B** – No explanation is available for this answer.

Back to Q 17 on page 189

18. The correct answer is **C** – No explanation is available for this answer.

Back to Q 18 on page 189

19. The correct answer is **C** – No explanation is available for this answer.

Back to Q 19 on page 189

20. The correct answer is **C** – No explanation is available for this answer.

Back to Q 20 on page 189

21. The correct answer is **C** – No explanation is available for this answer.

Back to Q 21 on page 189

22. The correct answer is **C** – No explanation is available for this answer.

Back to Q 22 on page 190

23. The correct answer is **B** – No explanation is available for this answer.

Back to Q 23 on page 190

24. The correct answer is **C** – No explanation is available for this answer.

Back to Q 24 on page 190

25. The correct answer is **C** – No explanation is available for this answer.

Back to Q 25 on page 190

26. The correct answer is **C** – No explanation is available for this answer.

Back to Q 26 on page 190

Chapter 12
Malignant Non-Odontogenic Tumors and Tumor-Like Lesions

Malignant tumors arising from the odontogenic tissues will be discussed in a separate chapter (on page 209).

12.1 MCQs Questions

Choose **one or more** of the most appropriate answers. Some questions may have **more than one** correct answer. You have to choose all the correct answers as best as you can.

1. Which type of melanoma is highly invasive because it lacks the radial growth phase?
   (a) Superficial spreading melanoma
   (b) Nodular melanoma
   (c) Lentigo maligna melanoma
   (d) Acral lentiginous melanoma
   Answer for Q 1 on page 204
2. Which of the following skin cancers is least likely to metastasize?
   (a) Basal cell carcinoma
   (b) Squamous cell carcinoma
   (c) Malignant melanoma
   (d) Fibrosarcoma
   Answer for Q 2 on page 204
3. The occurrence of cleft between the nests of soft tumor cells and stroma in basal cell carcinoma is known as:
   (a) Suprabasal clefting
   (b) Sub-basilar clefting
   (c) Max-Joseph cleft
   (d) Retraction artifact
   Answer for Q 3 on page 204

4. The most common malignancy found in the oral cavity is:
   (a) Basal cell carcinoma
   (b) Transitional cell carcinoma
   (c) Melanoma
   (d) Squamous cell carcinoma
   (e) Adenocarcinoma

   Answer for Q 4 on page 204

5. The features of multiple skeletal radiolucencies reversed A/G ratio, Bence Jones protein in the urine, and solid plasma cell infiltrate in the biopsy in a 50-year-old man indicate a diagnosis of:
   (a) Metastatic prostatic carcinoma
   (b) Multiple myeloma
   (c) Hyperparathyroidism
   (d) Miliary Tuberculosis
   (e) Basal cell Nevi Syndrome

   Answer for Q 5 on page 204

6. Intraoral carcinoma cannot present clinically as:
   (a) Ulcers
   (b) Nodule
   (c) Cauliflower-like growth
   (d) Growth with fungating margins
   (e) Abscess

   Answer for Q 6 on page 204

7. Squamous cell carcinoma (SCC) present on lateral margin of tongue of staging T2N0, options of treatment is:
   (a) SONHD (Supraomohyoid neck dissections)
   (b) Remove lymph node I-II along with
   (c) Remove lymph node I-V along with
   (d) Remove lymph node I-IV along with

   Answer for Q 7 on page 205

8. In composite excision of tumor according to Gold, Upton and Marx, there is:
   (a) Resection of tumor with entire wound
   (b) Resection of tumor leaving the marginal bone intact
   (c) Resection of tumor with unaffected neighboring tissue
   (d) Resection of tumor with wide margins excision

   Answer for Q 8 on page 205

9. Carcinoma of the lip:
   (a) Is equally common on the upper and lower vermilion borders
   (b) Is principally caused by reverse smoking
   (c) Usually arises in angular cheilitis
   (d) Has a generally better prognosis than intra-oral cancers

   Answer for Q 9 on page 205

10. Carcinoma of the lip:
   (a) Is more common on the lower vermilion borders than the upper lip
   (b) Is principally caused by reverse smoking
   (c) Usually arises in angular cheilitis
   (d) Often arises due to betel nut chewing

   Answer for Q 10 on page 205

11. Carcinoma of the lip:
   (a) Is equally common on the upper and lower vermilion borders
   (b) Is principally caused by reverse smoking
   (c) Usually arises in angular cheilitis
   (d) Often arises in a field of dysplastic change

   Answer for Q 11 on page 205

12. Squamous cell carcinoma of the floor of the mouth:
   (a) Infiltration of the submandibular duct can cause symptoms of obstructive sialadenitis
   (b) Can metastasize to both sides of the neck
   (c) Are often described as "Oyster carcinoma"
   (d) All of the above

   Answer for Q 12 on page 205

13. The classification based on TNM (tumor, nodes, metastasis) findings:
    (a) Is a system used for recording histopathological grading
    (b) Is a clinical staging of cancer
    (c) Stage I indicates spread to lymph nodes bilaterally
    (d) Stage II indicates intact basement membrane

    Answer for Q 13 on page 205

14. The classification based on TNM (tumor, nodes, metastasis) findings:
    (a) Is a system used for recording histopathological grading?
    (b) Stage III indicates a tumor less than 2 cm in its greatest diameter
    (c) Affection of epsilateral is not equivalent to unilateral lymph nodes
    (d) Stage IV indicates distant metastasis via blood

    Answer for Q 14 on page 205

15. One of the following is a well-differentiated variant of squamous cell carcinoma:
    (a) Spindle cell carcinoma
    (b) Keratoacanthoma
    (c) Verrucous carcinoma
    (d) Adenosquamous carcinoma

    Answer for Q 15 on page 205

16. Multiple basal cell carcinoma is one of the clinical manifestations of:
    (a) Melkersson Rosenthal syndrome
    (b) Gorlin syndrome
    (c) Treacher Collins syndrome
    (d) Crouzon syndrome

    Answer for Q 16 on page 205

17. Poorly differentiated squamous cell carcinoma is characterized Histologically by:
    (a) Nests of epithelial cells with keratin formation
    (b) Nests of epithelial cells without keratin formation
    (c) Scattered malignant epithelial cells
    (d) None of the above

    Answer for Q 17 on page 205

18. Staging of oral carcinoma is based on:
    (a) Histogenesis
    (b) Percentage of differentiated cells
    (c) Clinical parameters
    (d) All of the above

    Answer for Q 18 on page 205

19. Which of the following tumors is characterized by poor prognosis?
    (a) Well-differentiated squamous cell carcinoma
    (b) Verrucous carcinoma
    (c) Nasopharyngeal carcinoma
    (d) Keratoacanthoma

    Answer for Q 19 on page 205

20. Prolonged exposure to sun light is a major predisposing factor for the development of:
    (a) Basal cell carcinoma
    (b) Verrucous carcinoma
    (c) Squamous cell papilloma
    (d) Oral submucous fibrosis

    Answer for Q 20 on page 205

21. All the following are oncogenic viruses **except**:
    (a) Epstein-Barr virus
    (b) Herpes simplex virus type 1
    (c) Human papilloma virus
    (d) Herpes simplex virus type 2

    Answer for Q 21 on page 205

22. The most common malignant primary tumor of bone is:
    (a) Multiple myeloma
    (b) Burkitt's lymphoma
    (c) Osteogenic sarcoma
    (d) Central giant cell granuloma

    Answer for Q 22 on page 206

23. Starry sky appearance is a characteristic feature of:
    (a) Osteosarcoma
    (b) Burkitt's lymphoma
    (c) Giant cell fibroma
    (d) Congenital epulis of newborn

    Answer for Q 23 on page 206

24. Burkitt's lymphoma is associated with the proliferation of:
    (a) T-cell
    (b) B-cell
    (c) Lymph vessels
    (d) Lymph nodes

    Answer for Q 24 on page 206

25. Incidence of most common malignant tumors in men in India is in:
    (a) Lungs
    (b) Oral cavity
    (c) Prostate
    (d) Liver

    Answer for Q 25 on page 206

26. Rodent ulcer is most commonly seen on
    (a) Face below ala-tragus line
    (b) Face above ala-tragus line
    (c) Anywhere on hairless skin
    (d) All of the above

    Answer for Q 26 on page 206

27. The predisposing factor for squamous cell carcinoma
    (a) Solar keratosis
    (b) Chronic ulcers
    (c) Leukoplakia
    (d) All of the above

    Answer for Q 27 on page 206

28. Keratin pearls with downward proliferation of epithelial masses is characteristic feature of:
    (a) Squamous cell carcinoma
    (b) Basal cell carcinoma
    (c) Epidermoid carcinoma
    (d) Melanoma

    Answer for Q 28 on page 206

29. Which of the following is correct statement?
    (a) Grading is the degree of macroscopic and microscopic differentiation of tumor
    (b) Staging is the extent of spread of tumor
    (c) TNM and AJC systems can be used for staging malignant tumors
    (d) All of the above

    Answer for Q 29 on page 206

30. Onion skin appearance is seen in:
    (a) Ewing's sarcoma
    (b) Osteosarcoma
    (c) Osteoma
    (d) Fibrosarcoma

    Answer for Q 30 on page 206

31. From which of the following surfaces a basal cell carcinoma can develop?
    (a) Cutaneous side of lip
    (b) Mucosal side of lip
    (c) Lining mucosa of cheek
    (d) Palate

    Answer for Q 31 on page 206

32. Which of the following is true of basal cell carcinoma?
    (a) It is also called rodent ulcer and is a well differentiated tumor arising from adnexa of skin
    (b) It is common in middle third of face below canthal line and above ala tragus line
    (c) It hardly shows metastasis and is fixed to underlying skin
    (d) All of the above

    Answer for Q 32 on page 206

33. Squamous cell carcinoma of oral cavity closely resembles:
    (a) Cancer of cervix
    (b) Cancer of breast
    (c) Carcinoma of lung
    (d) Malignant lymphoma

    Answer for Q 33 on page 206

34. The most common malignancies found in males are:
    (a) Lung and oral cavity
    (b) Brain and parotid
    (c) Prostate and parotid
    (d) Brain and prostate

    Answer for Q 34 on page 206

35. A patient with a history of cigarette smoking develops weight loss, difficulty in swallowing, and sudden change in voice. The most likely diagnosis:
    (a) Carcinoma of larynx
    (b) Carcinoma of oropharynx
    (c) Laryngitis
    (d) Pharyngitis

    Answer for Q 35 on page 206

36. Which of the following has best prognosis?
    (a) Malignant melanoma
    (b) Squamous cell carcinoma
    (c) Basal cell carcinoma
    (d) Osteosarcoma

    Answer for Q 36 on page 207

37. Which of the following tumor shows formation of epithelial pearls and intercellular bridges?
    (a) Well differentiated squamous cell carcinoma
    (b) Osteosarcoma
    (c) Malignant melanoma
    (d) All of the above

    Answer for Q 37 on page 207

38. Which of the following is true of Hodgkin's lymphoma?
    (a) Malignant neoplasm commonly seen in young adults
    (b) Mirror imaged Reed-Sternberg cell is the diagnostic characteristic of the lymph node
    (c) Ingestion of alcohol elicits pain in involved lymph node
    (d) All of the above

    Answer for Q 38 on page 207

39. Burkitt's lymphoma is associated with the proliferation of:
    (a) T cells
    (b) B cells
    (c) Lymph vessels
    (d) Lymph nodes

    Answer for Q 39 on page 207

40. A tumor characterized by rapid rate of growth which almost doubles its size by next day is:
    (a) Hodgkin's lymphoma
    (b) Malignant melanoma
    (c) African Burkitt's jaw lymphoma
    (d) Squamous cell carcinoma

    Answer for Q 40 on page 207

41. It is a bone tumor containing plasma cells showing hyperimmunoglobulinaemia, light chain dimers (Bence-Jones proteins) in urine. The tumor we are talking about is:
    (a) Hodgkin's tumor
    (b) Leukemia
    (c) Multiple myeloma
    (d) Osteosarcoma

    Answer for Q 41 on page 207

42. Which of the following is related to grave prognosis of a malignant melanoma?
    (a) Degree of pigmentation
    (b) Depth of Invasion
    (c) Lymphadenopathy
    (d) Pallor

    Answer for Q 42 on page 207

43. A 43-year-old man comes to the physician because of a black growth on his right hand. He first noticed this "growth" about 6 months ago, and it has been getting progressively darker and larger. A biopsy is

taken from the center of the lesion and is sent to pathology for microscopic examination. Which of the following markers will be the most helpful in establishing the diagnosis?

(a) CD markers

(b) CA 19-9

(c) CA-125

(d) S 100

Answer for Q 43 on page 207

44. Nodular growth of alveolus is seen in:

(a) Paget's disease

(b) Osteomas

(c) Cementifying fibroma

(d) All of the above

Answer for Q 44 on page 207

45. How common is the squamous cell carcinoma of the head and neck?

(a) Squamous cell carcinoma accounts for 90% of all malignancy

(b) Squamous cell carcinoma accounts for 1% of all malignancy

(c) Squamous cell carcinoma accounts for 50% of all malignancy

(d) Squamous cell carcinoma is a very rare tumor

Answer for Q 45 on page 207

46. Which of the following is the earliest manifestation of oral cancer?

(a) Exophytic mass

(b) Endophytic mass

(c) Erythroplakia

(d) Pigmented papule

Answer for Q 46 on page 207

47. What is the prognosis of verrucous carcinoma?

(a) Excellent

(b) Fair

(c) Poor

(d) Unheard of

Answer for Q 47 on page 207

48. Which of the following is a predisposing factor of nasopharyngeal carcinoma?
    (a) Consumption of salty fish
    (b) Candida albicans
    (c) UV light
    (d) Smokeless tobacco

    Answer for Q 48 on page 207

49. Multiple basal cell carcinomas are seen in which of the following?
    (a) Peutz Jeghers syndrome
    (b) Plummer-Vinson Syndrome
    (c) Down syndrome
    (d) Nevoid basal cell carcinoma syndrome

    Answer for Q 49 on page 207

50. Melanoma is **more** common in which ethnic group?
    (a) Caucasian
    (b) Hispanic
    (c) African American
    (d) Indian

    Answer for Q 50 on page 207

51. What is the interpretation of clinical stage I squamous cell carcinoma?
    (a) The disease is localized and the tumor size is less than 2 cm
    (b) Tumor invades the subjacent tissue and bilateral palpable nodes are involved
    (c) Tumor invades the subjacent tissue with no lymph node involvement
    (d) Tumor invades the subjacent tissue with distance metastasis

    Answer for Q 51 on page 208

52. Evidence of distant metastasis is related to one of the following stages of the TNM system:
    (a) Stage 1
    (b) Stage 2
    (c) Stage 3
    (d) Stage 4

    Answer for Q 52 on page 208

53. The "ABCDE" system of evaluation is used for the diagnose of:
    (a) Nasopharyngeal carcinoma
    (b) Adenosquamous carcinoma
    (c) Basal cell carcinoma
    (d) Malignant melanoma

    Answer for Q 53 on page 208

12.2 Answers with Comments:

1. The correct answer is **B** – Nodular melanoma is highly invasive and has a poor prognosis because it lacks the radial growth phase. Think nodular as in NO radial growth phase. Remember that the radial growth phase is when the melanoma does not penetrate the basement membrane. The vertical growth phase is worrisome because it penetrates through the skin.

   Back to Q 1 on page 193

2. The correct answer is **A** – Basal cell carcinoma has a rare incidence of metastasis. Out of these three, melanoma is the most likely to metastasize, up to 20% of cases.

   Back to Q 2 on page 193

3. The correct answer is **D** – Histopathologically, basal cell carcinoma (BCC) is characterized by basaloid tumor nodules of varying size showing peripheral palisading of cells and nuclei, and **separation** from surrounding stroma by optically empty appearing clefts. These were traditionally regarded as an artifact, occurring during routine tissue processing. Recently, reflectance confocal microscopy (RCM) has been applied for evaluation of BCC. Besides other features, small areas of low refractility separating tumor islands from the surrounding tissue can be observed in vivo, suggesting that the presence of amorphous material like **mucin** might be the causal factor for these clefts. Source: [7]

   Back to Q 3 on page 193

4. The correct answer is **D** – No explanation is available for this answer.

   Back to Q 4 on page 194

5. The correct answer is **B** – Multiple myeloma (MM), also known as plasma cell myeloma is a malignant tumor of plasma cells characterized by multiple radiolucencies, Bence Jones protein and infiltrating malignant plasma cells in biopsies.

   Back to Q 5 on page 194

6. The correct answer is **E** – Abscess is a localized suppurative inflammation with clear signs and symptoms of inflammatory process.

   Back to Q 6 on page 194

7. The correct answer is **D** – No explanation is available for this answer.

   Back to Q 7 on page 194

8. The correct answer is **D** – No explanation is available for this answer.

   Back to Q 8 on page 195

9. The correct answer is **D** – Intraoral carcinomas have a richer blood supply and are more difficult to excise.

   Back to Q 9 on page 195

10. The correct answer is **A** – The lower vermilion borders of the lower lip is exposed to the sun-rays more than the upper lip. Also, the lower lip is more prone for chronic lip biting than the upper one.

    Back to Q 10 on page 195

11. The correct answer is **D** – No explanation is available for this answer.

    Back to Q 11 on page 195

12. The correct answer is **D** – No explanation is available for this answer.

    Back to Q 12 on page 195

13. The correct answer is **B** – No explanation is available for this answer.

    Back to Q 13 on page 196

14. The correct answer is **D** – No explanation is available for this answer.

    Back to Q 14 on page 196

15. The correct answer is **C** – Verrucous carcinoma is a well differentiated form of squamous cell carcinoma with favorable prognosis.

    Back to Q 15 on page 196

16. The correct answer is **B** – No explanation is available for this answer.

    Back to Q 16 on page 196

17. The correct answer is **B** – Lack of keratin is an indication of loss of function of cell. Loss of cellular function is one of the most important features of poor differentiation.

    Back to Q 17 on page 196

18. The correct answer is **C** – Staging of oral carcinoma depends mainly on the clinical parameters, while grading depends mainly on the histopathological features of the tumor.

    Back to Q 18 on page 197

19. The correct answer is **C** – No explanation is available for this answer.

    Back to Q 19 on page 197

20. The correct answer is **A** – No explanation is available for this answer.

    Back to Q 20 on page 197

21. The correct answer is **B** – No explanation is available for this answer.

    Back to Q 21 on page 197

22. The correct answer is **C** – No explanation is available for this answer.

    Back to Q 22 on page 197

23. The correct answer is **B** – No explanation is available for this answer.

    Back to Q 23 on page 198

24. The correct answer is **B** – No explanation is available for this answer.

    Back to Q 24 on page 198

25. The correct answer is **B** – This is probably might be due to betel nut and tobacco chewing which is widespread in India.

    Back to Q 25 on page 198

26. The correct answer is **B** – Face above ala-tragus line is more subjected to the harmful ultraviolet rays of the sun.

    Back to Q 26 on page 198

27. The correct answer is **D** – No explanation is available for this answer.

    Back to Q 27 on page 198

28. The correct answer is **A** – Epidermoid carcinoma is an obsolete and abandoned term for squamous cell carcinoma.

    Back to Q 28 on page 199

29. The correct answer is **D** – No explanation is available for this answer.

    Back to Q 29 on page 199

30. The correct answer is **A** – No explanation is available for this answer.

    Back to Q 30 on page 199

31. The correct answer is **A** – Basal cell carcinoma is essentially a skin tumor, its existence as a mucosal tumor is very rare.

    Back to Q 31 on page 199

32. The correct answer is **D** – No explanation is available for this answer.

    Back to Q 32 on page 199

33. The correct answer is **A** – Cervical carcinoma (carcinoma of cervix share some common features with oral carcinoma. Both of them can arise on top of preexisting epithelial dysplasia.

    Back to Q 33 on page 200

34. The correct answer is **A** – No explanation is available for this answer.

    Back to Q 34 on page 200

35. The correct answer is **A** – No explanation is available for this answer.

Back to Q 35 on page 200

36. The correct answer is **C** – Basal cell carcinoma is a locally invasive tumor that rarely metastasize to remote areas.

Back to Q 36 on page 200

37. The correct answer is **A** – No explanation is available for this answer.

Back to Q 37 on page 200

38. The correct answer is **D** – No explanation is available for this answer.

Back to Q 38 on page 201

39. The correct answer is **B** – No explanation is available for this answer.

Back to Q 39 on page 201

40. The correct answer is **C** – No explanation is available for this answer.

Back to Q 40 on page 201

41. The correct answer is **C** – No explanation is available for this answer.

Back to Q 41 on page 201

42. The correct answer is **C** – No explanation is available for this answer.

Back to Q 42 on page 201

43. The correct answer is **D** – No explanation is available for this answer.

Back to Q 43 on page 201

44. The correct answer is **C** – No explanation is available for this answer.

Back to Q 44 on page 202

45. The correct answer is **A** – No explanation is available for this answer.

Back to Q 45 on page 202

46. The correct answer is **A** – No explanation is available for this answer.

Back to Q 46 on page 202

47. The correct answer is **B** – The earliest manifestation of oral cancer is the formation of an exophytic mass which soon ulcerates.

Back to Q 47 on page 202

48. The correct answer is **A** – No explanation is available for this answer.

Back to Q 48 on page 203

49. The correct answer is **D** – No explanation is available for this answer.

Back to Q 49 on page 203

50. The correct answer is **A** – No explanation is available for this answer.

Back to Q 50 on page 203

51. The correct answer is **A** – No explanation is available for this answer.

Back to Q 51 on page 203

52. The correct answer is **D** – No explanation is available for this answer.

Back to Q 52 on page 203

53. The correct answer is **D** – No explanation is available for this answer.

Back to Q 53 on page 204

CHAPTER 13
ODONTOGENIC TUMORS AND TUMOR-LIKE LESIONS

Odontogenic tumors are tumors arising from odontogenic tissues. Although most of these tumors are true neoplasms, many of them are developmental disturbances (hamartomas).

Odontogenic tissues which may act as a source for these tumors are:

1. Ectodermal tissues
   (a) Dental lamina and its remnants (Serre's pearl).
   (b) Enamel organ and its remnants (reduced dental epithelium).
   (c) Epithelial root sheath of Hertwig and its remnants (epithelial rests of Malassez).
2. Ectomesenchyme tissues[1] (in old literature was termed mesenchymal tissues)
   (a) Dental papilla and its remnants are represented by the dental pulp.
   (b) Tooth sac and its remnants is represented by the periodontal ligament.

It is worthy to note that the incidence rates of odontogenic tumors mentioned in this chapter are subject to variations depending upon geographic, racial and ethnic factors.

13.1 MCQs Questions

Choose **one or more** of the most appropriate answers. Some questions may have **more than one** correct answer. You have to choose all the correct answers as best as you can.

1. Extensive squamous metaplasia inside ameloblastoma present in:
   (a) Follicular ameloblastoma
   (b) Plexiform ameloblastoma
   (c) Acanthomatous ameloblastoma
   (d) Granular cell ameloblastoma

   Answer for Q 1 on page 221

[1]Ectomesenchyme is a form of mesenchyme, in the embryo, consisting of neural crest cells; forms the tissues of the head and neck while mesenchyme is that part of the mesoderm of an embryo that develops into connective tissue, bone, cartilage, etc. other than that of the head and neck.

2. Which of the following surgery is indicated for the removal of the 3 cm ameloblastoma involving the inferior border of the mandible?
   (a) Enucleation
   (b) Fulguration
   (c) Cryosurgery
   (d) Resection

   Answer for Q 2 on page 221

3. Ameloblastoma is best managed by:
   (a) Chemotherapy
   (b) Radiotherapy
   (c) Gene Therapy
   (d) Surgical excision

   Answer for Q 3 on page 221

4. The most appropriate method to differentiate between a dentigerous cyst and an ameloblastoma is through:
   (a) Radiographic examination
   (b) Aspiration cytology
   (c) Microscopic examination
   (d) Clinical features

   Answer for Q 4 on page 221

5. Mandibular resection is the treatment of choice for ameloblastoma because:
   (a) It infiltrates the surrounding bone
   (b) It can metastasize fast
   (c) It is an aggressive tumor
   (d) It has abnormal histological pattern

   Answer for Q 5 on page 221

6. A man has 1 × 1.5 cm pedunculated lesion on the soft palate which has a rough, warty surface but is the same color as adjacent mucosa. Appropriate management of this lesion is to:
   (a) Perform an incisional therapy
   (b) Perform excisional biopsy
   (c) Scrape for exfoliative cytology
   (d) Observe for two weeks

   Answer for Q 6 on page 221

7. When treated with simple curettage, which odontogenic tumor is most likely to recur?
   (a) Complex odontome
   (b) Compound odontoma
   (c) Odontogenic myxoma
   (d) Ameloblastic fibroma

   Answer for Q 7 on page 221

8. Odontoma is treated by:
   (a) Excision
   (b) Resection
   (c) Curettage
   (d) Radiotherapy

   Answer for Q 8 on page 221

9. Treatment of ameloblastoma:
   (a) Excision of tumor
   (b) Resection of the mandible along with the tumor
   (c) Incisional biopsy and marsupialization
   (d) No active treatment is necessary

   Answer for Q 9 on page 222

10. Adenoameloblastoma (adenomatoid odontogenic tumor) treatment:
    (a) Enbloc resection of maxilla
    (b) Marsupialization
    (c) Enucleation
    (d) No treatment

    Answer for Q 10 on page 222

11. Locally invasive odontogenic tumors just 1 cm away from lower border:
    (a) Enbloc resection
    (b) Hemimandibulectomy
    (c) Enucleation
    (d) No treatment

    Answer for Q 11 on page 222

12. Solid (calcifying odontogenic cyst) COC is now termed as:
    - (a) Odontogenic ghost cell tumor
    - (b) Dentinogenic ghost cell tumor in the 2017 WHO classification
    - (c) Keratocystic odontogenic tumor
    - (d) A & C

    Answer for Q 12 on page 222

13. Nomenclature calcifying odontogenic cyst has been continuously changing, due to debate as to whether it is:
    - (a) Cyst
    - (b) Tumor
    - (c) Inflammatory nature
    - (d) Developmental condition
    - (e) A and B

    Answer for Q 13 on page 222

14. What is the most common mutation in calcifying odontogenic cyst?
    - (a) β catenin
    - (b) BRAF
    - (c) PPARγ
    - (d) PTCH
    - (e) RAS

    Answer for Q 14 on page 222

15. Which of the following is true regarding the most common clinical features associated with adenomatoid odontogenic tumor (AOT)?
    - (a) Anterior mandible, impacted central incisor tooth, elderly male
    - (b) Anterior maxilla, unerupted canine tooth, teenage female
    - (c) Posterior mandible, impacted first molar tooth, middle age female
    - (d) Posterior maxilla, impacted premolar tooth, teenage male

    Answer for Q 15 on page 222

16. Which of the following is true about the microscopic variants of ameloblastoma?
    (a) Multiple microscopic variants are possible in the same tumor
    (b) Multiple microscopic variants are unlikely to occur in the same tumor
    (c) Multiple microscopic variants within the same tumor is associated with hypercalcemia
    (d) Multiple microscopic variants within the same tumor suggest high grade transformation is more likely to occur

    Answer for Q 16 on page 222

17. Which of the following histological patterns of ameloblastoma is most likely to be misdiagnosed as an odontogenic cyst?
    (a) Extraosseous peripheral type of ameloblastoma with follicular growth
    (b) Granular cell variant of ameloblastoma
    (c) Unicystic type of ameloblastoma with luminal growth
    (d) Acanthomatous variant of ameloblastoma

    Answer for Q 17 on page 222

18. What odontogenic tumor most commonly is associated with a calcifying odontogenic cyst?
    (a) Craniopharyngioma
    (b) Adenomatoid odontogenic tumor
    (c) Ameloblastoma
    (d) Basal cell adenocarcinoma
    (e) Odontoma

    Answer for Q 18 on page 222

19. Which of the following features favors the term dentinogenic ghost cell tumor over a calcifying odontogenic cyst?
    (a) Ameloblast-like epithelium
    (b) Pink ghost cells with no nuclei
    (c) Islands of squamous differentiation
    (d) Predominantly solid pattern of growth
    (e) Stellate reticulum-like cells

    Answer for Q 19 on page 222

20. Which feature is most typical for a calcifying odontogenic cyst?
    (a) Cyst lining showing a well defined layer of palisading basal cells and a stellate reticulum-like suprabasalar layer
    (b) Uncapsulated infiltrative lesion with mitotic activity
    (c) No ameloblastic epithelium present
    (d) Sellar or suprasellar location

    Answer for Q 20 on page 223

21. Which radiographic features distinguishes an ameloblastoma from a dentinogenic ghost cell tumor?
    (a) Air fluid levels
    (b) Calcifications
    (c) Cystic spaces
    (d) Invasive features

    Answer for Q 21 on page 223

22. A 36-year-old man with an asymptomatic swelling in the body of the mandible with radiographic features of radiolucency with radiopaque flecks is suffering from:
    (a) Odontogenic keratocyst
    (b) Calcifying epithelial odontogenic tumor (CEOT)
    (c) Ameloblastoma
    (d) None of the above

    Answer for Q 22 on page 223

23. All of the following tumors might have calcification **except**:
    (a) Adenomatoid odontogenic tumor
    (b) Pindborg tumor
    (c) Ameloblastoma
    (d) Ameloblastic fibro-odontoma

    Answer for Q 23 on page 223

24. Compound odontoma shows:
    (a) Mixed tissue of dental origin with no resemblance to tooth structure
    (b) Numerous teeth like structure with denticles commonly found in maxillary lateral incisors
    (c) Haphazardly arranged calcified mass
    (d) All of the above

    Answer for Q 24 on page 223

25. Locally invasive and destructive lesions with rare metastasis:
    (a) Fibroma
    (b) Ameloblastoma
    (c) Adenomatoid odontogenic tumor
    (d) Odontome

    Answer for Q 25 on page 223

26. Lesions associated with vital tooth?
    (a) Condensing osteitis
    (b) Cementoma
    (c) Periapical abscess
    (d) Periapical granuloma

    Answer for Q 26 on page 223

27. All of the following lesions may be classified as odontogenic tumors **except**:
    (a) Acanthomatous ameloblastoma
    (b) Branchial cleft cyst
    (c) Myxoma
    (d) Simple ameloblastoma

    Answer for Q 27 on page 223

28. Ameloblastoma most frequently occurs in:
    (a) Mandibular molar region
    (b) Maxillary molar region
    (c) Mandibular premolar region
    (d) Maxillary premolar region

    Answer for Q 28 on page 223

29. Compound odontoma shows on a radiograph as:
    (a) Supernumerary teeth
    (b) Radiolucent and radiopaque areas
    (c) Masses of calcified areas
    (d) Distinguishable tooth like structures

    Answer for Q 29 on page 223

30. Which of the following is true neoplasm of functional cementoblasts?
    (a) Periapical cemental dysplasia
    (b) Familial cemental dysplasia
    (c) Benign cementoblastoma
    (d) Hypercementosis

    Answer for Q 30 on page 223

31. Liesegang rings are found in:
    (a) Calcifying epithelial odontogenic cyst
    (b) Primordial cyst
    (c) Calcifying epithelial odontogenic tumor
    (d) Odontoma

    Answer for Q 31 on page 224

32. Which of the following is an odontogenic tumor?
    (a) Arrhenoblastoma
    (b) Astrocytoma
    (c) Ameloblastoma
    (d) Granular cell tumor

    Answer for Q 32 on page 224

33. The most common odontogenic tumor which occurs in relation to an unerupted tooth in the anterior maxilla:
    (a) Adenomatoid odontogenic tumor
    (b) Odontoma
    (c) Myxoma
    (d) Cementifying fibroma

    Answer for Q 33 on page 224

34. Which of the following is the most common lesion of the mandible?
    (a) Ameloblastoma
    (b) Osteogenic sarcoma
    (c) Squamous cell carcinoma
    (d) Osteoclastoma

    Answer for Q 34 on page 224

35. Radiographic finding in Pindborg tumor is:
    (a) Sun-burst appearance
    (b) Onion-peel appearance
    (c) Driven - snow appearance
    (d) Cherry - blossom appearance

    Answer for Q 35 on page 224

36. None functional, locally aggressive, clinically persistent tumor is:
    (a) CEOT
    (b) Enameloma
    (c) Odontoma
    (d) Ameloblastoma

    Answer for Q 36 on page 224

37. A 40-year-old woman has ameloblastoma, the histomorphologic features will be:
    (a) Peripheral palisading cellular strand with central loose stellate reticulum
    (b) Peripheral palisading with central stromal retraction artifact
    (c) Peripheral palisading cellular strand with peripheral loose stellate reticulum
    (d) Central loose stellate reticulum shows marked nuclear atypia and numerous mitotic

    Answer for Q 37 on page 224

38. Adenomatoid odontogenic tumor is most commonly found in:
    (a) Anterior mandible
    (b) Posterior maxilla
    (c) Anterior maxilla
    (d) Ramus of the mandible

    Answer for Q 38 on page 224

39. Adamantinoma is:
    (a) An old term used to describe ameloblastoma
    (b) More common in long bones particularly the tibia
    (c) Rare, low-grade malignant tumors of unknown etiology
    (d) All of these

    Answer for Q 39 on page 224

40. Odontogenic tumor that has amyloid-like structure is:
    (a) Adenomatoid odontogenic tumor
    (b) Calcifying epithelial odontogenic tumor
    (c) Squamous odontogenic tumor
    (d) Compound odontoma

    Answer for Q 40 on page 224

41. The difference between squamous odontogenic tumor (SOT) and squamous cell carcinoma (SCC) is:
    (a) SOT has no dysplasia
    (b) SOT occur inside the bone while SCC occur in the soft tissue
    (c) SCC has no dysplasia
    (d) There is no difference

    Answer for Q 41 on page 224

42. In ameloblastic fibroma:
    (a) Epithelial component is neoplastic only
    (b) Mesenchymal component is neoplastic only
    (c) Both components are neoplastic
    (d) None of them are neoplastic

    Answer for Q 42 on page 224

43. The difference between ameloblastic fibroma and ameloblastoma:
    (a) Ameloblastoma occur in the posterior area of the mandible
    (b) Ameloblastic fibroma occur in the anterior area of the mandible
    (c) Ameloblastoma occur in young age
    (d) Ameloblastic fibroma occur in younger age

    Answer for Q 43 on page 224

44. The most common odontogenic tumor is:
    (a) Ameloblastic fibroma
    (b) Odontogenic fibroma
    (c) Odontoma
    (d) Cementoblastoma

    Answer for Q 44 on page 224

45. Malignant ameloblastoma:
    (a) Histologically appear completely benign
    (b) Has a lot of cytological dysplasia
    (c) Stay in the alveolar ridge without metastasis
    (d) Treated by local excision only

    Answer for Q 45 on page 224

46. The only difference in diagnosis between cementoblastoma and osteoblastoma is:
    (a) Osteoblastoma is larger in size
    (b) Cementoblastoma attached to the root
    (c) Cementoblastoma is larger in size
    (d) There is no difference between the two

    Answer for Q 46 on page 224

47. Mixed odontogenic tumors, has epithelial and ectomeschymal components and both are neoplastic:
    (a) First statement is true and the second is false
    (b) First statement is false and the second is true
    (c) Both statements are true
    (d) Both statements are false

    Answer for Q 47 on page 225

48. Acanthomatous pattern of ameloblastoma main feature is:
    (a) It has granular cell metaplasia
    (b) It has some keratin formation
    (c) It has columnar cell epithelium metaplasia
    (d) It has more aggressive behavior than other types

    Answer for Q 48 on page 225

49. The most common radiographic picture in ameloblastoma is:
    (a) Unilocular radiolucency
    (b) Multilocular radiolucency
    (c) Mixed radiopaque radiolucent
    (d) Pure radiopaque

    Answer for Q 49 on page 225

50. The most aggressive type of unicystic ameloblastoma is:
    - (a) Luminal type
    - (b) Intraluminal type
    - (c) Mural type
    - (d) Follicular type

    Answer for Q 50 on page 225

51. The most important feature of malignant ameloblastoma is:
    - (a) It is locally destructive
    - (b) It has cytological dysplasia
    - (c) It can recur
    - (d) It can metastasize

    Answer for Q 51 on page 225

52. The following tumor has snowflakes calcification:
    - (a) Adenomatoid odontogenic tumor
    - (b) Calcifying epithelial odontogenic tumor
    - (c) Clear cell odontogenic carcinoma
    - (d) Squamous odontogenic tumor

    Answer for Q 52 on page 225

53. The following tumor has gelatinous nature in gross section:
    - (a) Ameloblastoma
    - (b) Adenomatoid odontogenic tumor
    - (c) Odontogenic myxoma
    - (d) Odontogenic fibroma

    Answer for Q 53 on page 225

54. Ameloblastoma is an aggressive tumor because:
    - (a) It locally destroys adjacent vital structure
    - (b) It metastasizes to distant structures and destroy them
    - (c) It is severely painful
    - (d) It is associated with malignant tumors

    Answer for Q 54 on page 225

55. Which one of the following ameloblastoma has the worse prognosis?
    (a) Unicystic ameloblastoma
    (b) Conventional ameloblastoma
    (c) Peripheral ameloblastoma
    (d) Ameloblastic carcinoma

    Answer for Q 55 on page 225

56. Adenomatoid odontogenic tumor is characterized histologically by:
    (a) Polyhedral epithelial cells
    (b) Tubular / duct like cells
    (c) Stellate shaped cells
    (d) Stratified squamous epithelial cells

    Answer for Q 56 on page 225

13.2 Answers with Comments:

1. The correct answer is **C** – No explanation is available for this answer.

   Back to Q 1 on page 209

2. The correct answer is **D** – Involvement of the inferior border of the mandible necessitate resection.

   Back to Q 2 on page 210

3. The correct answer is **D** – Ameloblastoma is not responsive to radiotherapy, chemotherapy or gene therapy till now.

   Back to Q 3 on page 210

4. The correct answer is **C** – As ameloblastoma can arise on top of a preexisting dentigerous cysts, the only method to differentiated between them is the biopsy examination.

   Back to Q 4 on page 210

5. The correct answer is **A** – No explanation is available for this answer.

   Back to Q 5 on page 210

6. The correct answer is **B** – Small lesions are best treated and examined by excisional biopsy.

   Back to Q 6 on page 210

7. The correct answer is **C** – Odontogenic myxoma is a locally invasive and infiltrative lesion, therefore it should be treated by excision with safety margin rather than by curettage.

   Back to Q 7 on page 211

8. The correct answer is **A** – No explanation is available for this answer.

Back to Q 8 on page 211

9. The correct answer is **B** – Ameloblastoma is a locally invasive and infiltrative lesion, therefore it should be treated by excision with safety margin rather than by curettage.

   Back to Q 9 on page 211

10. The correct answer is **C** – Adenomatoid odontogenic tumor is a benign capsulated lesion that is best treated by enucleation to preserve the vital tissues around the tumor.

    Back to Q 10 on page 211

11. The correct answer is **A** – No explanation is available for this answer.

    Back to Q 11 on page 211

12. The correct answer is **B** – Solid lesions are designated dentinogenic ghost cell tumors in the 2017 WHO classification.

    Back to Q 12 on page 212

13. The correct answer is **E** – Nomenclature has been continuously changing, due to debate as to whether COC is a neoplasm or a developmental cyst:
    - In 1992, WHO classified this lesion as an odontogenic tumor but continued to use the term calcifying odontogenic cyst.
    - In 2005, WHO renamed the lesion as calcifying cystic odontogenic tumor (CCOT).
    - In 2017, the term calcifying odontogenic cyst was reapplied to this lesion and it was reclassified as a benign odontogenic cyst
    - Other old names include Gorlin cyst and keratinizing and calcifying odontogenic cyst.
    - COC belongs to odontogenic ghost cell family of lesions.
    - Solid lesions are designated dentinogenic ghost cell tumors in the 2017 WHO classification.

    Back to Q 13 on page 212

14. The correct answer is **A** – No explanation is available for this answer.

    Back to Q 14 on page 212

15. The correct answer is **B** – No explanation is available for this answer.

    Back to Q 15 on page 212

16. The correct answer is **A** – No explanation is available for this answer.

    Back to Q 16 on page 213

17. The correct answer is **C** – No explanation is available for this answer.

    Back to Q 17 on page 213

18. The correct answer is **E** – No explanation is available for this answer.

    Back to Q 18 on page 213

19. The correct answer is **D** – Dentinogenic ghost cell tumor and calcifying odontogenic cyst share significant histopathologic features. Both exhibit amelobastic-like epithelium, ghost cells, stellate reticulum, squamous differentiation, and varying levels of dentin and calcification; however, the dentinogenic ghost cell tumor is a solid neoplasm, whereas the calcifying odontogenic cyst has a single lumen "unilocular cyst" [8].

   Back to Q 19 on page 213

20. The correct answer is **A** – No explanation is available for this answer.

   Back to Q 20 on page 214

21. The correct answer is **B** – The radiographic and histopathologic features of ameloblastoma and dentinogenic ghost cell tumor are very similar. Ameloblastoma, on the other hand, rarely has calcifications on radiographs. Ameloblastoma often has a multilocular appearance on radiographs. The most prevalent and clinically important odontogenic tumour is ameloblastoma, which is significantly more common than dentinogenic ghost cell tumor.

   Back to Q 21 on page 214

22. The correct answer is **B** – As the tumor exhibits calcification, these appear in the radiograph as radiopaque flecks.

   Back to Q 22 on page 214

23. The correct answer is **C** – Calcification in ameloblastoma is very rare.

   Back to Q 23 on page 214

24. The correct answer is **B** – Compound odontome consists of multiple small denticles. The enamel, dentin, cementum, and pulp tissue are arranged in normal anatomical relationship to each other and not haphazard as in complex odontome.

   Back to Q 24 on page 214

25. The correct answer is **B** – Ameloblastoma is a locally invasive lesion.

   Back to Q 25 on page 215

26. The correct answer is **B** – Benign Cementoblastoma (True cementoma) is typically associated with vital teeth.

   Back to Q 26 on page 215

27. The correct answer is **B** – No explanation is available for this answer.

   Back to Q 27 on page 215

28. The correct answer is **A** – No explanation is available for this answer.

   Back to Q 28 on page 215

29. The correct answer is **D** – No explanation is available for this answer.

   Back to Q 29 on page 215

30. The correct answer is **C** – Benign cementoblastoma is considered as the true neoplasm of cementoblasts, other types of cementomas represent a dysplasia or a developmental disturbance.

    Back to Q 30 on page 216

31. The correct answer is **C** – No explanation is available for this answer.

    Back to Q 31 on page 216

32. The correct answer is **C** – No explanation is available for this answer.

    Back to Q 32 on page 216

33. The correct answer is **A** – No explanation is available for this answer.

    Back to Q 33 on page 216

34. The correct answer is **A** – No explanation is available for this answer.

    Back to Q 34 on page 216

35. The correct answer is **C** – No explanation is available for this answer.

    Back to Q 35 on page 217

36. The correct answer is **D** – No explanation is available for this answer.

    Back to Q 36 on page 217

37. The correct answer is **A** – No explanation is available for this answer.

    Back to Q 37 on page 217

38. The correct answer is **A** – No explanation is available for this answer.

    Back to Q 38 on page 217

39. The correct answer is **D** – No explanation is available for this answer.

    Back to Q 39 on page 217

40. The correct answer is **B** – No explanation is available for this answer.

    Back to Q 40 on page 218

41. The correct answer is **A** – No explanation is available for this answer.

    Back to Q 41 on page 218

42. The correct answer is **C** – No explanation is available for this answer.

    Back to Q 42 on page 218

43. The correct answer is **D** – No explanation is available for this answer.

    Back to Q 43 on page 218

44. The correct answer is **C** – No explanation is available for this answer.

    Back to Q 44 on page 218

45. The correct answer is **C** – No explanation is available for this answer.

    Back to Q 45 on page 219

46. The correct answer is **B** – No explanation is available for this answer.

Back to Q 46 on page 219

47. The correct answer is **C** – No explanation is available for this answer.

Back to Q 47 on page 219

48. The correct answer is **B** – No explanation is available for this answer.

Back to Q 48 on page 219

49. The correct answer is **B** – No explanation is available for this answer.

Back to Q 49 on page 219

50. The correct answer is **C** – No explanation is available for this answer.

Back to Q 50 on page 220

51. The correct answer is **D** – No explanation is available for this answer.

Back to Q 51 on page 220

52. The correct answer is **A** – No explanation is available for this answer.

Back to Q 52 on page 220

53. The correct answer is **C** – No explanation is available for this answer.

Back to Q 53 on page 220

54. The correct answer is **A** – No explanation is available for this answer.

Back to Q 54 on page 220

55. The correct answer is **D** – No explanation is available for this answer.

Back to Q 55 on page 221

56. The correct answer is **B** – No explanation is available for this answer.

Back to Q 56 on page 221

CHAPTER 14
DISEASES OF SALIVARY GLANDS

Salivary glands are exocrine glands that produce saliva through a system of ducts. There are three paired major salivary glands (parotid, submandibular, and sublingual) as well as many minor salivary glands scattered all over the oral cavity. Regarding to the type of secretion there are 3 types of salivary glands, serous, mucous or seromucous (mixed).

14.1 MCQs Questions

Choose **one or more** of the most appropriate answers. Some questions may have **more than one** correct answer. You have to choose all the correct answers as best as you can.

1. Which one of the following tumors can affect parotid gland bilaterally?
   (a) Basal cell adenoma
   (b) mucoepidermoid carcinoma
   (c) Acinic cell carcinoma
   (d) Papillary cystadenoma lymphomatosum
   Answer for Q 1 on page 242
2. One of the following tumors occurs most commonly in the minor salivary glands of the palate:
   (a) Pleomorphic adenoma
   (b) Warthin's tumor
   (c) Adenocystic carcinoma
   (d) Acinic cell carcinoma
   Answer for Q 2 on page 243
3. The cause of sicca syndrome is:
   (a) Hereditary
   (b) Environmental
   (c) Inflammatory
   (d) Autoimmune

Answer for Q 3 on page 243

4. The virus implicated in the etiology of mumps is the:
   (a) Herpes simplex virus
   (b) paramyxo virus
   (c) Herpes zoster virus
   (d) Cytomegalo virus

Answer for Q 4 on page 243

5. A 50-year-old male presented to the dental clinic complaining of an ulcer in the hard palate in the last two weeks after extraction of the upper first molar, the most likely diagnosis is:
   (a) Squamous cell carcinoma
   (b) Malignant pleomorphic adenoma
   (c) Necrotizing sialometaplasia
   (d) Adenoid cystic carcinoma

Answer for Q 5 on page 243

6. The cell present in the connective tissue stroma of Warthin's tumor is:
   (a) Lymphocyte
   (b) Plasma cell
   (c) Neutrophil
   (d) Basophil

Answer for Q 6 on page 243

7. Snow storm appearance is a radiographic term used to describe:
   (a) Sialolith
   (b) Chronic sialadenitis
   (c) Sicca syndrome
   (d) Acute suppurative parotitis

Answer for Q 7 on page 243

8. Invasion of perineural lymphatics by tumor cells is a characteristic feature of which of the following?
   (a) Adenoid cystic carcinoma
   (b) Mucoepidermoid carcinoma
   (c) Acinic cell carcinoma
   (d) Malignant pleomorphic adenoma

Answer for Q 8 on page 243

9. Epi-myoepithelial islands is a histological hallmark of:
   (a) Necrotizing sialometaplasia
   (b) Sialoadenosis
   (c) Sjogren's syndrome
   (d) Acute suppurative parotitis

   Answer for Q 9 on page 243

10. All of the following are growth patterns of adenoid cystic carcinoma **except**:
   (a) Cribriform
   (b) Follicular
   (c) Tubular
   (d) Solid

   Answer for Q 10 on page 243

11. Cigarette smoking is proposed to be an etiological factor of:
   (a) Mixed tumor
   (b) Papillary cystadenoma lymphomatosum
   (c) Oncocytoma
   (d) Basal cell adenoma

   Answer for Q 11 on page 243

12. The parotid, submandibular, and sublingual salivary glands contribute to:
   (a) 20% of total saliva secretions
   (b) 40% of total saliva secretions
   (c) 60% of total saliva secretions
   (d) 90 % of total saliva secretions

   Answer for Q 12 on page 243

13. In the resting (unstimulated) state, approximately two-thirds of the total volume of the whole saliva is produced by:
   (a) Submandibular salivary glands
   (b) Parotid gland
   (c) Sublingual salivary gland
   (d) Minor salivary gland

   Answer for Q 13 on page 243

14. Upon stimulation, the following gland is responsible for at least 50% of the total volume of saliva from the mouth:
    (a) Submandibular salivary glands
    (b) Parotid gland
    (c) Sublingual salivary gland
    (d) Minor salivary gland

    Answer for Q 14 on page 243

15. One of the following salivary gland is serous:
    (a) Submandibular salivary gland
    (b) Parotid gland
    (c) Sublingual salivary gland
    (d) Minor salivary glands

    Answer for Q 15 on page 243

16. One of the following facts is **untrue** regarding minor salivary glands:
    (a) They are exclusively mucous
    (b) Contribute significantly to the lubrication of the oral mucosa
    (c) They are exclusively serous
    (d) High protein content

    Answer for Q 16 on page 243

17. Microscopic examination of sialoadenosis reveals:
    (a) Accumulation of epimyoepithelial cells forming islands
    (b) Aggregation of lymphocytes with germinal centers to form lymphoepithelial masses
    (c) Hypertrophy of the acinar cells, sometimes two to three times greater than normal size with accumulation of zymogen granules
    (d) Multiple cystic spaces filled with mucin

    Answer for Q 17 on page 243

18. The normal daily production of saliva varies between:
    (a) 0.5 and 1.5 liters
    (b) 2 and 3 liters
    (c) 3 and 4 liters
    (d) 4 and 5 liters

    Answer for Q 18 on page 244

19. The whole unstimulated saliva flow rate is approximately:
    (a) 0.1–0.2 ml / min
    (b) 0.3–0.4 ml / min
    (c) 0.5–0.6 ml / min
    (d) 0.6–0.7 ml / min

    Answer for Q 19 on page 244

20. "leafless tree" pattern seen in sialography is a characteristic feature of:
    (a) Sialoadenosis
    (b) Sjogren's syndrome
    (c) Mikulicz disease
    (d) All of the above

    Answer for Q 20 on page 244

21. The whole stimulated saliva flow rate is approximately:
    (a) 1–2 ml / min
    (b) 2–3 ml / min
    (c) 4–5 ml / min
    (d) 7–8 ml / min

    Answer for Q 21 on page 244

22. The buffering system of saliva is mediated through:
    (a) Mucopolysaccharides
    (b) Glycoproteins
    (c) Sucrose and starch
    (d) Bicarbonate, phosphate and protein

    Answer for Q 22 on page 244

23. Sialadenosis is an unusual noninflammatory disorder characterized by enlargement of:
    (a) Parotid gland
    (b) Submandibular salivary gland
    (c) Sublingual salivary gland
    (d) Minor salivary glands

    Answer for Q 23 on page 244

24. Human saliva contains:
    (a) α amylase and lipase
    (b) Lysozyme
    (c) Lactoferrin
    (d) Peroxidase
    (e) All of the above

    Answer for Q 24 on page 244

25. IgG4-related disease is the new term applied to: [9]
    (a) Sjögren syndrome
    (b) Mikulicz disease
    (c) Mikulicz syndrome
    (d) Sarcoidosis

    Answer for Q 25 on page 244

26. IgG4-related sialadenitis occurs most frequently in:
    (a) Submandibular gland
    (b) Parotid gland
    (c) Sublingual gland
    (d) Minor salivary glands

    Answer for Q 26 on page 244

27. Küttner tumor is the lesions associated with:
    (a) Sjögren syndrome
    (b) Sarcoidosis
    (c) Mikulicz disease
    (d) Rheumatoid arthritis

    Answer for Q 27 on page 244

28. Microscopic examination revealing chronic sclerosing sialadenitis, characterized by a heavy lympho-plasmacytic infiltrate, hyperplastic lymphoid follicles, and acinar atrophy with prominent interlobular fibrosis and obliterative phlebitis is a characteristic feature of:
    (a) Küttner tumor and IgG4-related sialadenitis (Mikulicz disease)
    (b) Sjögren syndrome
    (c) Acute suppurative parotitis
    (d) Mikulicz syndrome

    Answer for Q 28 on page 244

29. Sjögren syndrome is:
    (a) More common in males than females in a ratio of 9:1
    (b) More common in females than males in a ratio of 9:1
    (c) Equally distributed in males and females
    (d) Shows a bimodal distribution

    Answer for Q 29 on page 244

30. "fruit-laden, branchless tree" pattern seen in sialographic examination is a characteristic feature of:
    (a) Sjögren syndrome
    (b) Chronic sialadenitis
    (c) Acute suppurative parotitis
    (d) Mumps

    Answer for Q 30 on page 245

31. The factor in the saliva, which enhances the speed of the oral mucosal healing is:
    (a) Epidermal growth factor
    (b) Cortisol
    (c) Glucose
    (d) Urea

    Answer for Q 31 on page 245

32. The burning mouth syndrome is a set of painful and burning sensations in the mouth experienced even when clinical investigation of the mucosa proves to be normal. The causative factors for this condition may be:
    (a) Local factors (e.g., dental materials used to restore teeth)
    (b) Systemic (including lack of minerals, vitamins, etc.).
    (c) Mental health problems.
    (d) Psycho-social difficulties
    (e) All of the above

    Answer for Q 32 on page 245

33. Benign lymphoepithelial lesion is a characteristic feature of:
    (a) Suppurative parotitis
    (b) Sjögren syndrome
    (c) Sarcoidosis
    (d) Cheilitis granulomatosa

    Answer for Q 33 on page 245

34. Saliva is always:

(a) Hypotonic to plasma

(b) Hypertonic to plasma

(c) Isotonic to plasma

(d) None of the above

Answer for Q 34 on page 245

35. Signs associated with common chronic salivary gland hypofunction (xerostomia) include:

(a) Dry, chapped lips; desiccated, dry and fissured tongue

(b) Angular cheilitis / pseudomembranous and erythematous candidiasis

(c) Dental caries (cervical and root caries in particular)

(d) Gingivitis

(e) All of the above

Answer for Q 35 on page 245

36. Which of the following is true about salivary gland canalicular adenoma?

(a) Cannot be multifocal

(b) Is a benign tumor

(c) Is rare in minor salivary glands

(d) Lacks stromal tissue

Answer for Q 36 on page 245

37. Patients with Sjögren syndrome have an increased risk for:

(a) Leukemia

(b) Fibrosarcoma

(c) Lymphoma

(d) Myeloma

Answer for Q 37 on page 245

38. Which of the following is true about salivary gland canalicular adenoma?

(a) Is a type of adenocarcinoma

(b) Is often associated with lymph node metastases

(c) May contain squamous balls

(d) May show vascular emboli

Answer for Q 38 on page 245

39. The preferred site for taking biopsy in case of Sjögren syndrome is:
    (a) Minor labial salivary glands
    (b) Minor palatal salivary glands
    (c) Parotid gland
    (d) Submandibular gland

    Answer for Q 39 on page 245

40. Acute suppurative parotitis is categorized as:
    (a) Viral infection
    (b) Specific bacterial infection
    (c) Non-specific bacterial infection
    (d) Fungal infection

    Answer for Q 40 on page 245

41. The increase in the flow of saliva is termed as:
    (a) Ptyalism
    (b) Xerostomia
    (c) Sialolith
    (d) Sialadenitis

    Answer for Q 41 on page 245

42. A cyst occurring in the floor of the mouth due to salivary duct obstruction is termed:
    (a) Dermoid cyst
    (b) Ranula
    (c) Epidermoid cyst
    (d) Sialoodontogenic cyst

    Answer for Q 42 on page 245

43. The increase in the flow of saliva with drooling is termed as:
    (a) Xerostomia
    (b) Sialolith
    (c) Sialorrhea
    (d) Sialadenitis

    Answer for Q 43 on page 245

44. An abnormal decrease in the flow of saliva is called:

(a) Ptyalism

(b) Trismus

(c) Xerostomia

(d) Salivation

(e) Sialadenitis

Answer for Q 44 on page 245

45. Enlargements of the salivary gland in the acute phase is due to hypertrophy of individual acinar cells and in chronic phase, due to replacement of normal gland parenchyma with fat are characteristic of:

(a) Chemical mumps

(b) Nutritional mumps

(c) Epidemic parotitis

(d) Acute postoperative parotitis

Answer for Q 45 on page 245

46. One of the following tumors occurs most commonly in the minor salivary glands of the palate:

(a) Pleomorphic adenoma

(b) Warthin tumor

(c) Adenocystic carcinoma

(d) Acinic cell carcinoma

Answer for Q 46 on page 246

47. The etiology of Sjögren syndrome is:

(a) Hereditary

(b) Environmental

(c) Autoimmune

(d) Inflammatory

Answer for Q 47 on page 246

48. A 45-year-old man presented to the clinic complaining of an ulcer in the hard palate in the last three weeks after palatal injection of a local anesthetic solution, the most probable diagnosis is:

(a) Squamous cell carcinoma

(b) Necrotizing sialometaplasia

(c) Malignant pleomorphic adenoma

(d) Adenoid cystic carcinoma

Answer for Q 48 on page 246

49. The cells that predominate in the connective tissue stroma of Warthin tumor affecting the parotid gland is:
    (a) Plasma cell
    (b) Lymphocyte
    (c) Neutrophil
    (d) Basophil

    Answer for Q 49 on page 246

50. Snow storm appearance is a radiographic term used to describe:
    (a) Sialolith
    (b) Chronic sialadenitis
    (c) Sjogren's syndrome
    (d) Acute suppurative parotitis

    Answer for Q 50 on page 246

51. Epimyoepithelial islands is a collection of epithelial and myoepithelial cells and is considered as a histological hallmark of:
    (a) Necrotizing sialometaplasia
    (b) Sjogren's syndrome
    (c) Sialoadenosis
    (d) Acute suppurative parotitis

    Answer for Q 51 on page 246

52. Cigarette smoking is proposed to be an etiological factor of:
    (a) Canalicular adenoma
    (b) Papillary cystadenoma lymphomatosum
    (c) Oncocytoma
    (d) Basal cell adenoma

    Answer for Q 52 on page 246

53. The preferred site for taking biopsy for the diagnosis of Sjögren syndrome is:
    (a) Minor palatal salivary glands
    (b) Minor labial salivary glands
    (c) Parotid gland
    (d) Submandibular gland

    Answer for Q 53 on page 246

54. Acute suppurative parotitis is considered as:
   (a) Viral infection
   (b) Non-specific bacterial infection
   (c) Specific bacterial infection
   (d) Fungal infection

   Answer for Q 54 on page 246

55. 3-year-old child came from kindergarten complaining of headache, malaise and fever. His mother gave him pain killer and ask him to have a nap to be OK. He wakes up with unilateral swelling in his face causing elevation of the lobule of the ear. The covering skin is slightly reddened. Laboratory investigation denote raised serum amylase enzyme. What is the possible diagnosis of this case?
   (a) Sialadenitis
   (b) Acute suppurative parotitis
   (c) Epidemic parotitis
   (d) Recurrent parotitis

   Answer for Q 55 on page 246

56. A cyst occurring in the floor of the mouth due to salivary duct obstruction is termed:
   (a) Dermoid cyst
   (b) Mucous retention/extravasation cyst
   (c) Epidermoid cyst
   (d) Sialoodontogenic cyst

   Answer for Q 56 on page 246

57. Papillary cystadenoma lymphomatosum, which occurs almost exclusive in the parotid gland, is commonly called:
   (a) Cylindroma
   (b) Pleomorphic adenoma
   (c) Warthin's tumor
   (d) Mikulicz's disease
   (e) Jaffy's syndrome

   Answer for Q 57 on page 246

58. A calculus in the submandibular gland duct can be removed by:
    (a) Dilatation of the duct
    (b) Excision of the opening of duct
    (c) Removal of the gland
    (d) Incision of the duct and removal of the calculus

Answer for Q 58 on page 246

59. Salivary calculus is more common in:
    (a) Submandibular gland
    (b) Sublingual gland
    (c) Parotid gland
    (d) Minor salivary gland

Answer for Q 59 on page 246

60. During removal of a parotid tumor, the auriculotemporal nerve is injured. This could result in:
    (a) Facial paralysis
    (b) Trigeminal neuralgia
    (c) Gustatory sweating
    (d) Orolingual Paresthesia

Answer for Q 60 on page 246

61. Submandibular duct is exposed via intraoral approach by incising the:
    (a) Buccinator
    (b) Mucous membrane
    (c) Masseter
    (d) All of the above

Answer for Q 61 on page 246

62. Excision of the submandibular gland for calculus or tumors is done by incision below angle of the jaw. Special care should be taken to avoid which nerve?
    (a) Ansa cervicalis
    (b) Mandibular branch of facial nerve
    (c) Posterior auricular nerve
    (d) Submandibular ganglion

Answer for Q 62 on page 247

63. Treatment of mucocele on lower lip:
    (a) Incision
    (b) Excision
    (c) Excision with adjacent glands
    (d) Biopsy

    Answer for Q 63 on page 247

64. Which of the following detects salivary gland duct diverticuli:
    (a) Ultrasonography
    (b) Plain radiography
    (c) Sialography
    (d) Xeroradiography

    Answer for Q 64 on page 247

65. During surgical excision of the parotid gland, the following structures may be damaged:
    (a) Lesser occipital nerve, hypoglossal nerve and chorda tympani
    (b) Facial nerve and auriculotemporal nerve
    (c) Submandibular duct
    (d) Cervical fascia

    Answer for Q 65 on page 247

66. During surgery on the submandibular gland:
    (a) Damage to the lingual nerve will cause loss of sensation to the posterior third of the tongue
    (b) The submandibular gland is seen to wrap around the posterior border of the mylohyoid
    (c) The facial artery and vein are usually divided as they course through the deep part of the gland.
    (d) The hypoglossal nerve is seen to loop under the submandibular duct

    Answer for Q 66 on page 247

67. The following gland is removed in surgery for a ranula:
    (a) Submandibular gland
    (b) Sublingual gland
    (c) Parotid gland
    (d) Lacrimal gland

    Answer for Q 67 on page 247

68. A 40-year-old woman reports the development of painful crater like ulcer on mucosa of left hard palate within one week following the extraction of maxillary left second premolar. What's the possible diagnosis?
    (a) Necrotizing sialometaplasia
    (b) Traumatic bone cyst
    (c) Acute parotitis
    (d) Mucoepidermoid carcinoma
    Answer for Q 68 on page 247
69. Treatment of calculus within the submandibular salivary gland is:
    (a) Removal of sinus
    (b) Removal of the gland
    (c) Dichotomy
    (d) Milking of the stone
    Answer for Q 69 on page 247
70. The plunging ranula is so called because of:
    (a) its size
    (b) lifting of tongue
    (c) Extension through mylohyoid
    (d) Involvement of lingual nerve
    Answer for Q 70 on page 247
71. Facial nerve paralysis is common with:
    (a) Pleomorphic adenoma
    (b) Oncocytoma
    (c) Warthin's tumor
    (d) Lymphoepithelial carcinoma
    Answer for Q 71 on page 247
72. An elderly woman presents with swelling of lateral aspect of left side of neck which was present for last ten months but start increasing in size for the last two months and is now painful. There is small ulcer-

ation of skin overlying the mass with distortion of left facial region when patient speaks. Differential diagnosis will include all of the following **except**:

(a) Adenoid cystic carcinoma

(b) Pleomorphic adenoma

(c) Mucoepidermoid carcinoma

(d) Malignant mixed tumor

Answer for Q 72 on page 247

73. 45-years-old male complains of slowly growing painless palatal swelling. The radiograph was normal. Biopsy shows capsulated mass composed of fibroid, mucinous and chondroid tissue. What is your possible diagnosis?

(a) Mucoepidermoid

(b) Warthin tumor

(c) Pleomorphic adenoma

(d) Oncocytoma

Answer for Q 73 on page 247

74. Mucoepidermoid carcinoma is a malignant salivary gland tumor characterized microscopically by 3 phasic patterns consisting of:

(a) Epidermoid, osteoblast and chondroblast

(b) Mucous, epidermoid and intermediate cells

(c) Epidermis, fibroblast and mucous cells

(d) Osteocytes, chondroblast and epidermis cells

Answer for Q 74 on page 247

75. Among the choices below, what is the most common site to find an oral cavity mucocele?

(a) Gingiva

(b) Intrabony, within the maxillary or mandibular bone

(c) Lower labial mucosa

(d) Parotid gland

(e) Upper labial mucosa

Answer for Q 75 on page 247

14.2 Answers with Comments:

1. The correct answer is **D** – No explanation is available for this answer.

Back to Q 1 on page 227

2. The correct answer is **C** – No explanation is available for this answer.

Back to Q 2 on page 227

3. The correct answer is **D** – No explanation is available for this answer.

Back to Q 3 on page 227

4. The correct answer is **B** – No explanation is available for this answer.

Back to Q 4 on page 228

5. The correct answer is **C** – No explanation is available for this answer.

Back to Q 5 on page 228

6. The correct answer is **A** – No explanation is available for this answer.

Back to Q 6 on page 228

7. The correct answer is **C** – No explanation is available for this answer.

Back to Q 7 on page 228

8. The correct answer is **A** – No explanation is available for this answer.

Back to Q 8 on page 228

9. The correct answer is **C** – No explanation is available for this answer.

Back to Q 9 on page 229

10. The correct answer is **B** – No explanation is available for this answer.

Back to Q 10 on page 229

11. The correct answer is **B** – No explanation is available for this answer.

Back to Q 11 on page 229

12. The correct answer is **D** – 90% of total saliva secretions are produced by the major salivary glands [10].

Back to Q 12 on page 229

13. The correct answer is **A** – No explanation is available for this answer [10].

Back to Q 13 on page 229

14. The correct answer is **B** – No explanation is available for this answer [10].

Back to Q 14 on page 230

15. The correct answer is **B** – Parotid glands are serous and produce water like secretions. Submandibular and sublingual glands are mixed. Source: [10]

Back to Q 15 on page 230

16. The correct answer is **C** – Minor salivary glands contribute significantly to the lubrication of the oral mucosa because of their high protein content. Source: [10].

Back to Q 16 on page 230

17. The correct answer is **C** – No explanation is available for this answer.

    Back to Q 17 on page 230

18. The correct answer is **A** – The normal daily production of saliva varies between 0.5 and 1.5 liters. Source: [10].

    Back to Q 18 on page 230

19. The correct answer is **B** – The whole unstimulated saliva flow rate is approximately 0.3–0.4 ml / min. This rate decreases to 0.1 ml / min during sleep and increases to about 4, 0–5, 0 ml / min during eating, chewing and other stimulating activities. Source: [10].

    Back to Q 19 on page 231

20. The correct answer is **A** – No explanation is available for this answer.

    Back to Q 20 on page 231

21. The correct answer is **C** – The whole unstimulated saliva flow rate is approximately 0.3–0.4 ml / min. This rate decreases to 0.1 ml / min during sleep and increases to about 4, 0–5, 0 ml / min during eating, chewing and other stimulating activities. Source: [10].

    Back to Q 21 on page 231

22. The correct answer is **D** – Saliva contains three buffer systems (bicarbonate, phosphate and protein) and helps in maintaining acceptable pH range of 6.0-7.5 within the mouth. Source: [10].

    Back to Q 22 on page 231

23. The correct answer is **A** – No explanation is available for this answer.

    Back to Q 23 on page 231

24. The correct answer is **E** – No explanation is available for this answer.

    Back to Q 24 on page 232

25. The correct answer is **B** – Mikulicz syndrome is the disease by which sarcoidosis, tuberculosis or lymphomas affects salivary glands. Sjögren syndrome is a condition by which the lacrimal and salivary glands are affected (primary) together with any other autoimmune disease e.g. lupus erythematosus or rheumatoid arthritis (secondary) [9].

    Back to Q 25 on page 232

26. The correct answer is **A** – No explanation is available for this answer.

    Back to Q 26 on page 232

27. The correct answer is **C** – No explanation is available for this answer.

    Back to Q 27 on page 232

28. The correct answer is **A** – No explanation is available for this answer.

    Back to Q 28 on page 232

29. The correct answer is **B** – No explanation is available for this answer.

Back to Q 29 on page 233

30. The correct answer is **A** – No explanation is available for this answer.

Back to Q 30 on page 233

31. The correct answer is **A** – No explanation is available for this answer.

Back to Q 31 on page 233

32. The correct answer is **E** – No explanation is available for this answer.

Back to Q 32 on page 233

33. The correct answer is **B** – No explanation is available for this answer.

Back to Q 33 on page 233

34. The correct answer is **A** – No explanation is available for this answer. Source: [10].

Back to Q 34 on page 234

35. The correct answer is **E** – No explanation is available for this answer. Source: [10]

Back to Q 35 on page 234

36. The correct answer is **B** – No explanation is available for this answer.

Back to Q 36 on page 234

37. The correct answer is **C** – Lymphoma. Patients with Sjögren syndrome have a lifetime risk for lymphoma of 5% to 15%, which is estimated to be about 20 times greater than the general population [9].

Back to Q 37 on page 234

38. The correct answer is **C** – No explanation is available for this answer.

Back to Q 38 on page 234

39. The correct answer is **A** – No explanation is available for this answer.

Back to Q 39 on page 235

40. The correct answer is **C** – No explanation is available for this answer.

Back to Q 40 on page 235

41. The correct answer is **A** – No explanation is available for this answer.

Back to Q 41 on page 235

42. The correct answer is **B** – No explanation is available for this answer.

Back to Q 42 on page 235

43. The correct answer is **C** – No explanation is available for this answer.

Back to Q 43 on page 235

44. The correct answer is **C** – No explanation is available for this answer.

Back to Q 44 on page 236

45. The correct answer is **B** – No explanation is available for this answer. Source: [11]

Back to Q 45 on page 236

46. The correct answer is **C** – No explanation is available for this answer.

Back to Q 46 on page 236

47. The correct answer is **C** – No explanation is available for this answer.

Back to Q 47 on page 236

48. The correct answer is **B** – No explanation is available for this answer.

Back to Q 48 on page 236

49. The correct answer is **B** – No explanation is available for this answer.

Back to Q 49 on page 237

50. The correct answer is **C** – No explanation is available for this answer.

Back to Q 50 on page 237

51. The correct answer is **B** – No explanation is available for this answer.

Back to Q 51 on page 237

52. The correct answer is **B** – No explanation is available for this answer.

Back to Q 52 on page 237

53. The correct answer is **B** – No explanation is available for this answer.

Back to Q 53 on page 237

54. The correct answer is **B** – No explanation is available for this answer.

Back to Q 54 on page 238

55. The correct answer is **C** – No explanation is available for this answer.

Back to Q 55 on page 238

56. The correct answer is **B** – No explanation is available for this answer.

Back to Q 56 on page 238

57. The correct answer is **C** – No explanation is available for this answer.

Back to Q 57 on page 238

58. The correct answer is **D** – No explanation is available for this answer.

Back to Q 58 on page 239

59. The correct answer is **A** – No explanation is available for this answer.

Back to Q 59 on page 239

60. The correct answer is **C** – No explanation is available for this answer.

Back to Q 60 on page 239

61. The correct answer is **B** – No explanation is available for this answer.

Back to Q 61 on page 239

62. The correct answer is **B** – No explanation is available for this answer.

    Back to Q 62 on page 239

63. The correct answer is **C** – No explanation is available for this answer.

    Back to Q 63 on page 240

64. The correct answer is **D** – No explanation is available for this answer.

    Back to Q 64 on page 240

65. The correct answer is **B** – No explanation is available for this answer.

    Back to Q 65 on page 240

66. The correct answer is **B** – No explanation is available for this answer.

    Back to Q 66 on page 240

67. The correct answer is **B** – No explanation is available for this answer.

    Back to Q 67 on page 240

68. The correct answer is **A** – No explanation is available for this answer.

    Back to Q 68 on page 241

69. The correct answer is **B** – No explanation is available for this answer.

    Back to Q 69 on page 241

70. The correct answer is **C** – No explanation is available for this answer.

    Back to Q 70 on page 241

71. The correct answer is **D** – No explanation is available for this answer.

    Back to Q 71 on page 241

72. The correct answer is **B** – No explanation is available for this answer.

    Back to Q 72 on page 241

73. The correct answer is **C** – No explanation is available for this answer.

    Back to Q 73 on page 242

74. The correct answer is **B** – No explanation is available for this answer.

    Back to Q 74 on page 242

75. The correct answer is **C** – No explanation is available for this answer.

    Back to Q 75 on page 242

Chapter 15
Bone Diseases

In this chapter, you will find some questions which are related to diseases of bone but not mentioned elsewhere in the chapters of infections and developmental diseases.

15.1 MCQs Questions

Choose **one or more** of the most appropriate answers. Some questions may have **more than one** correct answer. You have to choose all the correct answers as best as you can.

1. Which of the following bone disorders could present as either decreased or increased bone formation?
   (a) Osteogenesis imperfecta
   (b) Osteoporosis
   (c) Osteopetrosis
   (d) Osteitis deformans (Paget's disease)
   Answer for Q 1 on page 274
2. An otherwise healthy and normal appearing 1-year-old boy presents to your emergency room after a mild fall with a broken mandible and humerus. His parents say he just started taking his first steps a few days ago. They report a history of many broken bones in the family. What is the most likely fundamental problem in this family?
   (a) Defective type I collagen production
   (b) Defective type IV collagen production
   (c) Mutation in FGFR3
   (d) Vitamin D deficiency
   Answer for Q 2 on page 274

3. A cartilage tumor is more likely to be benign if:
   (a) It is large
   (b) It is peripheral
   (c) There are multiple masses
   (d) It is painful

   Answer for Q 3 on page 274

4. During healing of bone fractures or extraction sockets, the first laid down bone is:
   (a) Bundle bone
   (b) Compact bone
   (c) Cancellous bone
   (d) Woven bone

   Answer for Q 4 on page 274

5. Which of the following characteristically presents with nocturnal pain that is relieved by aspirin?
   (a) Acute osteomyelitis
   (b) Osteoblastoma
   (c) Osteosarcoma
   (d) Osteoid osteoma

   Answer for Q 5 on page 275

6. Widening of the fracture line in the first 3 weeks after bone fracture is due to:
   (a) Osteoblastic activity to lay down new osteoid tissue
   (b) Osteoclastic activity to remove bone debris and sharp edges
   (c) Migration of fibroblasts to the site of the fracture
   (d) Formation of new capillaries

   Answer for Q 6 on page 275

7. Replacement of blood clot into granulation tissue is termed:
   (a) Resorption
   (b) Organization
   (c) Involution
   (d) Osteoid formation

   Answer for Q 7 on page 275

8. Callus formation is:
   (a) Formation of the blood clot
   (b) Formation of granulation tissue at the site of fracture
   (c) Calcification of the osteoid tissue
   (d) Formation of lamellar bone

   Answer for Q 8 on page 275

9. Remodeling of the fracture site is:
   (a) Calcification of the osteoid tissue
   (b) Resorption of woven bone and replacement by lamellar bone
   (c) Formation of blood clot
   (d) Formation of woven bone

   Answer for Q 9 on page 275

10. Restoration of the epithelial continuity over the extraction socket occurs after:
    (a) 10–14 days after extraction
    (b) 1 –2 days after extraction
    (c) 4 –8 days after extraction
    (d) 3 –6 months after extraction

    Answer for Q 10 on page 275

11. Regarding the etiology of Facial fibrous dysplasia, the following cause is the most correct:
    (a) Hereditary and transmitted through a dominant gene
    (b) Environmental and results from hypoxia or drugs during pregnancy
    (c) Spontaneous gene mutation at the post zygotic stage of embryo formation
    (d) Trauma in the late stages of pregnancy

    Answer for Q 11 on page 275

12. *Café au lait* (coffee with milk) pigmentation of the skin is a characteristic feature of:
    (a) Cherubism
    (b) Marble bone disease
    (c) Maccune-Albright syndrome
    (d) Paget's disease of bone

    Answer for Q 12 on page 275

13. Sexual precocity (premature puberty) is a characteristic feature of:
    - (a) Cherubism
    - (b) Maccune-Albright syndrome
    - (c) Marble bone disease
    - (d) Paget's disease of bone

    Answer for Q 13 on page 275

14. The differential diagnosis of facial fibrous dysplasia is problematic with one of the following conditions:
    - (a) Osteogenic sarcoma
    - (b) Ossifying fibroma (calcifying fibroma
    - (c) Marble bone disease
    - (d) Paget's disease of bone

    Answer for Q 14 on page 275

15. Presence of multinucleated giant cells in great quantities is a hallmark (characteristic for:
    - (a) Ossifying fibroma
    - (b) Cherubism
    - (c) Facial fibrous dysplasia
    - (d) Paget's disease of bone

    Answer for Q 15 on page 275

16. The etiologic factor for cherubism is:
    - (a) Environmental
    - (b) Hereditary, autosomal recessive
    - (c) Hereditary, autosomal dominant
    - (d) X-linked mode of inheritance

    Answer for Q 16 on page 275

17. One of the following is **not** a feature of Marble bone disease:
    - (a) Osteopetrosis
    - (b) Delayed formation of sequestrum
    - (c) May be treated by bone marrow transplantation
    - (d) Osteoporosis

    Answer for Q 17 on page 276

18. One of the following lesions could be treated by intralesional injection of corticosteroids (triamcinolone acetonide) weekly for 6 weeks:
    (a) Central giant cell granuloma
    (b) Traumatic bone cyst
    (c) Brown nodes of hyperparathyroidism
    (d) Facial fibrous dysplasia

    Answer for Q 18 on page 276

19. One of the following conditions usually affects multiple bones
    (a) Facial fibrous dysplasia
    (b) Central giant cell granuloma
    (c) Brown nodes of hyperparathyroidism
    (d) Ossifying fibroma

    Answer for Q 19 on page 276

20. One of the following is a characteristic microscopic feature of the newly formed bone in both mono and polystotic fibrous dysplasia of bone:
    (a) Mosaic
    (b) Chinese-letter pattern
    (c) Liesegang rings
    (d) brushborder

    Answer for Q 20 on page 276

21. If the mutation in the GNAS1 gene occurs during embryonic life, the clinical result is:
    (a) Monostotic fibrous dysplasia
    (b) Maccune-Albright syndrome
    (c) Cherubism
    (d) A and B

    Answer for Q 21 on page 276

22. Which of the following microscopic features is valuable to differentiate fibrous dysplasia from ossifying fibroma?
    (a) Detection of peripheral osteoclasts
    (b) Detection of peripheral osteoblasts
    (c) Absence of peripheral osteoclasts
    (d) absence of peripheral osteoblasts

    Answer for Q 22 on page 276

23. Features of multiple bone radiolucencies, hypercalcemia and partial loss of lamina dura are indicative of:
    (a) Hyperparathyroidism
    (b) Polystotic fibrous dysplasia
    (c) Paget's disease of bone
    (d) Florid cementosseous dysplasia

    Answer for Q 23 on page 276

24. The bilateral presentation of a multilocular mandibular giant cell lesion in a 5 years old child is indicative of:
    (a) Ossifying fibroma
    (b) Central giant cell granuloma
    (c) Cherubism
    (d) Florid cement-osseous dysplasia

    Answer for Q 24 on page 276

25. Dry socket is a form of:
    (a) Osteomyelitis
    (b) Osteitis
    (c) Osteoma
    (d) Periostitis
    (e) Granuloma

    Answer for Q 25 on page 276

26. The most likely diagnosis in a 23-year-old, mentally alert, male dwarf with disproportionate arm and leg to body growth, prominent forehead, and retruded maxilla is:
    (a) Cretinism
    (b) Pituitary dwarfism
    (c) Acromegaly
    (d) Achondroplasia
    (e) Eagle's syndrome

    Answer for Q 26 on page 276

27. Osteosarcoma characteristically may develop in cases of:
    (a) Osteopetrosis
    (b) Osteogenesis imperfecta
    (c) Acromegaly
    (d) Osteitis deformans
    (e) All of above

    Answer for Q 27 on page 276

28. Histiocystosis X (Tumors of Langerhans Cell Histiocytes), sometimes referred to as non-lipid reticuloendotheliosis, includes:
    (a) Letterer–Swie's disease
    (b) Hand–Schüller–Christian disease
    (c) Eosinophilic Granuloma
    (d) Histiocytoma
    (e) All of above

    Answer for Q 28 on page 276

29. A 12-year-old boy came to your clinic because of increasing pain and swelling in the anterior area of the maxilla that was first experienced a month ago. He had no history of previous trauma to the area of concern. Physical examination revealed mild swelling with tenderness in the area above the upper left canine. A dental examination of the teeth was apparently normal, with no caries or periodontal disease. Radiographs showed a radiolucent zone and a surrounding sclerotic zone. Computed tomography (CT) revealed a 10 mm circumscribed osteolytic area in the cortex of the maxilla with surrounding sclerosis. Histopathological examination of the biopsy excluded malignancy. The most probable diagnosis is:
    (a) Chondrosarcoma
    (b) Osteoid osteoma
    (c) Osteosarcoma
    (d) Osteoma

    Answer for Q 29 on page 276

30. The classic triad of Hand–Schüller–Christian disease includes lesions of bone, exopthalmos and:
    (a) Diabetes insipidus
    (b) Hepatosplenomegaly
    (c) Diabetes mellitus
    (d) Albuminuria
    (e) Hypothyroidism

Answer for Q 30 on page 276

31. Best timing for the cosmetic treatment of fibrous dysplasia is:
    (a) Immediately
    (b) At puberty
    (c) After cessation of skeletal growth unless the lesion is interfering with normal functions.
    (d) After the age of 40 unless the lesion is interfering with normal functions.

Answer for Q 31 on page 276

32. Treatment of fibrous dysplasia is:
    (a) Radical resection of the lesion
    (b) Radiation therapy
    (c) If the lesion is small, dissection is done. If the lesion is large, cosmetic surgery has to be carried out.
    (d) Cryosurgery

Answer for Q 32 on page 276

33. Enucleation of palatal tumor can result in:
    (a) Excessive bleeding from nasopalatine vessels
    (b) Tearing of nasal mucosa
    (c) Damage to nasopalatine nerve
    (d) Alteration of speech

Answer for Q 33 on page 277

34. Treatment of solitary Langerhans histiocytoma of the mandible is by:
    (a) Curettage
    (b) Radiotherapy
    (c) No treatment is required
    (d) Chemotherapy

Answer for Q 34 on page 277

35. Treatment of fibrous dysplasia in a young 25 years old patient involving maxilla is best treated by:
    (a) Enbloc resection
    (b) Cosmetic contouring
    (c) Maxillary resection
    (d) Radiation therapy

Answer for Q 35 on page 277

36. Enbloc resection of the segment of the bone:
    (a) Complete resection of the jaw bone
    (b) Resection of half of the affected jaw
    (c) Resection of the tumor only
    (d) The entire tumor removed intact with a rim of uninvolved bone while

    Answer for Q 36 on page 277

37. Garre's osteomyelitis is:
    (a) Chronic focal sclerosis and non-suppurative osteomyelitis
    (b) Chronic focal sclerosis and suppurative osteomyelitis
    (c) Characterized by suppuration and acute pain
    (d) Chronic diffuse sclerosing osteomyelitis

    Answer for Q 37 on page 277

38. Osteoradionecrosis is due to:
    (a) Infection
    (b) Endarteritis of blood vessels
    (c) Sepsis
    (d) None of the above

    Answer for Q 38 on page 277

39. Treatment of Garre's osteomyelitis is:
    (a) Incision and drainage
    (b) Sequestrectomy
    (c) Saucerization
    (d) Surgical recontouring

    Answer for Q 39 on page 277

40. Involucrum is:
    (a) Dead bone
    (b) New live bone surrounding dead bone or in the opposite site of infected bone
    (c) Previous live bone
    (d) Sclerotic bone

    Answer for Q 40 on page 277

41. Osteomyelitis:
    (a) Never occurs in infants
    (b) In acute cases fracture of the mandible is very common
    (c) Of mandible can show symptoms of lip paresthesia
    (d) Produces no lymphadenopathy

    Answer for Q 41 on page ??

42. Dead bone is seen on the radiograph as:
    (a) More radiolucent
    (b) More radiopaque
    (c) With osteophytes growing out
    (d) Soap bubble appearance

    Answer for Q 42 on page ??

43. Hyperbaric oxygen is indicated for:
    (a) Obstructive lung disease
    (b) Osteoradionecrosis
    (c) Cardiac failure
    (d) Renal disease

    Answer for Q 43 on page ??

44. Osteomyelitis of the jaw can be cured by:
    (a) Resection
    (b) Physiotherapy
    (c) Sequestrectomy with antibiotic treatment
    (d) Drainage

    Answer for Q 44 on page ??

45. After incision and drainage of an abscess, the infectious process has failed to regress in spite of the patient being on high doses of an antibiotic. It would be wise to:
    (a) Insert a large drain
    (b) Repeat culture and sensitivity tests
    (c) Debride and irrigate the area with a fibrinolytic agent
    (d) Begin the parenteral administration of proteolytic enzymes to augment the antibiotics

    Answer for Q 45 on page ??

46. Which of the following features is **not** associated with acute osteomyelitis of mandible?
    - (a) Severe pain
    - (b) Purulent exudate
    - (c) Paresthesia of lower lip
    - (d) Radiographic evidence of bone destruction

    Answer for Q 46 on page ??

47. Sequestrum means:
    - (a) Necrosed bone, separated from its surrounding by granulation tissue
    - (b) A broken tooth pieces
    - (c) Is new bone formed in osteomyelitis
    - (d) Is necrosed tooth

    Answer for Q 47 on page ??

48. Which of the following infection is the cause for multiple sites of osteomyelitis of the jaw:
    - (a) Peritonsillar abscess
    - (b) Local Trauma
    - (c) Hematogenous infection
    - (d) Buccal space infection

    Answer for Q 48 on page ??

49. In osteomyelitis, the necrotic bone is termed:
    - (a) Cloacae
    - (b) Involucrum
    - (c) Sequestrum
    - (d) Diverticulum

    Answer for Q 49 on page ??

50. Focal sclerosing osteomyelitis could be misdiagnosed as:
    - (a) Cementomas
    - (b) Periapical granuloma
    - (c) Denticles
    - (d) Periodontal cyst

    Answer for Q 50 on page 278

51. Numbness of the lower lip is an early feature of:
    (a) Chronic periapical abscess
    (b) Periapical granuloma
    (c) Osteomyelitis
    (d) Acute periapical abscess

    Answer for Q 51 on page 278

52. In acute osteomyelitis, the radiographic change in the first two weeks is:
    (a) Moth eaten appearance
    (b) Nothing could be detected radiographically
    (c) Radiolucency intermingled with radiopacities
    (d) A large radiopaque mass representing the sequestrum

    Answer for Q 52 on page 278

53. Garre's osteomyelitis is frequently termed:
    (a) Focal sclerosing osteomyelitis
    (b) Chronic osteomyelitis with proliferative periostitis
    (c) Diffuse sclerosing osteomyelitis
    (d) Chemical osteomyelitis

    Answer for Q 53 on page 278

54. In Garre's osteomyelitis, the newly formed sclerotic bone is formed in the following location:
    (a) Diffuse inside the involved bone
    (b) Under the apex of the involved tooth
    (c) Subperiosteal
    (d) Supraperiosteal

    Answer for Q 54 on page 278

55. Diffuse Sclerosing Osteomyelitis is common in:
    (a) Old age
    (b) Young age
    (c) No specific age groups
    (d) None of the above

    Answer for Q 55 on page 278

56. Cotton wool appearance is a characteristic feature of:
    (a) Periapical granuloma
    (b) Garre's osteomyelitis
    (c) Diffuse sclerosing osteomyelitis
    (d) Focal sclerosing osteomyelitis

    Answer for Q 56 on page 278

57. Pyogenic Osteomyelitis of the jaw is more common in:
    (a) No specific site predilection
    (b) Both mandible and maxilla
    (c) Maxilla
    (d) Mandible

    Answer for Q 57 on page 278

58. Sequestrum is:
    (a) Old bone formed under the endosteum
    (b) Necrotic bone not surrounded by granulation tissue
    (c) Necrotic bone surrounded by granulation tissue
    (d) New bone formed under the periosteum

    Answer for Q 58 on page 278

59. In which of the following conditions serum acid phosphatase levels are increased?
    (a) Prostate gland carcinoma
    (b) Oat cell carcinoma
    (c) Squamous cell carcinoma of oral cavity
    (d) All of the above

    Answer for Q 59 on page 278

60. Onion skin appearance is seen in:
    (a) Ewing's sarcoma
    (b) Osteosarcoma
    (c) Osteoma
    (d) Fibrosarcoma

    Answer for Q 60 on page 278

61. Sequestrum is a term reserved for:
    (a) Newly formed bone
    (b) Necrotic bone
    (c) Vital bone
    (d) Granulation tissue

    Answer for Q 61 on page 278

62. Garre's osteomyelitis, pulp polyp, and focal sclerosing osteomyelitis have one factor in common:
    (a) Old age
    (b) Young age
    (c) Immunocompromised condition
    (d) Hereditary pattern

    Answer for Q 62 on page 278

63. The mode of inheritance of the three major forms of osteopetrosis are:
    (a) Autosomal dominant
    (b) Autosomal recessive
    (c) X-linked recessive
    (d) A & B
    (e) None of the above

    Answer for Q 63 on page 278

64. Small round cell tumor of bone is:
    (a) African jaw lymphoma
    (b) Multiple myeloma
    (c) Ewing's sarcoma
    (d) Osteogenic Sarcoma

    Answer for Q 64 on page 278

65. Sunburst appearance and Codman's triangle are seen in:
    (a) Osteosarcoma
    (b) Fibrosarcoma
    (c) Chondrosarcoma
    (d) None of the above

    Answer for Q 65 on page 278

66. The most common non-primary malignant lesion of bone is:
    (a) Osteosarcoma
    (b) Osteochondroma
    (c) Ewing's sarcoma
    (d) Metastatic carcinoma

    Answer for Q 66 on page 279

67. Usually metastatic lesions are osteolytic, but osteoblastic secondaries occur in cancer of:
    (a) Thyroid
    (b) Prostate
    (c) Kidney
    (d) Uterus

    Answer for Q 67 on page 279

68. The lesion of bone which is expansile and eccentrically ballooned out is:
    (a) Ossifying fibroma
    (b) Aneurysmal bone cyst
    (c) Fibrous dysplasia
    (d) None of the above

    Answer for Q 68 on page 279

69. Cotton Wool appearance on a radiograph may be indicative of:
    (a) Acute suppurative osteomyelitis
    (b) Chronic suppurative osteomyelitis
    (c) Diffuse sclerosing osteomyelitis
    (d) Proliferative periostitis

    Answer for Q 69 on page 279

70. One of the following modalities is used for the treatment of osteopetrosis:
    (a) Non-steroidal anti inflammatory drugs (NSAIDs)
    (b) Antibiotics
    (c) Antibiotics combined with antifungal drugs
    (d) Bone marrow transplantation

    Answer for Q 70 on page 279

71. One of the following is **not** a feature of cleidocranial dysplasia:
    (a) Caused by mutations in the RUNX2 (or CBFA1) gene
    (b) Caused by Tabby gene
    (c) Affects odontogenesis
    (d) Affects bones developed in membranes and to a lesser extent bones developed in cartilage
    (e) 40% of cases may be caused by spontaneous mutations.

    Answer for Q 71 on page 279

72. The causes of delayed or failure of eruption of permanent teeth in cleidocranial dysplasia are:
    (a) Crowding of permanent and supernumerary teeth where the number of supernumerary teeth can be impressive, with some patients demonstrating more than 60 such teeth
    (b) Lack of secondary cementum in unerupted teeth
    (c) insufficient alveolar bone resorption, possibly resulting from altered periodontal ligament cells with reduced capacity to induce osteoclastogenesis.
    (d) All of the above

    Answer for Q 72 on page 279

73. What is correct about focal osteoporotic marrow defect:
    (a) No sex predilection
    (b) Approximately 75% of cases occur in adult males
    (c) Approximately 75% of cases occur in adult females
    (d) More common in the anterior area of the mandible

    Answer for Q 73 on page 279

74. The histological feature of focal osteoporotic marrow defect is:
    (a) Empty cavity with little straw-colored fluid
    (b) Cellular hematopoietic, fatty marrow and little normal bone trabeculae
    (c) Multinucleated giant cells within a fibrovascular stroma
    (d) Normal salivary tissue entrapped in the jaw bones

    Answer for Q 74 on page 279

75. Focal osteoporotic marrow defect is:
    (a) Tender
    (b) Painless
    (c) Painful
    (d) Can cause massive bony expansion

    Answer for Q 75 on page 279

76. The most common site for focal osteoporotic marrow defect is:
   (a) Incisor area of the mandible
   (b) Molar area of the maxilla
   (c) Molar area of the mandible
   (d) Incisor area of the maxilla

   Answer for Q 76 on page 279

77. The etiology of focal osteoporotic marrow defect is:
   (a) Hereditary, autosomal dominant pattern
   (b) Of unknown etiology with many speculations
   (c) Developmental and congenital
   (d) Infectious process

   Answer for Q 77 on page 279

78. The proposed treatment of focal osteoporotic marrow defect is:
   (a) Irradiation
   (b) No treatment is required
   (c) Chemotherapy
   (d) Massive doses of antibiotics for a protracted time

   Answer for Q 78 on page 279

79. Idiopathic osteosclerosis represents focally increased bone density which is due to:
   (a) Localized infection of the jaw
   (b) Unknown cause
   (c) As a consequence of hyperparathyroidism
   (d) Neoplastic disorder
   (e) Systemic disorder

   Answer for Q 79 on page 279

80. Idiopathic osteosclerosis vs focal chronic sclerosing osteomyelitis (condensing osteitis):
   (a) Both conditions are of unknown etiology
   (b) The former is of unknown etiology, while the later is inflammatory
   (c) Both are benign neoplasms of bone
   (d) Both conditions are painful

   Answer for Q 80 on page 280

81. The differential diagnosis of idiopathic osteosclerosis from focal sclerosing osteomyelitis depends on:

    (a) Absence of cortical expansion

    (b) Biopsy in which the idiopathic osteosclerosis shows massive inflammatory cell infiltration

    (c) Absence of pain

    (d) Tooth vitality and the absence of a deep restoration or caries in cases of idiopathic osteosclerosis

    Answer for Q 81 on page 280

82. Medication-related osteonecrosis is more common in:

    (a) Mandible more than maxilla

    (b) Maxilla more than mandible

    (c) Equally distributed between mandible and maxilla

    (d) Never occurs in the mandible and maxilla because of their high vascularity

    Answer for Q 82 on page 280

83. The treatment of choice for idiopathic osteosclerosis is:

    (a) No treatment is required except for periodic examination

    (b) Surgical curettage

    (c) Irradiation followed by chemotherapy

    (d) Resection of the affected area

    Answer for Q 83 on page 280

84. An 84-year-old woman referred to your clinic for routine checkup. Intraoral examination revealed healthy mucosa no sign of infection. Her past medical history was unremarkable. The radiography of the molar region showed an ill-defined radiolucent area with irregular borders. The condition was asymptomatic with no bony expansion. The histopathological examination revealed normal hematopoietic bone marrow characterized by erythroid, granulocytic, monocytic, and lymphocytic series. In addition, megakaryocytes, fat cells, and bone trabeculae were also observed. The most probable diagnosis is:

    (a) Idiopathic osteosclerosis

    (b) Osteoid osteoma

    (c) focal osteoporotic marrow defect

    (d) Traumatic bone cyst (simple bone cyst)

Answer for Q 84 on page 280

85. One of the following is **not** a feature of massive osteolysis:
   (a) Progressive destruction of one or more bones
   (b) Occurs exclusively in jaw bones
   (c) The destroyed bone is replaced by a vascular proliferation and, ultimately, dense fibrous tissue without bone regeneration
   (d) About 50% of patients recall prior trauma

   Answer for Q 85 on page 280

86. Increased recurrence potential of simple bone cyst (traumatic bone cyst) affecting the jaw bones is more probable if:
   (a) The cyst exhibit scalloped margins
   (b) The cyst shows resorption of the lamina dura
   (c) The cyst exhibit nodular bone expansion
   (d) The cyst consists of multiple cavities.
   (e) All of the above

   Answer for Q 86 on page 280

87. One or more of the following modalities are used for the treatment of simple bone cyst (traumatic bone cyst) affecting the jaw bones:
   (a) Surgical exploration without curettage
   (b) Surgical exploration with curettage
   (c) Bone marrow injection
   (d) A & B

   Answer for Q 87 on page 280

88. The "blood-soaked sponge" appearance during surgery is a typical feature of:
   (a) Aneurysmal bone cyst
   (b) Simple bone cyst
   (c) Benign cystic lymph node
   (d) Latent bone cyst

   Answer for Q 88 on page 280

89. One of the following is a member of the family of polystotic fibrous dysplasia:
   (a) Multiple neurofibromatosis
   (b) Cemento-ossifying fibroma
   (c) Mazabraud syndrome
   (d) Cherubism

Answer for Q 89 on page 280

90. Osteomyelitis most commonly occurs in:
    (a) Mandible
    (b) Maxilla
    (c) Maxilla and mandible are equally affected
    (d) Sella turcica

Answer for Q 90 on page 280

91. About cherubism, one of the following statements is correct:
    (a) It is considered as a sub type of fibrous dysplasia
    (b) It is presented clinically as a firm unilateral swelling of the jaw
    (c) It might cause failure of eruption of teeth
    (d) It is a hereditary autosomal recessive disorder

Answer for Q 91 on page 280

92. Which of the following lesions is characterized histologically by presence of multinucleated giant cells:
    (a) Simple bone cyst
    (b) Familial fibrous dysplasia (cherubism)
    (c) Facial fibrous dysplasia
    (d) Osteoporosis

Answer for Q 92 on page 280

93. Proptosis of the eye is a common clinical feature of:
    (a) Cherubism
    (b) Facial fibrous dysplasia
    (c) Globulomaxillary cyst
    (d) Adenomatoid odontogenic tumor

Answer for Q 93 on page 280

94. Central giant cell granuloma is a true neoplasm. It is presented clinically as firm sessile lesion on the gingiva:
    (a) The two statements are correct
    (b) The first statement is incorrect while the second statement is correct
    (c) The first statement is correct while the second statement is incorrect
    (d) The two statements are incorrect

Answer for Q 94 on page 280

95. Which of the following conditions is commonly associated with dry socket after extraction?
    (a) Facial fibrous dysplasia
    (b) Familial fibrous dysplasia
    (c) Osteoradionecrosis
    (d) Central giant cell granuloma

    Answer for Q 95 on page 280

96. Delayed formation of sequestra is a feature of:
    (a) Osteoporosis
    (b) Cherubism
    (c) Osteopetrosis
    (d) Cleidocranial dysplasia

    Answer for Q 96 on page 281

97. A young girl presents with and expansile mass in the left maxillary region which was seen as a poorly demarcated, finely trabeculated mass on radiographic examination. Histopathologic examination revealed randomly distributed spicules of woven bone scattered through a fibrous connective tissue. Most suggestive diagnosis of the lesion is:
    (a) Fibrous dysplasia
    (b) Osteoma
    (c) Osteogenic sarcoma
    (d) Osteopetrosis

    Answer for Q 97 on page 281

98. Café au lait pigmentation of skin is a feature of:
    (a) Neurolemmoma
    (b) Fibrous dysplasia
    (c) Granular cell myoblastoma
    (d) Congenital epulis of newborn

    Answer for Q 98 on page 281

99. A 3-year-old boy shows only bilateral symmetric enlargement of the posterior mandibular areas. The most probable diagnosis is:
    (a) Osteitis deformans
    (b) Allbright syndrome
    (c) Cherubism
    (d) Facial fibrous dysplasia

Answer for Q 99 on page 281

100. The juvenile ossifying fibroma is a controversial lesion that has been distinguished from conventional ossifying fibroma on the basis of:

(a) Age

(b) Clinical behavior

(c) Site predilection

(d) failure to detect GNAS or HRPT2 mutations in juvenile ossifying fibromas suggesting that these lesions are distinct from fibrous dysplasia and conventional ossifying fibromas

(e) All of the above

Answer for Q 100 on page 281

101. One of the following is **not** a sub-type of juvenile ossifying fibroma:

(a) Trabecular

(b) Psammomatoid

(c) Trabecular and psammomatoid

(d) Hemorrhagic

Answer for Q 101 on page 281

102. Mosaic pattern of bone is a characteristic histologic feature of:

(a) cherubism

(b) fibrous dysplasia of bone

(c) hyperparathyroidism

(d) Paget's disease of bone

Answer for Q 102 on page 281

103. A child with bowing long bones, loss of hearing, history of multiple bone fracture and brown opalescent dentin could be diagnosed as:

(a) Cherubism

(b) Osteogenesis imperfect

(c) Hyperparathyroidism

(d) Allbright syndrome

Answer for Q 103 on page 281

104. The condition of polyostotic fibrous dysplasia presenting with multiple bone lesions in conjunction with cutaneous and endocrinal abnormalities is diagnosed as:
   (a) Allbright syndrome
   (b) Jaffe's syndrome
   (c) Gorlin syndrome
   (d) Craniofacial dysplasia

   Answer for Q 104 on page 281

105. Osteoma cutis is the term used to describe:
   (a) Endosteal or central osteomas
   (b) Periosteal osteoma
   (c) Extraskeletal osteomas located within muscle or the dermis of the skin
   (d) All of the above

   Answer for Q 105 on page 281

106. For the differential diagnosis of osteoblastoma from osteoid osteoma:
   (a) Osteoblastoma is painful while osteoid osteoma is painless
   (b) Osteoblastoma is painless while osteoid osteoma is painful
   (c) Both lesions are painful but the pain induced by osteoid osteoma is relieved by NSAIDs like aspirin
   (d) Both lesions are painful but the pain induced by osteoblastoma is relieved by NSAIDs like aspirin

   Answer for Q 106 on page 281

107. One of the following features is useful for the differential diagnosis of osteoblastoma from osteoid osteoma:
   (a) Osteoblastoma can reach a larger size, while osteoid osteoma cannot
   (b) Both lesions can attain the same size if left untreated
   (c) Osteoid osteoma can reach a larger size, while osteoblastoma cannot
   (d) Size is not a feature for the differential diagnosis

   Answer for Q 107 on page 281

108. Markedly raised serum alkaline phosphatase level is seen with:
   (a) Paget's disease
   (b) Hyperparathyroidism
   (c) Cherubism
   (d) central giant cell granuloma

   Answer for Q 108 on page 281

109. The diagnosis of periapical cement-osseous dysplasia is confirmed by:
   (a) the vitality of the involved teeth
   (b) the associating bone expansion
   (c) the florid distribution affecting more than one quarter of the jaws.
   (d) the posterior location of the involved tooth.

   Answer for Q 109 on page 281

110. The dental anomaly that usually accompanies osteogenesis imperfecta is termed:
   (a) Dentinogenesis imperfecta
   (b) Brown opalescent dentin
   (c) Dilaceration
   (d) Gemination

   Answer for Q 110 on page 281

111. One of the following features characterizes fibrous dysplasia and helps to differentiate it from ossifying fibroma.
   (a) Scattered radiopacities
   (b) Expansion of bone
   (c) Fibrous tissue component
   (d) Radiographically ill-defined border

   Answer for Q 111 on page 282

112. Which of the following best matches with the term dry socket?
   (a) A type of osteitis resulting from early loss of blood clot following tooth extraction
   (b) A lesion of an asymptomatic focal sclerosing osteomyelitis
   (c) A sequel of a pulpitis
   (d) A type of drug induced osteomyelitis

   Answer for Q 112 on page 282

113. Medication-related osteonecrosis of the jaw includes:
   (a) Bisphosphonates medication
   (b) Antiangiogenic therapy
   (c) Monoclonal antibody designed to prevent osteoclastic maturation
   (d) All of the above

   Answer for Q 113 on page 282

114. One or more of the following features are useful for the differential diagnosis of aggressive osteoblastoma from low-grade osteosarcoma:
   (a) Infiltrative growth of low-grade osteosarcoma
   (b) Marked cytologic atypia of low-grade osteosarcoma
   (c) Atypical mitotic figures are more prominent in low-grade osteosarcoma.
   (d) All of the above

   Answer for Q 114 on page 282

115. The diagnosis of chondroma in the craniofacial bones should be viewed with great skepticism because:
   (a) Many cases of craniofacial chondromas show a high recurrence rate with the tendency of the recurring tumors to turn into malignancy
   (b) Many cases of chondrosarcomas were misdiagnosed as chondromas
   (c) The differential diagnosis of chondromas from chondrosarcomas is difficult and problematic
   (d) All of the above

   Answer for Q 115 on page 282

116. Chondromyxoid fibroma appears histologically as:
   (a) A well-circumscribed, lobular mass of mature hyaline cartilage, which consists of well-formed lacunae containing small chondrocytes with pale cytoplasm and small, round nuclei
   (b) Lobules of spindle-shaped or stellate cells with abundant myxoid or chondroid inter-cellular substance and scattered multinucleated giant cells
   (c) Hyaline cartilage lobules admixed with bone trabeculae
   (d) Osteoid tissue intermingled with hyaline lobules of cartilage

   Answer for Q 116 on page 282

117. Synovial chondromatosis (chondrometaplasia) is:
   (a) Painless and asymptomatic
   (b) Painful with crepitus, periarticular swelling and limitation of joint motion
   (c) Never occurs in the TMJ but may occurs in other large joints
   (d) Occurs usually bilaterally if it will affects the TMJ

   Answer for Q 117 on page 282

118. Fibrous dysplasia is:
   (a) A hereditary disease
   (b) Not hereditary but results from gene mutation
   (c) Environmental disease
   (d) A Neoplastic disorder

Answer for Q 118 on page 282

119. The cause of café au lait pigmentation in fibrous dysplasia might be due to:
    (a) Excessive exposure to sun ray
    (b) Mutation in the GNAS gene at an early stage of development results in alteration of endocrine cells
    (c) Mutation in the GNAS gene at an early stage of development results in alteration of melanocytes functions
    (d) Unknown

    Answer for Q 119 on page 282

120. Mutations in the GNAS gene, which encodes the alpha subunit of a stimulatory G protein is detected in:
    (a) Ossifying fibroma
    (b) Cemento-osseous dysplasia
    (c) Osteoid osteoma and osteoblastoma
    (d) Fibrous dysplasia of bone

    Answer for Q 120 on page 282

15.2 Answers with Comments:

1. The correct answer is **D** – Paget's disease has an early phase of bone resorption and a late phase of bone formation. The end result is that there is a large amount of weak bone produced. Paget's may be triggered by a viral infection. Osteogenesis imperfecta is caused by defective type I collagen (decreased bone). Osteopetrosis is the result of decreased bone resorption by osteoclasts (increased bone).

   Back to Q 1 on page 249

2. The correct answer is **A** – Osteogenesis imperfecta is the result of deficient type I collagen production. There are many variants of the disease. Another reasonable answer is vitamin D deficiency. However, rickets does not generally present with broken bones upon minor trauma. It is much more likely to believe a genetic inheritance pattern as there are many affected individuals in the same family. Moreover, vitamin D supplementation in milk and cereal largely avoids this condition.

   Back to Q 2 on page 249

3. The correct answer is **B** – Benign cartilage tumors tend to be small, peripheral, solitary, and painless.

   Back to Q 3 on page 250

4. The correct answer is **D** – During the healing of bones, the first bone to be formed is the woven bone, which is termed callus. Later on, during the process of healing, this woven bone is resorbed and replaced by the lamellar type of bone.

   Back to Q 4 on page 250

5. The correct answer is **D** – Osteoid osteoma is generally painful and its pain can be relieved by aspirin. Other NSAIDs such as ibuprofen can be used. Pain caused by osteoid osteomas can be relieved with aspirin and NSAIDS, which inhibit the prostaglandins released by the tumor cells. Prostaglandins cause changes in vascular pressure, which stimulates sensory nerve endings locally, causing pain. Inhibition of these prostaglandins relieves pain. Few studies have shown lasting affects of symptom relief after long term use of NSAIDS, some studies have shown without surgical management there is a probability of evolution into a osteoblastoma.

   Back to Q 5 on page 250

6. The correct answer is **B** – No explanation is available for this answer.

   Back to Q 6 on page 250

7. The correct answer is **B** – Organization is the process in which granulation tissue invades the blood clot and replace it during the healing process.

   Back to Q 7 on page 250

8. The correct answer is **C** – No explanation is available for this answer.

   Back to Q 8 on page 251

9. The correct answer is **B** – No explanation is available for this answer.

   Back to Q 9 on page 251

10. The correct answer is **A** – No explanation is available for this answer.

    Back to Q 10 on page 251

11. The correct answer is **C** – No explanation is available for this answer.

    Back to Q 11 on page 251

12. The correct answer is **C** – No explanation is available for this answer.

    Back to Q 12 on page 251

13. The correct answer is **B** – No explanation is available for this answer.

    Back to Q 13 on page 252

14. The correct answer is **B** – No explanation is available for this answer.

    Back to Q 14 on page 252

15. The correct answer is **B** – No explanation is available for this answer.

    Back to Q 15 on page 252

16. The correct answer is **C** – No explanation is available for this answer.

Back to Q 16 on page 252

17. The correct answer is **D** – No explanation is available for this answer.

Back to Q 17 on page 252

18. The correct answer is **A** – No explanation is available for this answer.

Back to Q 18 on page 253

19. The correct answer is **C** – No explanation is available for this answer.

Back to Q 19 on page 253

20. The correct answer is **B** – No explanation is available for this answer.

Back to Q 20 on page 253

21. The correct answer is **D** – No explanation is available for this answer.

Back to Q 21 on page 253

22. The correct answer is **D** – No explanation is available for this answer.

Back to Q 22 on page 253

23. The correct answer is **A** – No explanation is available for this answer.

Back to Q 23 on page 254

24. The correct answer is **C** – No explanation is available for this answer.

Back to Q 24 on page 254

25. The correct answer is **B** – No explanation is available for this answer.

Back to Q 25 on page 254

26. The correct answer is **D** – No explanation is available for this answer.

Back to Q 26 on page 254

27. The correct answer is **E** – No explanation is available for this answer.

Back to Q 27 on page 255

28. The correct answer is **E** – No explanation is available for this answer.

Back to Q 28 on page 255

29. The correct answer is **B** – No explanation is available for this answer.

Back to Q 29 on page 255

30. The correct answer is **A** – No explanation is available for this answer.

Back to Q 30 on page 255

31. The correct answer is **C** – No explanation is available for this answer.

Back to Q 31 on page 256

32. The correct answer is **C** – No explanation is available for this answer.

Back to Q 32 on page 256

33. The correct answer is **B** – No explanation is available for this answer.

Back to Q 33 on page 256

34. The correct answer is **A** – No explanation is available for this answer.

Back to Q 34 on page 256

35. The correct answer is **B** – No explanation is available for this answer.

Back to Q 35 on page 256

36. The correct answer is **D** – No explanation is available for this answer.

Back to Q 36 on page 257

37. The correct answer is **A** – No explanation is available for this answer.

Back to Q 37 on page 257

38. The correct answer is **B** – No explanation is available for this answer.

Back to Q 38 on page 257

39. The correct answer is **D** – No explanation is available for this answer.

Back to Q 39 on page 257

40. The correct answer is **B** – No explanation is available for this answer.

Back to Q 40 on page 257

41. The correct answer is **C** – No explanation is available for this answer.

Back to Q 41 on page 258

42. The correct answer is **B** – Due to dystrophic calcification of the sequestrum.

Back to Q 42 on page 258

43. The correct answer is **B** – No explanation is available for this answer.

Back to Q 43 on page 258

44. The correct answer is **C** – No explanation is available for this answer.

Back to Q 44 on page 258

45. The correct answer is **B** – No explanation is available for this answer.

Back to Q 45 on page 258

46. The correct answer is **D** – No explanation is available for this answer.

Back to Q 46 on page 259

47. The correct answer is **A** – No explanation is available for this answer.

Back to Q 47 on page 259

48. The correct answer is **C** – No explanation is available for this answer.

Back to Q 48 on page 259

49. The correct answer is **C** – No explanation is available for this answer.

Back to Q 49 on page 259

50. The correct answer is **A** – No explanation is available for this answer.

Back to Q 50 on page 259

51. The correct answer is **C** – No explanation is available for this answer.

Back to Q 51 on page 260

52. The correct answer is **D** – No explanation is available for this answer.

Back to Q 52 on page 260

53. The correct answer is **B** – No explanation is available for this answer.

Back to Q 53 on page 260

54. The correct answer is **C** – No explanation is available for this answer.

Back to Q 54 on page 260

55. The correct answer is **B** – No explanation is available for this answer.

Back to Q 55 on page 260

56. The correct answer is **C** – No explanation is available for this answer.

Back to Q 56 on page 261

57. The correct answer is **D** – No explanation is available for this answer.

Back to Q 57 on page 261

58. The correct answer is **C** – No explanation is available for this answer.

Back to Q 58 on page 261

59. The correct answer is **A** – No explanation is available for this answer.

Back to Q 59 on page 261

60. The correct answer is **A** – No explanation is available for this answer.

Back to Q 60 on page 261

61. The correct answer is **B** – No explanation is available for this answer.

Back to Q 61 on page 262

62. The correct answer is **B** – No explanation is available for this answer.

Back to Q 62 on page 262

63. The correct answer is **D** – No explanation is available for this answer.

Back to Q 63 on page 262

64. The correct answer is **C** – No explanation is available for this answer.

Back to Q 64 on page 262

65. The correct answer is **A** – No explanation is available for this answer.

Back to Q 65 on page 262

66. The correct answer is **D** – No explanation is available for this answer.

Back to Q 66 on page 263

67. The correct answer is **B** – No explanation is available for this answer.

Back to Q 67 on page 263

68. The correct answer is **B** – No explanation is available for this answer.

Back to Q 68 on page 263

69. The correct answer is **C** – No explanation is available for this answer.

Back to Q 69 on page 263

70. The correct answer is **D** – Bone marrow transplantation potentially may cure bone marrow failure and may improve the phenotype. The rationale for this procedure is based on the hematopoietic origin of osteoclasts [9].

Back to Q 70 on page 263

71. The correct answer is **B** – Studies suggest that RUNX2 additionally plays an important role in odontogenesis via participation in odontoblast differentiation, enamel organ formation, and dental lamina proliferation. Disruption of these functions might explain the distinct dental anomalies associated with this disorder [9].

Back to Q 71 on page 264

72. The correct answer is **D** – No explanation is available for this answer [9].

Back to Q 72 on page 264

73. The correct answer is **C** – No explanation is available for this answer.

Back to Q 73 on page 264

74. The correct answer is **B** – No explanation is available for this answer.

Back to Q 74 on page 264

75. The correct answer is **C** – No explanation is available for this answer.

Back to Q 75 on page 264

76. The correct answer is **C** – No explanation is available for this answer.

Back to Q 76 on page 265

77. The correct answer is **B** – No explanation is available for this answer.

Back to Q 77 on page 265

78. The correct answer is **B** – No explanation is available for this answer.

Back to Q 78 on page 265

79. The correct answer is **B** – Idiopathic osteosclerosis represents focally increased bone density of unknown cause. It cannot be attributed to any inflammatory, dysplastic, neoplastic, or systemic disorder.

Idiopathic osteosclerosis also has been termed dense bone island, bone eburnation, bone whorl, bone scar, enostosis, and focal periapical osteopetrosis [9].

Back to Q 79 on page 265

80. The correct answer is **B** – No explanation is available for this answer.

Back to Q 80 on page 265

81. The correct answer is **D** – No explanation is available for this answer.

Back to Q 81 on page 266

82. The correct answer is **A** – No explanation is available for this answer.

Back to Q 82 on page 266

83. The correct answer is **A** – No explanation is available for this answer.

Back to Q 83 on page 266

84. The correct answer is **C** – No explanation is available for this answer.

Back to Q 84 on page 266

85. The correct answer is **B** – No explanation is available for this answer.

Back to Q 85 on page 267

86. The correct answer is **E** – No explanation is available for this answer.

Back to Q 86 on page 267

87. The correct answer is **D** – No explanation is available for this answer.

Back to Q 87 on page 267

88. The correct answer is **A** – No explanation is available for this answer.

Back to Q 88 on page 267

89. The correct answer is **C** – Characterized by fibrous dysplasia and intramuscular myxomas [9].

Back to Q 89 on page 267

90. The correct answer is **A** – No explanation is available for this answer.

Back to Q 90 on page 268

91. The correct answer is **C** – No explanation is available for this answer.

Back to Q 91 on page 268

92. The correct answer is **B** – No explanation is available for this answer.

Back to Q 92 on page 268

93. The correct answer is **B** – No explanation is available for this answer.

Back to Q 93 on page 268

94. The correct answer is **D** – No explanation is available for this answer.

Back to Q 94 on page 268

95. The correct answer is **C** – No explanation is available for this answer.

    Back to Q 95 on page 269

96. The correct answer is **C** – No explanation is available for this answer.

    Back to Q 96 on page 269

97. The correct answer is **A** – No explanation is available for this answer.

    Back to Q 97 on page 269

98. The correct answer is **B** – No explanation is available for this answer.

    Back to Q 98 on page 269

99. The correct answer is **C** – No explanation is available for this answer.

    Back to Q 99 on page 269

100. The correct answer is **E** – No explanation is available for this answer.

    Back to Q 100 on page 270

101. The correct answer is **D** – No explanation is available for this answer.

    Back to Q 101 on page 270

102. The correct answer is **D** – No explanation is available for this answer.

    Back to Q 102 on page 270

103. The correct answer is **B** – No explanation is available for this answer.

    Back to Q 103 on page 270

104. The correct answer is **A** – No explanation is available for this answer.

    Back to Q 104 on page 271

105. The correct answer is **C** – No explanation is available for this answer.

    Back to Q 105 on page 271

106. The correct answer is **C** – Unlike the pain associated with osteoid osteoma, the pain associated with osteoblastoma usually is not relieved by NSAIDs [9].

    Back to Q 106 on page 271

107. The correct answer is **A** – Most osteoblastomas are between 2 and 4 cm, but they may be as large as 10 cm, while osteoid osteomas rarely exceed 2 cm in diameter [9].

    Back to Q 107 on page 271

108. The correct answer is **A** – No explanation is available for this answer.

    Back to Q 108 on page 271

109. The correct answer is **A** – No explanation is available for this answer.

    Back to Q 109 on page 272

110. The correct answer is **A** – No explanation is available for this answer.

Back to Q 110 on page 272

111. The correct answer is **D** – No explanation is available for this answer.

Back to Q 111 on page 272

112. The correct answer is **A** – No explanation is available for this answer.

Back to Q 112 on page 272

113. The correct answer is **D** – No explanation is available for this answer.

Back to Q 113 on page 272

114. The correct answer is **D** – No explanation is available for this answer.

Back to Q 114 on page 273

115. The correct answer is **D** – No explanation is available for this answer.

Back to Q 115 on page 273

116. The correct answer is **B** – No explanation is available for this answer.

Back to Q 116 on page 273

117. The correct answer is **B** – No explanation is available for this answer.

Back to Q 117 on page 273

118. The correct answer is **B** – No explanation is available for this answer.

Back to Q 118 on page 273

119. The correct answer is **C** – During early embryonic development, mutation of a pluripotent stem cell can cause abnormalities in multiple cell types, including osteoblasts, melanocytes, and endocrine cells [9].

Back to Q 119 on page 274

120. The correct answer is **D** – GNAS gene mutations have not been detected in ossifying fibroma, other bone tumors or cemento-osseous dysplasia [9].

Back to Q 120 on page 274

CHAPTER 16
INFECTIONS OF THE ORAL AND PARA-ORAL TISSUES

Infections of the oral cavity are common. They might be caused by viruses, bacteria or fungi.

16.1 MCQs Questions

Choose **one or more** of the most appropriate answers. Some questions may have **more than one** correct answer. You have to choose all the correct answers as best as you can.

1. The cells most frequently found in a granuloma are:
   (a) Mast cells
   (b) Giant cells
   (c) Lymphocytes
   (d) Neutrophils
   (e) RBCs

   Answer for Q 1 on page 305

2. A patient with severe mycotic infection of the head characterized by the classical syndrome of uncontrolled diabetes, cellulitis, ophthalmoplegia[1] and meningoencephalitis:
   (a) Rhinosporidiosis
   (b) Candidiasis
   (c) Phycomycosis (Mucormycosis)
   (d) Actinomycosis

   Answer for Q 2 on page 305

[1] double or blurred vision resulting from paralysis of the extraocular muscles that control the movements of the eye.

3. Mucormycosis is noted especially in uncontrolled insulin-dependent diabetics due to:
   (a) Ketoacidosis inhibits the binding of iron to transferrin, allowing serum iron levels to rise
   (b) The growth of these fungi is enhanced by iron
   (c) Diabetes in general compromise the immune system
   (d) All of the above

   Answer for Q 3 on page 305

4. The most common route of infection in AIDS is:
   (a) Organ transplant
   (b) Blood transfusion
   (c) From mother to child
   (d) Sexual transmission

   Answer for Q 4 on page 305

5. Koplik's spots are an early intraoral manifestation of:
   (a) Varicella
   (b) Variola
   (c) Rubella
   (d) AIDS
   (e) Mumps

   Answer for Q 5 on page 305

6. Least common type of chronic mucocutaneous candidiasis is:
   (a) Chronic familial mucocutaneous candidiasis
   (b) Chronic localized mucocutaneous candidiasis
   (c) Chronic diffuse mucocutaneous candidiasis
   (d) Candidiasis endocrinopathy syndrome

   Answer for Q 6 on page 305

7. A patient with oral moniliasis that does not respond to nystatin therapy should be evaluated for the following **except**:
   (a) Diabetes insipidus
   (b) Diabetes mellitus
   (c) Hyperparathyroidism
   (d) Malignant lymphoma
   (e) Raised Ca^{+} in serum

   Answer for Q 7 on page 305

8. All of the following are examples of chronic atrophic candidiasis **except**:
   (a) Angular cheilitis
   (b) Denture sore mouth
   (c) Lip chewing
   (d) Median rhomboid glossitis

   Answer for Q 8 on page 305

9. The classic stigmata of congenital syphilis do not include:
   (a) Saber shins[2]
   (b) Interstitial keratitis
   (c) Eighth nerve deafness
   (d) Rhagades
   (e) Cleft lip

   Answer for Q 9 on page 306

10. The "Ghon's complex" is associated with:
   (a) Primary of childhood tuberculosis
   (b) The adrenogenital syndrome
   (c) Uveoparotid fever or Heerfordt's syndrome
   (d) Histiocystosis
   (e) AIDS

   Answer for Q 10 on page 306

11. Which of the following types of candidiasis resemble leukoplakia in clinical appearance:
   (a) Chronic hyperplastic candidiasis
   (b) Acute pseudomembranous candidiasis
   (c) Acute atrophic candidiasis
   (d) Chronic atrophic candidiasis

   Answer for Q 11 on page 306

12. Pericoronitis is seen in relation to:
   (a) Impacted third molars only
   (b) Around incompletely erupted crown
   (c) Completely erupted crowns only
   (d) None of the above

[2] Saber shin is a malformation of the tibia. It presents as a sharp anterior bowing, or convexity, of the tibia that can result from syphilis, Paget's disease of bone and vitamin D deficiency. Saber refers to the tibia's resemblance to the curve of a saber sword.

Answer for Q 12 on page 306

13. All of the following statements are true regarding cervicofacial actinomycosis **except**:
    (a) 10-20% of actinomycosis cases occur in cervicofacial region
    (b) The discharging pus contains visible sulfur granules
    (c) Cultures on blood agar often produce a typical molar tooth morphology
    (d) There is usually history of trauma such as tooth extraction or a blow to the jaw

Answer for Q 13 on page 306

14. Herpes simplex is caused by:
    (a) RNA virus
    (b) DNA virus
    (c) Retrovirus
    (d) Pox virus

Answer for Q 14 on page 306

15. All of the following infections exhibits pseudo epitheliomatous hyperplasia **except**:
    (a) North American blastomycosis
    (b) South American blastomycosis
    (c) Sporotrichosis
    (d) Histoplasmosis

Answer for Q 15 on page 306

16. Herpes simplex virus type I causes infection in:
    (a) Skin of the upper part of the body
    (b) Skin of the lower part of the body
    (c) Genitals
    (d) None of the above

Answer for Q 16 on page 306

17. The most common route of spread of mycobacterium tuberculosis is:
    (a) Urinary tract cells
    (b) Sexual contact
    (c) Respiratory droplets
    (d) Insects

Answer for Q 17 on page 306

18. A debilitated patient on oral penicillin has white lesions that can be stripped away from tongue, leaving a raw surface. This patient probably has:
    (a) Candidiasis
    (b) Lichen planus
    (c) Histoplasmosis
    (d) Mucosal dysplasia

    Answer for Q 18 on page 306
19. A 15-year-old boy has multiple vesiculating oral ulcers, severe pain, malaise, lymphadenopathy and an oral temperature of 39.5 °C of 3 days duration. The most likely diagnosis:
    (a) Herpes zoster
    (b) Acute herpetic gingivostomatitis
    (c) Periadenitis aphthae
    (d) Mumps

    Answer for Q 19 on page 306
20. The primary lesion of granulomatous infection of tuberculosis is called as:
    (a) Gumma
    (b) Lepra
    (c) Tubercle
    (d) Simon's focus

    Answer for Q 20 on page 306
21. All of the following statements about oral thrush are true **except**:
    (a) It is caused by Gram-negative fungus
    (b) It is characterized by a white plaque
    (c) It is a complication of immunosuppression systemic disease
    (d) It can affect neonates in an epidemic fashion

    Answer for Q 21 on page 306
22. A tubercle is made up of:
    (a) Caseous necrosis
    (b) Epitheloid and Langhans giant cell
    (c) Plasma cells and fibroblasts
    (d) All of the above

    Answer for Q 22 on page 306

23. Which of the following disorders is characterized by inflammation of dorsal root ganglia and vesicular eruption of the skin and mucous membranes in areas supplied by the affected sensory nerves:
    (a) Herpes zoster
    (b) Uveoparotid fever[3]
    (c) Herpes simplex
    (d) Aphthous stomatitis

    Answer for Q 23 on page 306

24. Clinical diagnosis of candidiasis is confirmed by:
    (a) Response to vitamin B12 therapy
    (b) Demonstration of mycelia and spores on histologic examination of surface scrap
    (c) Sun ray arrangement of fungal hyphae
    (d) Presence of sulfur granules

    Answer for Q 24 on page 306

25. Rhagades in syphilis is:
    (a) Corrugated lateral border of tongue
    (b) Scars radiating from mouth corners
    (c) Circumoral pigmentation
    (d) Drooping of oral commissure

    Answer for Q 25 on page 307

26. The differentiating features between Rubella and Rubeola (Measles) are that in rubella:
    (a) Koplik's spots do not occur
    (b) Oral mucous membranes are not usually affected
    (c) Complication following diseases are rare
    (d) All of the above

    Answer for Q 26 on page 307

27. Lues maligna is a form of:
    (a) Severe malignant melanoma
    (b) Lyell's disease
    (c) Secondary syphilis
    (d) Hansen's disease

    Answer for Q 27 on page 307

[3] Uveoparotid fever, also known as Heerfordt-Waldenström syndrome, is an uncommon acute presentation of systemic sarcoidosis. Patients may have features of complete/classic or incomplete disease.

28. Site specificity is characteristic manifestation of:
    (a) Syphilis
    (b) Candidiasis
    (c) Recurrent herpes simplex
    (d) Histoplasmosis

    Answer for Q 28 on page 307

29. Fournier's molars are associated with:
    (a) Congenital Syphilis
    (b) Fabry Anderson Syndrome
    (c) Apert Syndrome
    (d) Progeria

    Answer for Q 29 on page 307

30. Most patients infected with Mycobacterium tuberculosis develop a positive
    (a) type I hypersensitive skin test reaction
    (b) type II hypersensitive skin test reaction
    (c) type III hypersensitive skin test reaction
    (d) type IV hypersensitive skin test reaction

    Answer for Q 30 on page 307

31. Isoniazid, an anti-mycobacterial agent, can be used for a period of six months to 1 year in
    (a) active tuberculosis disease
    (b) positive tuberculin test with no active disease
    (c) close contacts of patients who have tuberculosis
    (d) all of the above

    Answer for Q 31 on page 307

32. A periapical granuloma may show clusters of lightly basophilic particles in association with plasmacytic infiltrate which are referred to as:
    (a) Rushton Bodies
    (b) Pyronine bodies
    (c) Russel Bodies
    (d) Hyaline bodies

    Answer for Q 32 on page 307

33. The infections associated with the following teeth generally drain through the lingual/palatal cortical plate:
    (a) Maxillary central incisors, mandibular lateral incisors and maxillary first molar
    (b) Maxillary lateral incisors, palatal roots of maxillary molars, mandibular second and third molars
    (c) Mandibular central incisors, palatal roots of maxillary molars, mandibular canines
    (d) Maxillary central incisors, maxillary canines, palatal roots of maxillary molars

    Answer for Q 33 on page 307

34. What is the most common location for AIDS related oral hairy leukoplakia?
    (a) Hard palate
    (b) Buccal mucosa
    (c) Lateral border of tongue
    (d) Floor of mouth

    Answer for Q 34 on page 307

35. Donovan bodies and pseudobubo[4]
    (a) Gonorrhea
    (b) Pyostomatitis vegetans[5]
    (c) Granuloma inguinale
    (d) Cat scratch disease

    Answer for Q 35 on page 307

36. SAPHO syndrome is:
    (a) Synovitis, Acromegaly, Psoriasis, Hypohidrosis, Osteitis
    (b) Synovitis, Acne, Pustulosis, Hyperostosis, Osteitis
    (c) Synovitis, Actinic cheilitis, Palatal cysts, Hairy tongue, Osteitis
    (d) Synovitis, Ankyloglossia, Periodontitis, Hairy tongue, Osteitis

    Answer for Q 36 on page 307

[4] Pseudobubo is an inguinal mass that represents subcutaneous extension to the inguinal area and mimics inguinal lymphadenopathy.

[5] Pyostomatitis vegetans is a rare and unusual disorder of the oral cavity, characterized by erythema and edema of the mucosa and numerous small, superficial yellow pustules. Its significance lies in its association with inflammatory disease of the bowel, either ulcerative colitis or Crohn's disease.

37. All are true about herpes infection **except**:
    (a) Infection is mostly subclinical
    (b) Ectodermal tissue is involved by the virus
    (c) PCR technique is the most sensitive and accurate method for diagnosis
    (d) Primary infection is seen in person with circulating antibodies

    Answer for Q 37 on page 307

38. Infectious conditions that exhibit sulfur granules are:
    (a) Actinomycosis and Botryomycosis[6]
    (b) Actinomycosis and Aspergillosis
    (c) Actinomycosis and Mucormycosis
    (d) Actinomycosis and Histoplasmosis

    Answer for Q 38 on page 307

39. Diagnostic tests for HIV:
    (a) Polymerized chain reaction
    (b) P24 antigen detection
    (c) Western blot analysis
    (d) All of the above

    Answer for Q 39 on page 307

40. Extra pulmonary tuberculosis is best diagnosed using the following imaging modality:
    (a) Ultrasonography
    (b) Computed axial tomography
    (c) Chest x ray
    (d) Magnetic resonance imaging

    Answer for Q 40 on page 308

41. Most common site of occurrence of oral lesions of hand, foot and mouth disease is:
    (a) Lips
    (b) Gingiva
    (c) Hard palate
    (d) Soft palate and pharynx

---

[6]Botryomycosis is a rare chronic granulomatous bacterial (pseudomycosis) infection that affects the skin, and rarely viscera. it is usually described in individuals with impaired immunity. The disease is caused usually by *Staphylococcus aureus*, however it can also be caused by *Pseudomonas aeruginosa, Pneumocystis carinii, Proteus spp.* and *Actinobacillus lignieresii.* The anatomic structure of its lesion is similar to that of actinomycosis and eumycetoma, and its granules resemble the sulfur granules of actinomycosis. Botryo means a cluster or bunch of grapes.

Answer for Q 41 on page 308

42. Trismus due to spasm of masseter in tetanus is called:

    (a) Lock jaw

    (b) opisthotonos[7] tonus

    (c) Risus Sardonicus[8]

    (d) All of the above

Answer for Q 42 on page 308

43. Lupus vulgaris is:

    (a) Tuberculosis of the skin

    (b) Tuberculosis of bone

    (c) Autoimmune disease

    (d) Actinomycosis

Answer for Q 43 on page 308

44. Higouménakis' sign is a feature of:

    (a) Trisomy 22

    (b) Congenital syphilis

    (c) Cretinism

    (d) Hypothyroidism

Answer for Q 44 on page 308

45. The bacteria which cause diphtheria is:

    (a) Clostridium

    (b) Corynebacterium

    (c) Mycobacterium

    (d) Pasteurella

Answer for Q 45 on page ??

46. Complication of diphtheria includes:

    (a) Myocarditis

    (b) Polyneuritis

    (c) Acute interstitial nephritis

    (d) All of the above

---

[7] Spasm of the muscles causing backward arching of the head, neck, and spine, as in severe tetanus, some kinds of meningitis, and strychnine poisoning.

[8] Risus sardonicus or rictus grin is a highly characteristic, abnormal, sustained spasm of the facial muscles that appears to produce grinning. It may be caused by tetanus, strychnine poisoning, or Wilson's disease, and has been reported after judicial hanging.

Answer for Q 46 on page 308

47. The virus involved in the pathogenesis of Kaposi sarcoma:
    (a) Epstein Barr virus
    (b) Lentivirus
    (c) Human herpesvirus
    (d) None of the above

Answer for Q 47 on page 308

48. Tuberculosis of lymph nodes is known as:
    (a) Phthisis[9]
    (b) Scrofula
    (c) Miliary tuberculosis
    (d) Lupus vulgaris

Answer for Q 48 on page 308

49. Non-plaque induced gingivitis with distinct erythematous band on marginal gingiva seen in HIV patient:
    (a) Linear gingival erythema
    (b) Necrotizing ulcerative gingivitis
    (c) Necrotizing stomatitis
    (d) Necrotizing ulcerative periodontitis

Answer for Q 49 on page 308

50. Lupus vulgaris is:
    (a) Paraneoplastic pemphigus
    (b) Familial benign pemphigus
    (c) Superficial form of pemphigus foliaceus
    (d) Begins as painless reddish-brown nodules which slowly enlarge to form irregularly shaped red plaque

Answer for Q 50 on page 308

51. Most frequent intraoral site of occurrence of tuberculous lesion is:
    (a) Gingiva
    (b) Tongue
    (c) Buccal mucosa
    (d) Palate

[9] Pulmonary tuberculosis or a similar progressive wasting disease.

Answer for Q 51 on page 308

52. *Borellia* vincenti, *Fusobacterium necrophorum* and *Prevotella intermedia* are the organisms responsible for:
    (a) Intestinal tuberculosis
    (b) Actinomycosis
    (c) Necrotizing ulcerative stomatitis (Noma)
    (d) Syphilis

Answer for Q 52 on page 308

53. Mantoux (Mendel–Mantoux) test is considered strongly positive when the maximum diameter of induration is:
    (a) More than 10 mm
    (b) More than 2 mm
    (c) Between 5 to 9mm
    (d) More than 15 mm

Answer for Q 53 on page 308

54. The identification of mycobacteria on a smear, a positive Z-N staining is reported when a minimum of:
    (a) Three acid-fast bacilli are seen
    (b) Eight acid-fast bacilli are seen
    (c) Ten acid-fast bacilli are seen
    (d) Fifteen acid-fast bacilli are seen

Answer for Q 54 on page 309

55. Most common form of actinomycosis is:
    (a) Cervicofacial
    (b) Pulmonary
    (c) Abdominal
    (d) Skeletal

Answer for Q 55 on page 309

56. The drug of choice for the treatment of acute necrotizing ulcerative gingivitis is:
    (a) Metronidazol
    (b) Oxytetracycline
    (c) Penicillin
    (d) Chlortetracycline
    (e) Doxycycline

Answer for Q 56 on page 309

57. The characteristic lesion of primary stage of acquired syphilis is:
    (a) Chancre
    (b) Gumma
    (c) Mucous patches
    (d) Rhagades

Answer for Q 57 on page 309

58. The lesion which are highly infective and mimics leukoplakia is:
    (a) Chancre
    (b) Gumma
    (c) Mucous patches
    (d) Lues Maligna[10]

Answer for Q 58 on page 309

59. All of the following are the sources of HIV transmission **except**:
    (a) Breast milk
    (b) Blood
    (c) Saliva
    (d) None of the above

Answer for Q 59 on page 309

60. Hutchinson's s triad consist of all of the following **except**:
    (a) Eight nerve deafness
    (b) Higoumenakis sign[11]
    (c) Hypoplasia of incisors and molars
    (d) Interstitial keratitis

Answer for Q 60 on page 309

61. A form of acute osteomyelitis that is seen in infants is termed:
    (a) Maxillitis neonatorum
    (b) Osteomyelitis neonatorum
    (c) Neonatal maxillitis
    (d) Natal osteomyelitis

Answer for Q 61 on page 309

[10] An unusual and severe, ulcerative nodular form of secondary syphilis
[11] Irregular thickening of the sternoclavicular portion of the clavicle seen in congenital syphilis.

62. Cicatrization is one of the most common manifestations of:

    (a) Rhinoscleroma[12]

    (b) Granuloma inguinale

    (c) Botryomycosis[13]

    (d) Syphilis

    Answer for Q 62 on page 309

63. Crater shape interdental papilla is a characteristic feature of:

    (a) diphtheria

    (b) Acute necrotizing ulcerative gingivitis

    (c) Scarlet fever

    (d) Recurrent intraoral herpes

    Answer for Q 63 on page 309

64. The most common route for furcation involvement in the maxillary permanent first molar is:

    (a) From palatal side

    (b) From buccal side

    (c) From mesial side

    (d) From distal side

    Answer for Q 64 on page 309

65. Garre's osteomyelitis is said to be commonly seen in young age as, in these individuals:

    (a) Periosteum is loosely attached to bone surface

    (b) Higher serum calcium level in young adults

    (c) More prone to trauma and infections

    (d) All of the above

    Answer for Q 65 on page 309

66. Lepra cells are seen in:

    (a) Leprosy

    (b) Cephalic tetanus

    (c) Cat scratch disease

    (d) Scarlet fever

    Answer for Q 66 on page 309

[12] Rhinoscleroma is a chronic granulomatous disease caused by *Klebsiella rhinoscleromatis.* It commonly affects the nasal cavity and nasopharynx, but it can also involve the larynx, trachea, bronchi, middle ear, and orbit.

[13] Botryomycosis is a rare chronic bacterial granulomatous disease that usually involves skin and rarely viscera. Main etiological agent is Staphylococcus aureus and less commonly Pseudomonas spp., Escherichia coli, Proteus spp., Streptococcus spp.

67. An "inverted J shadow" radiographic appearance may be representative of:
    (a) Superimposition of nasolabial fold over maxillary canine
    (b) Ala of the nose over crowns of maxillary lateral and canine
    (c) Mesial or distal furcation involvement of maxillary molars
    (d) Arch shaped bone destruction in aggressive periodontitis

Answer for Q 67 on page 310

68. A 6-years-old child cam to your clinic suffering from sever sore throat with pharyngitis and tonsillitis. Upon clinical examination, the patient was feverish. Pinpoint petechiae in the palate were seen. Submandibular, submental and cervical lymphadenitis was evident. Complete blood picture reveals atypical lymphocytes. The most probable diagnosis is:
    (a) Infectious mononucleosis
    (b) Primary herpetic gingivostomatitis
    (c) Herpangina
    (d) Recurrent intraoral herpes

Answer for Q 68 on page 310

69. The causative organisms for acute necrotizing ulcerative gingivitis are:
    (a) *Mycobacteria*
    (b) *Fusiform bacilli* and *Borellia vincenti*
    (c) *Treponema Pallidium* and *bacilli*
    (d) *Corynebacterium*

Answer for Q 69 on page 310

70. Imaging method of choice for evaluating periosteal new bone and sequestra in osteomyelitis is:
    (a) Magnetic resonance imaging
    (b) Computed Tomography
    (c) Technetium bone scan
    (d) Gallium citrate scan

Answer for Q 70 on page 310

71. Periapical inflammatory lesions are capable of laying a thin layer of bone within the maxillary antrum. This periosteal reaction may be termed:
    (a) inverted dome shadow
    (b) halo shadow
    (c) moon shadow
    (d) dome shadow

Answer for Q 71 on page 310

72. A 30-year-old patient presets with an asymptomatic doughy, soft, 2cm swelling of the lateral neck which has been present for months. Histopathological examination of the biopsy revealed presence of chronic inflammatory cells with hyphae that showed club-shaped termination. The most likely diagnosis is:
    (a) Tuberculous lymphadenitis
    (b) Cat scratch fever
    (c) Hodgkin lymphoma
    (d) Cervicofacial actinomycosis

    Answer for Q 72 on page 310

73. A patient presents with small yellow spots, present bilaterally on buccal mucosa opposite to posterior teeth without any other associated complaint. Most probable diagnosis of the condition is:
    (a) Koplik's spot
    (b) Fordyce's granules
    (c) melanotic macule
    (d) white sponge nevus

    Answer for Q 73 on page 310

74. A patient presented with asymptomatic, smooth, circumscribed red area in midline anterior to foramen caecum on the dorsum of tongue with microscopic evidence of inflammatory hyperplasia. The most probable diagnosis of the condition is:
    (a) hairy tongue
    (b) geographic tongue
    (c) lingual thyroid nodule
    (d) median rhomboid glossitis

    Answer for Q 74 on page 310

75. Acute necrotizing ulcerative gingivitis (ANUG) usually starts at:
    (a) Tip of the interdental papilla
    (b) Attached gingiva only
    (c) Attached gingiva and lateral borders of the tongue
    (d) Marginal gingiva only

    Answer for Q 75 on page 310

76. Acute streptococcal gingivitis is caused by:

(a) *Staphylococcus aureus*

(b) *Streptococcus gingivalis*

(c) *Streptococcus haemolyticus* (group A)

(d) *Streptococcus pneumoniae*

(e) B & C

Answer for Q 76 on page 310

77. In immunocompromised patients, acute necrotizing ulcerative gingivitis (ANUG) can progress into:

(a) Vincent's angina

(b) Maxillofacial gangrene (noma)

(c) Necrotizing stomatitis

(d) All of the above

Answer for Q 77 on page 310

78. A 12-year-old boy, was referred to your clinic for severe bleeding gums, gingival edema, fever, and halitosis. Upon clinical examination, soar throat with severe tonsillitis was evident. No gingival necrosis or ulceration was seen. No contributory medical history was detected. The most probable diagnosis is:

(a) Acute necrotizing ulcerative gingivitis

(b) Acute streptococcal gingivitis

(c) Primary herpetic gingivostomatitis

(d) Recurrent intraoral herpes infection

Answer for Q 78 on page 310

79. Pericoronitis is the termed applied to:

(a) Inflammation of the gingiva covering a completely impacted tooth

(b) Inflammation of the gingiva in relation to the crown of a partially erupted tooth

(c) Inflammation and necrosis of the interdental papilla

(d) A severe periapical infection discharging pus

Answer for Q 79 on page 310

80. Strawberry tongue is a characteristic feature of:

(a) Scarlet fever

(b) Primary herpetic gingivostomatitis

(c) Recurrent intraoral herpes infection

(d) Mumps

Answer for Q 80 on page 310

81. An infection that is characterized by a necrotic lesions in the pharynx covered by grayish white pseudomembrane, which may extend to the mouth and caused by Corynebacterium is:
    (a) Syphilis
    (b) Measles
    (c) Diphtheria
    (d) Acute necrotizing ulcerative gingivitis

    Answer for Q 81 on page 310

82. Chancre which is the primary stage of syphilis appears histologically as:
    (a) Chronic granulomatous lesion with gummatous necrosis
    (b) Chronic granulomatous lesion with caseous necrosis
    (c) Non-specific inflammation with perivascualr infiltration
    (d) Pseudomembranous inflammation

    Answer for Q 82 on page 310

83. One of the following stages of syphilis is not highly contagious:
    (a) Chancre of the primary stage
    (b) Mucocutaneous patches of the secondary stage
    (c) Gumma of the tertiary stage
    (d) All of them are highly contagious

    Answer for Q 83 on page 311

84. Diffuse syphilitic glossitis is:
    (a) Precancerous condition
    (b) Produces bald tongue
    (c) Accompanied by endarteritis obliterans
    (d) All of the above

    Answer for Q 84 on page 311

85. Caseating granuloma is a characteristic feature of:
    (a) *Mycobacterium tuberculosis*
    (b) *Mycobacterium bovis*
    (c) *Treponema pallidium* infection
    (d) A & B
    (e) A & C

    Answer for Q 85 on page 311

86. Scrofula is:
    (a) Tuberculous lymphadenitis
    (b) Tuberculosis of the skin
    (c) Tuberculosis of the vertebrae (Pott's disease)
    (d) The early lesions of tuberculosis affecting the apex of the lung

    Answer for Q 86 on page 311

87. The treatment of choice for tuberculous lymphadenitis is:
    (a) Incision and drainage
    (b) Surgical excision
    (c) Anti-tuberculous drugs
    (d) A & C
    (e) B & C

    Answer for Q 87 on page 311

88. Ray fungus is an obsolete name given for:
    (a) *Mycobacterium bovis*
    (b) *Mycobacterium tuberculosis*
    (c) *Actinomyces bovis*
    (d) *Mycobacterium Leprae*

    Answer for Q 88 on page 311

89. One of the following is **not** a member of orofacial granulomatosis:
    (a) Cheilitis granulomatosa
    (b) Cheilitis glandularis
    (c) Melkersson Rosenthal syndrome
    (d) Sarcoidosis
    (e) Oral lesions of Crohn's disease

    Answer for Q 89 on page 311

90. Astroid bodies are eosinophilic star-shaped cytoplasmic inclusions seen within the cytoplasm of multinucleated giant cell in one or more of the following:
    (a) Sarcoidosis
    (b) Tuberculosis
    (c) Syphilis
    (d) Actinomycosis

    Answer for Q 90 on page 311

91. Astroid bodies are eosinophilic star-shaped cytoplasmic inclusions seen within the cytoplasm of multinucleated giant cell in one or more of the following:
    (a) Tuberculosis
    (b) Syphilis
    (c) Tuberculoid leprosy
    (d) Actinomycosis

    Answer for Q 91 on page 311

92. Schaumann bodies are concentric lamellated calcified bodies seen within the cytoplasm of multinucleated cells usually seen in:
    (a) Leprosy
    (b) Syphilis
    (c) Actinomycosis
    (d) Sarcoidosis and Crohn's disease

    Answer for Q 92 on page 311

93. Oral thrush is:
    (a) Acute pseudomembranous candidiasis
    (b) Acute erythematous candidiasis
    (c) Angular cheilitis
    (d) Chronic hyperplastic candidosis

    Answer for Q 93 on page 311

94. One of the following stains are the best in detecting candidal hyphae in tissue smears or in histological sections:
    (a) Hematoxylin and Eosin (H&E)
    (b) Congo red
    (c) Alcian blue
    (d) Periodic acid Schiff (PAS)
    (e) A modified version of periodic acid Schiff (PAS) with a light green counter stain

    Answer for Q 94 on page 311

95. The thymoma associated candidiasis is a subtype of:
    (a) Chronic mucocutaneous candidosis syndromes
    (b) Chronic hyperplastic candidosis
    (c) Chronic erythematous candidosis
    (d) Acute erythematous candidiasis

Answer for Q 95 on page 311

96. In your opinion, median rhomboid glossitis (central papillary atrophy) is:
    (a) A developmental disturbance
    (b) Caused by *Candida albicans* fungus
    (c) A developmental disturbance on which candidal infection superimpose
    (d) A type of psoriasis

Answer for Q 96 on page 311

97. One of the following diseases is transmitted by sandflies (Phlebotomus species) and the infective agent is an intracellular parasite that infect the mononuclear phagocytes:
    (a) Tuberculosis
    (b) Leishmaniasis
    (c) Mucormycosis
    (d) Cryptococcosis

Answer for Q 97 on page 311

98. Pseudoepitheliomatous hyperplasia is a characteristic feature of ulcers resulting from one of the following infections:
    (a) Blastomycosis
    (b) Cryptococcosis
    (c) Mucormycosis
    (d) Syphilis

Answer for Q 98 on page 311

99. "Captain's wheel" or "steering wheel" appearance in histological sections is a characteristic feature of:
    (a) Coccidioidomycosis
    (b) Paracoccidioidomycosis (Paracocccidioides brasiliensis)
    (c) Cryptococcosis
    (d) Blastomycosis

Answer for Q 99 on page 312

100. One of the following infection is caused by a fungus from the genus "mucor"
    (a) Paracoccidioidomycosis
    (b) Cryptococcosis
    (c) Zygomycosis (phycomycosis)
    (d) Blastomycosis

Answer for Q 100 on page 312

101. Herpetic whitlow refers to:

(a) Viral infection of fingers

(b) Viral infection of gingiva

(c) Recurrent herpes labials

(d) Recurrent intraoral herpes

Answer for Q 101 on page 312

102. Ramsay-Hunt Syndrome is:

(a) The recurrent form of herpes simplex affecting the lip

(b) The primary infection of herpes simplex affecting the oral cavity

(c) Herpes zoster affecting the facial nerve via the geniculate ganglion

(d) Disease caused by Coxsackie virus type A16

Answer for Q 102 on page 312

103. Herpangina is caused by:

(a) Herpes simplex virus

(b) Herpes zoster virus

(c) Epstein-Barr virus

(d) Coxsackie virus type A16

Answer for Q 103 on page 312

104. One or more of the following features are useful in differentiating herpangina from primary herpetic gingivostomatitis:

(a) Herpangina is of shorter duration

(b) Herpangina usually affects the posterior part of the mouth (soft palate and nasopharynx)

(c) Ulcers of herpangina are more painful

(d) A & B

(e) A & C

Answer for Q 104 on page 312

105. One of the following viral infection can cause developmental disturbances (birth defects):

(a) Herpes simplex infection

(b) Varicella zoster infection

(c) Rubella (German measles)

(d) Coxsackie viral infection

Answer for Q 105 on page 312

106. Infectious mononucleosis is caused by:

   (a) Epstein-Barr virus

   (b) Herpes simplex virus

   (c) Herpes zoster virus

   (d) Rubella virus

   Answer for Q 106 on page 312

107. After the primary infection with Epstein-Barr virus, the virus remains latent in the following cells:

   (a) Plasma cells and endothelial cells

   (b) Oral epithelial cells and lymphocytes

   (c) Fibroblasts and nerve fibers

   (d) Osteoblasts and Osteocytes

   Answer for Q 107 on page 312

16.2 Answers with Comments:

1. The correct answer is **C** – Lymphocytes are the predominate cells in chronic granuloma.

   Back to Q 1 on page 283

2. The correct answer is **C** – No explanation is available for this answer.

   Back to Q 2 on page 283

3. The correct answer is **D** – Mucormycosis is noted especially in insulin-dependent diabetics who have uncontrolled diabetes and are ketoacidotic; ketoacidosis inhibits the binding of iron to transferrin, allowing serum iron levels to rise. The growth of these fungi is enhanced by iron [9].

   Back to Q 3 on page 284

4. The correct answer is **D** – No explanation is available for this answer.

   Back to Q 4 on page 284

5. The correct answer is **C** – No explanation is available for this answer.

   Back to Q 5 on page 284

6. The correct answer is **C** – No explanation is available for this answer.

   Back to Q 6 on page 284

7. The correct answer is **A** – No explanation is available for this answer.

   Back to Q 7 on page 284

8. The correct answer is **C** – Median rhomboid glossitis is controversial.

   Back to Q 8 on page 285

9. The correct answer is **E** – No explanation is available for this answer.

   Back to Q 9 on page 285

10. The correct answer is **A** – No explanation is available for this answer.

    Back to Q 10 on page 285

11. The correct answer is **A** – Appearing as plaques resembling milk curd.

    Back to Q 11 on page 285

12. The correct answer is **B** – No explanation is available for this answer.

    Back to Q 12 on page 285

13. The correct answer is **A** – No explanation is available for this answer.

    Back to Q 13 on page 286

14. The correct answer is **B** – No explanation is available for this answer.

    Back to Q 14 on page 286

15. The correct answer is **D** – See reference [[12]] for detailed discussion on pseudo epitheliomatous hyperplasia.

    Back to Q 15 on page 286

16. The correct answer is **D** – No explanation is available for this answer.

    Back to Q 16 on page 286

17. The correct answer is **C** – No explanation is available for this answer.

    Back to Q 17 on page 286

18. The correct answer is **A** – No explanation is available for this answer.

    Back to Q 18 on page 287

19. The correct answer is **B** – No explanation is available for this answer.

    Back to Q 19 on page 287

20. The correct answer is **C** – No explanation is available for this answer.

    Back to Q 20 on page 287

21. The correct answer is **A** – Caused by Gram positive fungus.

    Back to Q 21 on page 287

22. The correct answer is **D** – No explanation is available for this answer.

    Back to Q 22 on page 287

23. The correct answer is **A** – No explanation is available for this answer.

    Back to Q 23 on page 288

24. The correct answer is **B** – Albeit the clinical diagnosis of oral candidiasis is relatively simple, its confirmation may be problematic. However, the diagnosis can be made by the microscopic observation of Candida in oral lesion samples (microscopic morphological criteria) and by isolation in culture.

Back to Q 24 on page 288

25. The correct answer is **B** – No explanation is available for this answer.

Back to Q 25 on page 288

26. The correct answer is **D** – No explanation is available for this answer.

Back to Q 26 on page 288

27. The correct answer is **C** – No explanation is available for this answer.

Back to Q 27 on page 288

28. The correct answer is **C** – No explanation is available for this answer.

Back to Q 28 on page 289

29. The correct answer is **A** – No explanation is available for this answer.

Back to Q 29 on page 289

30. The correct answer is **D** – No explanation is available for this answer.

Back to Q 30 on page 289

31. The correct answer is **D** – No explanation is available for this answer.

Back to Q 31 on page 289

32. The correct answer is **B** – No explanation is available for this answer.

Back to Q 32 on page 289

33. The correct answer is **B** – No explanation is available for this answer.

Back to Q 33 on page 290

34. The correct answer is **C** – No explanation is available for this answer.

Back to Q 34 on page 290

35. The correct answer is **C** – No explanation is available for this answer.

Back to Q 35 on page 290

36. The correct answer is **B** – No explanation is available for this answer.

Back to Q 36 on page 290

37. The correct answer is **D** – No explanation is available for this answer.

Back to Q 37 on page 291

38. The correct answer is **A** – No explanation is available for this answer.

Back to Q 38 on page 291

39. The correct answer is **D** – No explanation is available for this answer.

Back to Q 39 on page 291

40. The correct answer is **D** – No explanation is available for this answer.

Back to Q 40 on page 291

41. The correct answer is **D** – No explanation is available for this answer.

Back to Q 41 on page 291

42. The correct answer is **A** – No explanation is available for this answer.

Back to Q 42 on page 292

43. The correct answer is **A** – No explanation is available for this answer.

Back to Q 43 on page 292

44. The correct answer is **B** – A unilateral enlargement of the sternoclavicular portion of the clavicle, seen in congenital syphilis. It is an end result of neonatal periostitis.

Back to Q 44 on page 292

45. The correct answer is **B** – No explanation is available for this answer.

Back to Q 45 on page 292

46. The correct answer is **D** – No explanation is available for this answer.

Back to Q 46 on page 292

47. The correct answer is **C** – Human herpes virus type 8, also known as he Kaposi sarcoma--associated herpesvirus (KSHV).

Back to Q 47 on page 293

48. The correct answer is **B** – No explanation is available for this answer.

Back to Q 48 on page 293

49. The correct answer is **A** – No explanation is available for this answer.

Back to Q 49 on page 293

50. The correct answer is **D** – No explanation is available for this answer.

Back to Q 50 on page 293

51. The correct answer is **B** – No explanation is available for this answer.

Back to Q 51 on page 293

52. The correct answer is **C** – No explanation is available for this answer.

Back to Q 52 on page 294

53. The correct answer is **D** – The Mantoux test or Mendel–Mantoux test (also known as the Mantoux screening test, tuberculin sensitivity test, Pirquet test, or PPD test for **P**urified **P**rotein **D**erivative) is a valuable tool for screening for tuberculosis (TB) and for tuberculosis diagnosis. It is one of the common tuberculin skin tests used around the world.

Back to Q 53 on page 294

54. The correct answer is **A** – No explanation is available for this answer.

Back to Q 54 on page 294

55. The correct answer is **A** – No explanation is available for this answer.

Back to Q 55 on page 294

56. The correct answer is **A** – No explanation is available for this answer.

Back to Q 56 on page 294

57. The correct answer is **A** – No explanation is available for this answer.

Back to Q 57 on page 295

58. The correct answer is **C** – No explanation is available for this answer.

Back to Q 58 on page 295

59. The correct answer is **C** – Evidence shows that the HIV virus is spread through the exchange of bodily fluids such as blood, semen and vaginal fluids, and breast milk but not saliva.

Back to Q 59 on page 295

60. The correct answer is **B** – No explanation is available for this answer.

Back to Q 60 on page 295

61. The correct answer is **C** – No explanation is available for this answer.

Back to Q 61 on page 295

62. The correct answer is **B** – No explanation is available for this answer.

Back to Q 62 on page 296

63. The correct answer is **B** – No explanation is available for this answer.

Back to Q 63 on page 296

64. The correct answer is **C** – There is a great controversy, some authors believe that the buccal site is the most common. From a periodontal perspective, furcations of the maxillary first molars are more commonly involved than those of the mandibular first molars. Additionally, the buccal furcations of the maxillary first molars are the most frequently affected, followed by the mesiopalatal and distopalatal furcations. However, fortunately, the buccal furcation is the most accessible one for both patients and clinicians. The access to the periodontal lesion in proximal furcations represents a challenge for maintaining good oral hygiene and performing an optimal periodontal treatment [13].

Back to Q 64 on page 296

65. The correct answer is **A** – No explanation is available for this answer.

Back to Q 65 on page 296

66. The correct answer is **A** – No explanation is available for this answer.

Back to Q 66 on page 296

67. The correct answer is **C** – No explanation is available for this answer.

Back to Q 67 on page 297

68. The correct answer is **A** – Presence of lymphocytosis and petechiae in the palate together with high fever are suggestive for infectious mononucleosis.

Back to Q 68 on page 297

69. The correct answer is **B** – No explanation is available for this answer.

Back to Q 69 on page 297

70. The correct answer is A – No explanation is available for this answer.

Back to Q 70 on page 297

71. The correct answer is **B** – No explanation is available for this answer.

Back to Q 71 on page 297

72. The correct answer is **D** – No explanation is available for this answer.

Back to Q 72 on page 298

73. The correct answer is **B** – No explanation is available for this answer.

Back to Q 73 on page 298

74. The correct answer is **D** – No explanation is available for this answer.

Back to Q 74 on page 298

75. The correct answer is **A** – No explanation is available for this answer.

Back to Q 75 on page 298

76. The correct answer is **C** – No explanation is available for this answer.

Back to Q 76 on page 299

77. The correct answer is **D** – No explanation is available for this answer.

Back to Q 77 on page 299

78. The correct answer is **B** – No explanation is available for this answer.

Back to Q 78 on page 299

79. The correct answer is **B** – No explanation is available for this answer.

Back to Q 79 on page 299

80. The correct answer is **A** – No explanation is available for this answer.

Back to Q 80 on page 299

81. The correct answer is **C** – No explanation is available for this answer.

Back to Q 81 on page 300

82. The correct answer is **C** – No explanation is available for this answer.

Back to Q 82 on page 300

83. The correct answer is **C** – No explanation is available for this answer.

Back to Q 83 on page 300

84. The correct answer is **D** – No explanation is available for this answer.

Back to Q 84 on page 300

85. The correct answer is **D** – No explanation is available for this answer.

Back to Q 85 on page 300

86. The correct answer is **A** – No explanation is available for this answer.

Back to Q 86 on page 301

87. The correct answer is **E** – No explanation is available for this answer.

Back to Q 87 on page 301

88. The correct answer is **C** – No explanation is available for this answer.

Back to Q 88 on page 301

89. The correct answer is **B** – No explanation is available for this answer.

Back to Q 89 on page 301

90. The correct answer is **A** – No explanation is available for this answer.

Back to Q 90 on page 301

91. The correct answer is **C** – No explanation is available for this answer.

Back to Q 91 on page 302

92. The correct answer is **D** – No explanation is available for this answer.

Back to Q 92 on page 302

93. The correct answer is **A** – No explanation is available for this answer.

Back to Q 93 on page 302

94. The correct answer is **E** – See [14].

Back to Q 94 on page 302

95. The correct answer is **A** – No explanation is available for this answer.

Back to Q 95 on page 302

96. The correct answer is **C** – No explanation is available for this answer.

Back to Q 96 on page 303

97. The correct answer is **B** – No explanation is available for this answer.

Back to Q 97 on page 303

98. The correct answer is **A** – No explanation is available for this answer.

Back to Q 98 on page 303

99. The correct answer is **B** – No explanation is available for this answer.

    Back to Q 99 on page 303

100. The correct answer is **C** – No explanation is available for this answer.

    Back to Q 100 on page 303

101. The correct answer is **A** – No explanation is available for this answer.

    Back to Q 101 on page 304

102. The correct answer is **C** – No explanation is available for this answer.

    Back to Q 102 on page 304

103. The correct answer is **D** – No explanation is available for this answer.

    Back to Q 103 on page 304

104. The correct answer is **D** – No explanation is available for this answer.

    Back to Q 104 on page 304

105. The correct answer is **C** – No explanation is available for this answer.

    Back to Q 105 on page 304

106. The correct answer is **A** – No explanation is available for this answer.

    Back to Q 106 on page 305

107. The correct answer is **B** – No explanation is available for this answer.

    Back to Q 107 on page 305

Chapter 17
White and Red Lesions of the Oral Cavity

Most of the lesions to be mentioned herein have been questioned and discussed in their relevant chapters, and the reader is advised to refer to these chapters for further details.

17.1 MCQs Questions

Choose **one or more** of the most appropriate answers. Some questions may have **more than one** correct answer. You have to choose all the correct answers as best as you can.

1. White lesions of the oral cavity appear as such due to one of the following:
   (a) Epithelial atrophy
   (b) Increased keratinization
   (c) Deposition of white pigment
   (d) Inflammation
   Answer for Q 1 on page 318
2. White lesions of the oral cavity appear as such due:
   (a) Hyperkeratosis
   (b) Hyperparakeratosis
   (c) Acanthosis
   (d) All of the above
   Answer for Q 2 on page 318
3. Red lesions of the oral mucosa occur as a result of:
   (a) Decreased thickness of epithelium due to atrophy
   (b) Alteration of the color of the connective tissue due to increased vascularity
   (c) Inflammation
   (d) All of the above
   Answer for Q 3 on page 318

4. Leukoedema:
   (a) Treated by vitamin B12 supplementation
   (b) Require surgical excision
   (c) Treated by removal of the cause
   (d) Require no treatment

   Answer for Q 4 on page 318

5. Leukoedema is:
   (a) Normal variation, more in black population
   (b) Potentially malignant
   (c) Unilateral
   (d) Results from reverse smoking

   Answer for Q 5 on page 318

6. Leukoedema is:
   (a) Often accompanied by red speckling
   (b) Area of atrophic epithelium
   (c) Diffuse white to grey opacification on the buccal mucosa – disappears when you stretch the cheek
   (d) Should be treated promptly for the fear of malignancy

   Answer for Q 6 on page 318

7. A-57-year-old female presented complaining of a "painful mouth". Clinical examination revealed multiple, irregular whitish plaques mixed with areas of erythema. The lesion can be wiped off. What is your most probable diagnosis?
   (a) Acute pseudomembranous Candidiasis
   (b) Leukoplakia
   (c) Erythoplakia
   (d) Lichen planus

   Answer for Q 7 on page 318

8. Leukoedema is:
   (a) Hereditary
   (b) A result of betel nut chewing
   (c) Symmetrical on both cheeks and asymptomatic
   (d) A variant of lichen planus that appears as a white patch

   Answer for Q 8 on page 318

9. White spongy nevus:
   (a) Mutations in genes producing keratin type 4 and/or 13
   (b) Can be wiped off
   (c) Unilateral
   (d) Painful

   Answer for Q 9 on page 318

10. A patient with history of tobacco chewing presents with an asymptomatic, exophytic papillary growth on right buccal mucosa. Histologic examination of the lesion reveal marked epithelial proliferation without invasion into the connective tissue and parakeratin plugging. Most probable diagnosis is:
    (a) Epidermoid carcinoma
    (b) basal cell carcinoma
    (c) Papilloma
    (d) verrucous carcinoma

    Answer for Q 10 on page 318

11. White spongy nevus:
    (a) Burning sensation
    (b) With areas of erythema
    (c) Similar in etiology to candidiasis
    (d) Require no treatment

    Answer for Q 11 on page 318

12. White spongy nevus:
    (a) Due to tobacco chewing
    (b) Ulcerative
    (c) Hereditary
    (d) Treatment is mandatory

    Answer for Q 12 on page 318

13. White lesions which are usually bilateral:
    (a) Hereditary benign intra-epithelial dyskeratosis
    (b) Dyskeratosis congenita
    (c) Pachyonychia congenita
    (d) Candidosis
    (e) All of the above

    Answer for Q 13 on page 318

14. White spongy nevus:
    (a) Thin and atrophied
    (b) Most common site is at the oral commissure
    (c) An autosomal dominant condition
    (d) Should be treated by topical corticosteroids and antifungal drugs

    Answer for Q 14 on page 319

15. A patient reported with a symptomless white patch on buccal mucosa which cannot be rubbed off. The patch was present for the last 3 months. Patient is a heavy cigarette smoker. Most probable diagnosis of the lesion is:
    (a) Leukoplakia
    (b) Candidiasis
    (c) Erythroplakia
    (d) White sponge nevus

    Answer for Q 15 on page 319

16. White spongy nevus shows histologically:
    (a) Hyperkeratosis
    (b) Acanthosis
    (c) Inter and intra-cellular edema of the prickle cell layer
    (d) All of the above

    Answer for Q 16 on page 319

17. One of the following lesions is developmental in nature **except**:
    (a) Candidiasis
    (b) Hereditary benign intraepithelial dyskeratosis
    (c) White spongy nevus
    (d) Dyskeratosis congenita
    (e) Pachyonychia congenita

    Answer for Q 17 on page 319

18. Hereditary benign intraepithelial dyskeratosis:
    (a) Also known as Witkop's disease
    (b) Hereditary
    (c) Treatment is unnecessary but reassurance may be required
    (d) All of the above

    Answer for Q 18 on page 319

19. White lesions which are usually bilateral:
    (a) Fordyce's spots
    (b) Lichen planus
    (c) Leukoedema
    (d) White spongy nevus
    (e) All of the above

    Answer for Q 19 on page 319

20. Dyskeratosis congenita is:
    (a) X-linked dominant
    (b) Autosomal dominant
    (c) X-linked recessive
    (d) Vitamin B12 deficiency

    Answer for Q 20 on page 319

21. One of the following is not a feature of Fanconi's syndrome:
    (a) Hereditary
    (b) Hypersplenism
    (c) Dyskeratosis Congenita
    (d) Lesions can be treated with corticosteroids and antibiotics

    Answer for Q 21 on page 319

22. Plummer-Vinson syndrome is characterized by:
    (a) Iron deficiency anemia
    (b) Atrophy of the mucosa of the oral cavity, pharynx and esophagus
    (c) Atrophy of tongue papillae with glossitis
    (d) Dysphagia due to atrophy causing burning sensation of the esophagus
    (e) All of the above

    Answer for Q 22 on page 319

17.2 Answers with Comments:

1. The correct answer is **B** – White lesions of the oral mucosa occur as a result of:
   (a) Increased thickness of epithelium which may result from:
      i. Hyperkeratosis
      ii. Acanthosis
      iii. Spongiosis resulting form intra and/or inter-cellular edema
   (b) Alteration of the color of the connective tissue such as decreased vascularity and increased fibrosis

   Back to Q 1 on page 313
2. The correct answer is **D** – See answer for Q 1.

   Back to Q 2 on page 313
3. The correct answer is **D** – – No explanation is available for this answer.

   Back to Q 3 on page 313
4. The correct answer is **D** – No explanation is available for this answer.

   Back to Q 4 on page 314
5. The correct answer is **A** – No explanation is available for this answer.

   Back to Q 5 on page 314
6. The correct answer is **C** – No explanation is available for this answer.

   Back to Q 1 on page 314
7. The correct answer is **A** – No explanation is available for this answer.

   Back to Q 7 on page 314
8. The correct answer is **C** – No explanation is available for this answer.

   Back to Q 8 on page 314
9. The correct answer is **A** – No explanation is available for this answer.

   Back to Q 9 on page 315
10. The correct answer is **D** – No explanation is available for this answer.

    Back to Q 10 on page 315
11. The correct answer is **D** – No explanation is available for this answer.

    Back to Q 11 on page 315
12. The correct answer is **C** – No explanation is available for this answer.

    Back to Q 12 on page 315
13. The correct answer is **E** – No explanation is available for this answer.

Back to Q 13 on page 315

14. The correct answer is **C** – No explanation is available for this answer.

Back to Q 14 on page 316

15. The correct answer is **A** – No explanation is available for this answer.

Back to Q 15 on page 316

16. The correct answer is **D** – No explanation is available for this answer.

Back to Q 16 on page 316

17. The correct answer is **A** – No explanation is available for this answer.

Back to Q 17 on page 316

18. The correct answer is **D** – No explanation is available for this answer.

Back to Q 18 on page 316

19. The correct answer is **E** – No explanation is available for this answer.

Back to Q 19 on page 317

20. The correct answer is **C** – No explanation is available for this answer.

Back to Q 20 on page 317

21. The correct answer is **D** – No explanation is available for this answer.

Back to Q 21 on page 317

22. The correct answer is **E** – No explanation is available for this answer.

Back to Q 22 on page 317

CHAPTER 18
PERIODONTAL DISEASES

Periodontal diseases are the second most common diseases affecting the oral cavity, the first being dental caries. They are one of the major causes of tooth loss. Therefore, every effort should be made for early detection of periodontal disease.

18.1 MCQs Questions

Choose **one or more** of the most appropriate answers. Some questions may have **more than one** correct answer. You have to choose all the correct answers as best as you can.

1. Attachment of teeth to bone is termed as:
   (a) Ankylosis
   (b) Gomphosis[1]
   (c) Synostosis
   (d) Synchondrosis
   Answer for Q 1 on page 350
2. A thin dark bluish line along the gingival margin is due to the absorption of:
   (a) Silver
   (b) Mercury
   (c) Drugs like tetracycline or minocycline
   (d) Lead
   Answer for Q 2 on page 350

[1] Fixed or immovable joints between bones and teeth or bones and other bones through tough fibrous tissue. Gomphosis can allow a very tiny movements between parts.

3. The number of epithelial rests of Malassez will:
   (a) Decreases with age
   (b) Increases with age
   (c) Remains constant
   (d) Increase or decrease based on function

   Answer for Q 3 on page 350

4. McCall's festoons are:
   (a) also called Stillman's clefts
   (b) due to poor oral hygiene
   (c) Congenital abnormality
   (d) Due to trauma from occlusion

   Answer for Q 4 on page 350

5. Most objective sign of gingivitis is:
   (a) Increase in gingival size
   (b) Increase in crevicular fluid
   (c) Increase in gingival redness
   (d) Bleeding on probing

   Answer for Q 5 on page 350

6. Acquired pellicle is fully formed in:
   (a) 30 minutes
   (b) 60 minutes
   (c) 12 hours
   (d) 24 hours

   Answer for Q 6 on page 350

7. Life-saver shaped enlargements of the marginal gingiva are called:
   (a) Gingival crater
   (b) McCall festoons
   (c) Stillman's cleft
   (d) Window peaks

   Answer for Q 7 on page 350

8. Which of the following cells are predominant in the stage I of gingivitis?
   (a) Plasma cells
   (b) Neutrophils
   (c) Mast cells
   (d) Lymphocytes

   Answer for Q 8 on page 350

9. The most common form of gingival disease is:
   (a) Gingivitis
   (b) Periodontitis
   (c) Gingival recession
   (d) Gingival hyperplasia

   Answer for Q 9 on page 350

10. Earliest clinical sign of gingivitis is:
    (a) Bleeding on probing
    (b) Change in color
    (c) Change in contour
    (d) Change in size

    Answer for Q 10 on page 350

11. Which single factor could contribute most of the development of simple gingivitis in children?
    (a) High fever
    (b) Poor oral hygiene
    (c) Oral habits
    (d) Physical nature of food ingested

    Answer for Q 11 on page 350

12. When periodontal probing in gingivitis is done, depth is measured from:
    (a) Base of pocket to cementoenamel junction
    (b) Base of pocket to free marginal gingiva
    (c) marginal gingiva to cementoenamel junction
    (d) Junctional epithelium

    Answer for Q 12 on page 351

13. Which of the following tooth stain is associated with low incidence of dental caries:
    - (a) Orange stain
    - (b) Green stain
    - (c) Black stain
    - (d) Brown stain

    Answer for Q 13 on page 351

14. Bacteria found in gingivitis are localized mainly in:
    - (a) Connective tissue fibers
    - (b) Gingival sulcus
    - (c) Alveolar bone
    - (d) Periodontal ligament

    Answer for Q 14 on page 351

15. All indices are used to evaluate calculus formation in long-term clinical trials **except**:
    - (a) The simplified calculus indexes
    - (b) The probe method of calculus assessment
    - (c) Calculus surface index
    - (d) Probing depth

    Answer for Q 15 on page 351

16. The histopathologic picture of chronic gingivitis shows:
    - (a) Leukocytic infiltration with increased neutrophils
    - (b) Widening of capillaries and venules
    - (c) Increased plasma cells and neutrophils
    - (d) Infiltration of neutrophils, lymphocytes and plasma cells

    Answer for Q 16 on page 351

17. Calculus is composed of:
    - (a) 5-10% water
    - (b) 10-15% water
    - (c) 0-5%water
    - (d) 15-25% water

    Answer for Q 17 on page 351

18. Gingivitis:
    (a) Inevitably progresses to periodontitis
    (b) Affects approximately 50% of adolescents
    (c) Is characterized by true pocketing
    (d) Is a reversible lesion

    Answer for Q 18 on page 351

19. Gingivitis is initiated most frequently by:
    (a) Pregnancy
    (b) Malocclusion
    (c) Vitamin deficiency
    (d) Local irritating factors

    Answer for Q 19 on page 351

20. The most common sequelae of gingivitis are:
    (a) Pericoronitis
    (b) Periodontitis
    (c) Periodontosis
    (d) Periapical pathology

    Answer for Q 20 on page 351

21. The hardening of the soft dental plaque will start between:
    (a) 1-7days
    (b) 7-14 days
    (c) 1-14 days
    (d) 14-28 days

    Answer for Q 21 on page 351

22. McCall Festoons are seen in which of the following teeth?
    (a) Central incisors
    (b) Canine and premolars
    (c) Lateral incisors
    (d) Molars

    Answer for Q 22 on page 351

23. Clinical signs of gingivitis appear in:
    (a) Initial gingivitis
    (b) Early gingivitis
    (c) Late gingivitis
    (d) Advanced gingivitis

    Answer for Q 23 on page 351

24. The most favorable type of pocket for reattachment to occur is the one with:
    (a) Three osseous walls
    (b) Two osseous walls
    (c) One osseous wall
    (d) Absence of osseous walls

    Answer for Q 24 on page 351

25. A key feature that differentiates stage III gingivitis from the stage II lesion is an increase in the number of:
    (a) Lymphocytes
    (b) Plasma Cells
    (c) Mast cells
    (d) Polymorphs

    Answer for Q 25 on page 351

26. McCall's Festoons result from:
    (a) Normal physiological process
    (b) Tooth brush trauma
    (c) Inflammation
    (d) Food lodgement

    Answer for Q 26 on page 351

27. Apostrophe shaped area:
    (a) Stillman's cleft
    (b) McCall's Festoons
    (c) Gingival sulcus
    (d) None of the above

    Answer for Q 27 on page 351

28. Radiographic appearance of gingivitis typically shows:
    (a) Horizontal bone loss
    (b) Vertical bone loss
    (c) Crestal type defects
    (d) No bony deformity

    Answer for Q 28 on page 352

29. Bleeding on probing will tell us that:
    (a) Gingival health of a child
    (b) Status of gingival health on the day of examination
    (c) 7 days has passed since last prophylaxis
    (d) 14 days has passe since last prophylaxis

    Answer for Q 29 on page 352

30. Pocket without destruction of underlying periodontal tissues:
    (a) Pseudo pocket
    (b) Infrabony pocket
    (c) Suprabony pocket
    (d) True pocket

    Answer for Q 30 on page 352

31. Periodontal pockets are not found in cases of:
    (a) Lateral periodontal abscess
    (b) Aggressive periodontitis
    (c) Chronic periodontitis
    (d) Necrotising ulcerative gingivitis

    Answer for Q 31 on page 352

32. Which of the following is a feature of gingivitis?
    (a) Inflamed tissue
    (b) Bleeding on probing
    (c) Increased gingival fluid
    (d) All of the above

    Answer for Q 32 on page 352

33. The true causative agent of necrotizing ulcerative gingivitis:

  (a) *Bacteroides melaninogenica (Prevotella melaninogenica)*

  (b) *Bacteroides intermedius*

  (c) *Capnocytophaga*

  (d) All of the above

  Answer for Q 33 on page 352

34. In aggressive periodontitis, an arc shaped alveolar bone loss can be seen extending from:

  (a) Distal surface of central incisor to mesial surface of canine

  (b) Distal surface of lateral incisor to mesial surface of first premolar

  (c) Distal surface of second premolar to mesial surface of first molar

  (d) Distal surface of second premolar to mesial surface of second molar

  Answer for Q 34 on page 352

35. All are features of Papillon–Lefèvre syndrome (PLS) **except**:

  (a) Keratotic lesion of the palmar and plantar surface

  (b) Hyperhidrosis

  (c) Associated with generalized aggressive periodontitis of primary and permanent teeth

  (d) Associated with localized aggressive periodontitis

  Answer for Q 35 on page 352

36. Gingival recession is most commonly due to:

  (a) Toothbrush trauma

  (b) Trauma from occlusion

  (c) Defective contacts

  (d) ANUG

  Answer for Q 36 on page 352

37. Papillon–Lefèvre syndrome (PLS) is:

  (a) Autosomal recessive

  (b) Autosomal dominant

  (c) X-linked dominant

  (d) X-linked recessive

  Answer for Q 37 on page 352

38. Plasma cells are most commonly seen in one of the stages of gingivitis:
    (a) Initial lesion
    (b) Early lesion
    (c) Established lesion
    (d) Advanced lesion

    Answer for Q 38 on page 352

39. Which of the following fungal infection is related to periodontal membrane:
    (a) Lutz's disease (South American Blastomycosis, Paracoccidioidomycosis)
    (b) Gilchrist's disease
    (c) Darling's disease
    (d) Coccidioidomycosis

    Answer for Q 39 on page 352

40. In gingivitis, the immunoglobulins are consistent with the increase in number of:
    (a) Fibroblasts
    (b) Neutrophils
    (c) Lymphocytes
    (d) Plasma cells

    Answer for Q 40 on page 352

41. Confirmation of the diagnosis of Papillon–Lefèvre syndrome (PLS) is made through:
    (a) Increased levels of urinary enzyme cathepsin C
    (b) Decreased levels of urinary enzyme cathepsin C
    (c) Elevated level of the urinary vanillylmandelic acid (VMA)
    (d) Decreased level of the urinary vanillylmandelic acid (VMA)

    Answer for Q 41 on page 352

42. The following condition **do not** create gingival defects necessitating gingivoplasty **except**:
    (a) Acute necrotizing ulcerative gingivitis
    (b) Desquamative gingivitis
    (c) Erosive lichen planus
    (d) Acute Herpetic gingivostomatitis

    Answer for Q 42 on page 352

43. One common radiographic finding in clinical gingivitis is:

    (a) Vertical bone loss

    (b) Normal bone pattern

    (c) Horizontal bone loss

    (d) Increase in bone density

    Answer for Q 43 on page 352

44. The most important cell which contributes to the severity of periodontal disease is:

    (a) Lymphocyte

    (b) Neutrophil

    (c) Mast cell

    (d) Plasma cell

    Answer for Q 44 on page 353

45. The change in color, shape, and texture of gingiva are seen in:

    (a) Stage 1 gingivitis

    (b) Stage 2 gingivitis

    (c) Stage 3 gingivitis

    (d) Stage 4 gingivitis

    Answer for Q 45 on page 353

46. One of the following bacterial species is **not** associated with adult periodontitis:

    (a) *Fusobacterium nucleatum*

    (b) *Bacteroides forsythus*

    (c) *Porphyromonas gingivalis*

    (d) *Shigella sonnei*

    (e) *Prevotella intermedia*

    Answer for Q 46 on page 353

47. Collagen fibrils have a transverse striation with a characteristic periodicity of:

    (a) 64 centimeters

    (b) 64 nanometers

    (c) 640 micrometers

    (d) 640 nanometers

    Answer for Q 47 on page 353

48. Early and established stage of gingivitis is differentiated by increase in number of:
    (a) Plasma cells
    (b) Neutrophil
    (c) B cells
    (d) Macrophages

    Answer for Q 48 on page 353

49. Which stage of gingivitis is also called subclinical gingivitis?
    (a) Initial stage
    (b) Advanced stage
    (c) Early stage
    (d) Established stage

    Answer for Q 49 on page 353

50. When looking at the notes of a patient, you see annotation for a Basic Periodontal Examination (BPE). What does a score of 3 mean on this particular index?
    (a) Gingival bleeding, no overhangs or calculus, pockets > 3.5 mm
    (b) Pockets within color-coded area, 4.5–6.5 mm
    (c) Color-coded area disappears, pockets > 5.5 mm
    (d) Pockets within color-coded area, 3.5–5.5 mm
    (e) Color-coded area disappears, pockets > 5.5 mm

    Answer for Q 50 on page 353

51. Pregnancy gingivitis is caused by:
    (a) *Bacteroides melaninogenicus*
    (b) *Actinobacillus actinomycetemcomitans*
    (c) *Streptococcus sanguis*
    (d) *Fusobacterium*

    Answer for Q 51 on page 353

52. When the dental plaque is allowed to accumulate in the absence of any plaque control procedures, it results in gingivitis within:
    (a) 1 to 3 days
    (b) 7 to 21 days
    (c) 2 months to 3 months
    (d) 24 hours to 48 hours

    Answer for Q 52 on page 353

53. Atypical gingivitis is:

(a) Other name of plasma cell gingivitis

(b) gingivitis seen in HIV patients

(c) gingivitis seen in Leukemia patients

(d) Gingivitis seen in aggressive periodontitis

Answer for Q 53 on page 353

54. Which one of the following statements regarding acute necrotizing ulcerative gingivitis (ANUG) is **true**?

(a) It is caused by Gram-positive anaerobic bacteria

(b) It is characterized by chronic onset

(c) It affects non-smokers more than smokers

(d) It is caused by acid fast bacilli

(e) It is characterized by interproximal necrosis (crater-shaped interdental papilla)

Answer for Q 54 on page 353

55. The predominant cell type in gingival crevicular fluid is the:

(a) Mast cell

(b) Plasma cell

(c) Macrophage

(d) Polymorphonuclear leukocyte

Answer for Q 55 on page 353

56. Gingival crevicular fluid is measured using:

(a) Whatman's filter paper

(b) pH paper

(c) Mylar strip

(d) Litmus paper

Answer for Q 56 on page 353

57. Correct treatment of a patient with ANUG is:

(a) 20% chlorhexidine mouthwashes twice daily

(b) Amoxicillin 500 mg three times daily for 5 days and 20% chlorhexidine mouth washes twice daily

(c) Erythromycin 250 mg four times daily for 5 days and 20% chlorhexidine mouthwashes twice daily

(d) Scaling and oral hygiene instruction

(e) Metronidazole 400 mg three times daily for 5 days and hydrogen peroxide mouthwash twice daily

Answer for Q 57 on page 353

58. The predominant immunoglobulin in sulcular fluid is:
    (a) IgA
    (b) IgG
    (c) IgM
    (d) IgE

    Answer for Q 58 on page 354

59. Which one of the following statements about tooth mobility is **incorrect**?
    (a) Movement of a crown of the tooth in the horizontal plane of less than 0.2 mm is considered normal
    (b) Grade 1 means movement of the crown of a tooth in the horizontal plane is 0.2–1 mm
    (c) Grade 2 means movement of the crown of a tooth in the horizontal plane is greater than 1 mm
    (d) Grade 3 means movement of the crown of a tooth in the horizontal plane is greater than 3 mm
    (e) Grade 3 means movement of the crown of a tooth in the vertical plane

    Answer for Q 59 on page 354

60. Orogranulocytes are:
    (a) Granulocytes present in the gingival connective tissue
    (b) Mast cells present in the GCF
    (c) PMNs reaching the oral cavity through subepithelium
    (d) All of the above

    Answer for Q 60 on page 354

61. Drug which reaches maximum concentration in gingival fluid is:
    (a) Tetracycline
    (b) Penicillin
    (c) Erythromycin
    (d) Sulfonamides

    Answer for Q 61 on page 354

62. Which one of the following clinical conditions predispose patients with impaired/defective neutrophil function to severe periodontitis?
    (a) Patterson–Brown–Kelly syndrome
    (b) Chediak–Higashi disease
    (c) Hypothyroidism
    (d) Hyperthyroidism
    (e) Gardner's syndrome

    Answer for Q 62 on page 354

63. Which cell type migrates into the gingival sulcus in large numbers in response to dental plaque?

    (a) Mast cells
    (b) Neutrophils
    (c) Lymphocytes
    (d) Plasma cells

    Answer for Q 63 on page 354

64. Sulcular fluid **<u>does not</u>** perform one of the following functions:

    (a) Contains plasma proteins which may improve adhesion
    (b) Possess antimicrobial properties
    (c) Exerts antibody activity
    (d) Provides nutrition to junctional epithelium via diffusion

    Answer for Q 64 on page 354

65. Which one of the following is associated with abnormal collagen formation leading to periodontal disease?

    (a) Type 1 diabetes mellitus
    (b) Papillon–Lefèvre syndrome
    (c) Hypophosphatasia
    (d) Type 2 diabetes mellitus
    (e) Hyperphosphatasia

    Answer for Q 65 on page 354

66. Glucose levels in gingival crevicular fluid (GCF) are:

    (a) Equal to glucose levels in serum
    (b) Zero
    (c) 3–4 times greater than serum levels
    (d) more than 10 times the serum levels

    Answer for Q 66 on page 354

67. It is likely that cell mediated immune reactions (delayed hypersensitivity) occur in periodontitis because subjects with periodontitis have:

    (a) High levels of histamine in involved gingival tissue
    (b) IgG antibodies reactive with plaque bacterial antigens
    (c) T lymphocytes sensitized to bacterial plaque antigens
    (d) High levels of collagenase in gingival fluids

    Answer for Q 67 on page 354

68. What is the name of the probe shown in the figure?

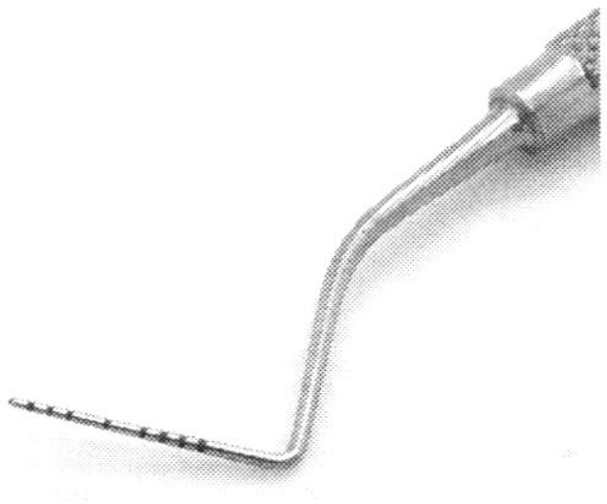

(a) Briault's

(b) Community Periodontal Index of Treatment Needs (CPITN)

(c) World Health Organization (WHO)

(d) Williams probe

(e) Florida

Answer for Q 68 on page 354

69. Leukotoxin:

(a) kills neutrophils

(b) attracts neutrophils

(c) aggregates neutrophils

(d) enhances phagocyte activity

Answer for Q 69 on page 354

70. The most potent bone resorbing interleukin is:

(a) IL-8

(b) IL-1B

(c) IL-5

(d) IL-3

Answer for Q 70 on page 354

71. In juvenile periodontitis, which bacterium is the recognized etiological agent?

(a) *Porphyromonas gingivalis*

(b) *Prevotella intermedia*

(c) *Actinobacillus actinomycetemcomitans*

(d) *Borrelia burgdorferi*

(e) *Fusobacterium intermedium*

Answer for Q 71 on page 355

72. Leukotoxin is released by:

    (a) *P. nucleatum*

    (b) *naeslundii*

    (c) *Forsythia*

    (d) *Actinomycetemcomitans*

    Answer for Q 72 on page 355

73. Which teeth are most commonly affected in juvenile periodontitis?

    (a) Incisors and first permanent molars

    (b) Incisors and canines

    (c) Canines and premolars

    (d) Premolars and first permanent molars

    (e) Canines and first permanent molars

    Answer for Q 73 on page 355

74. Plaque is considered as infection because:

    (a) Antibiotics prevent its formation

    (b) Its presence is evidence of bacterial growth

    (c) It is communicable between experimental animals and probably humans

    (d) Absent in germ-free animals

    (e) All of the above

    Answer for Q 74 on page 355

75. The gingival crevicular fluid is increased in all **except**:

    (a) Gingivitis

    (b) Smoking

    (c) Periodontal pocket

    (d) Trauma from occlusion

    Answer for Q 75 on page 355

76. The inorganic component of subgingival plaque is derived from:

    (a) Saliva

    (b) Gingival crevicular fluid

    (c) Inorganic matter of tooth

    (d) Food Debris

    Answer for Q 76 on page 355

77. Gingival fluid is a:
    (a) Transudate[2]
    (b) Can be either of the two (transudate and exudate)
    (c) Exudate
    (d) Neither of the two (transudate and exudate)

    Answer for Q 77 on page 355

78. What are the cells that produce PGE2 in the periodontium?
    (a) Macrophages
    (b) Fibroblasts
    (c) Neutrophils
    (d) Both Macrophages and Fibroblasts

    Answer for Q 78 on page 355

79. For which teeth surfaces would you use a Gracey no #1 or no #2 curette when scaling?
    (a) All teeth
    (b) All surfaces of anterior teeth
    (c) Mesial surfaces of anterior teeth
    (d) All surfaces of posterior teeth
    (e) Mesial surfaces of posterior teeth

    Answer for Q 79 on page 355

80. To identify oral microorganism in periodontal disease, Koch's postulate has been modified by:
    (a) Glickman
    (b) Socransky
    (c) Russel
    (d) Vermillion

    Answer for Q 80 on page 355

81. A parulis, is a localized accumulation of pus located within the
    (a) pulp
    (b) skin
    (c) fascial spaces
    (d) gum

    Answer for Q 81 on page 355

[2] An ultrafiltrate of plasma that contains few, if any, cells and does not contain large plasma proteins, such as fibrinogen. Transudate results from increased hydrostatic or reduced osmotic pressure.

82. One or more of the following syndromes are associated with gingival enlargement:
    (a) Elephantiasis gingivae
    (b) Plummer-Vinson syndrome
    (c) Rutherford syndrome
    (d) A & C
    (e) A & B

    Answer for Q 82 on page 355

83. One or more of the following conditions are associated with the premature loss of teeth:
    (a) Chédiak-Higashi syndrome
    (b) Plummer-Vinson syndrome
    (c) Papillon-Lefèvre syndrome
    (d) A & B
    (e) A & C

    Answer for Q 83 on page 355

84. In CPITN:
    (a) The dentition is divided into seven segments
    (b) Pocketing of 4–5 mm, that is, when the gingival margin is on the clear area is code no. #3
    (c) Pocketing of 6 mm or more, that is when the gingival margin is on the black area of the probe is code no
    (d) For appropriate treatment plan code 2 requires improvement in home care
    (e) For appropriate treatment plan code 3 require supra and subgingival scaling and improvement in home care

    Answer for Q 84 on page 355

85. U.S. food and drug administration for the adjunctive therapy of periodontitis has approved doxycycline hyclate:
    (a) Available as 100 mg capsule for use twice daily
    (b) Available as 20 mg capsule for use twice daily [15]
    (c) Available 200 mg capsule for use twice daily
    (d) Available as 40 mg capsule for use twice daily
    (e) Available as 20 mg capsule for once daily use

    Answer for Q 85 on page 355

86. Root planning is:
    (a) Removal of material Alba and stains from root surface
    (b) Removal of soft tissue wall of the periodontal pocket
    (c) Removal of calculus & plaque from root surface
    (d) Removal of food debris from tooth surface
    (e) Removal of diseased cementum along with other root deposits

    Answer for Q 86 on page 356

87. Greater occlusal pressure on the periodontium produces:
    (a) Increased resorption of alveolar bone and formation of cementum
    (b) A gradation of changes in periodontal ligament starting with tension of fibers which produce areas of fibrosis
    (c) Injury to fibroblasts and other connective tissue cells lead to necrosis of areas of the ligament
    (d) Disintegration of blood vessels within 30 minutes
    (e) Disintegration of blood vessels within 05 minutes

    Answer for Q 87 on page 356

88. Endocarditis prophylaxis is recommended in:
    (a) Mitral valve prolapse without valvular regurgitation
    (b) Previous coronary artery bypass graft surgery
    (c) Cardiac pacemakers
    (d) Implanted defibrillators
    (e) Tetralogy of Fallot

    Answer for Q 88 on page 356

89. The mobility of the teeth is graded 3 if:
    (a) The mobility is 1 mm
    (b) The mobility is less than 1 mm
    (c) The mobility is in apicoocclusal direction and 1 mm in labiolingual direction
    (d) The mobility is in apicoocclusal direction and mobility is less than 1 mm in labio-lingual direction
    (e) The mobility is in apicoocclusal direction and mobility in labiolingual direction is more than 2 mm

    Answer for Q 89 on page 356

90. The wavelength of the CO_2 laser used for gingivectomy is:
   (a) 10,600 nm
   (b) 1064 nm
   (c) 10 nm
   (d) 100 nm
   (e) 500 nm

   Answer for Q 90 on page 356

91. Localized aggressive periodontitis is best treated in early stage by:
   (a) Tetracycline 250 mg 4 times daily for fourteen days
   (b) Tetracycline 250 mg once daily for 7 days
   (c) Tetracycline 250 mg twice daily for 7 days
   (d) Tetracycline 250 mg 4 times daily for 3 days
   (e) Tetracycline 250 mg 4 times daily for 5 days

   Answer for Q 91 on page 356

92. Furcation involvement is measured by:
   (a) WHO probe
   (b) CPITN probe
   (c) Naber's probe
   (d) Michigan "O" probe
   (e) Periodontal explorer

   Answer for Q 92 on page 356

93. Classically the epithelial rete pegs show a saw tooth appearance, hyperkeratosis or parakeratosis, hydropic degeneration of basal layer and a dense band like infiltrate of T lymphocytes microscopically in:
   (a) Pemphigus
   (b) Pemphigoid
   (c) Linear IgA disease
   (d) Lichen planus
   (e) Chronic ulcerative stomatitis

   Answer for Q 93 on page 356

94. Vincent's angina is a fusispirochetal infection of:
   (a) Marginal gingival
   (b) Oropharynx and throat
   (c) Heart
   (d) Larynx and colon
   (e) Middle ear and small intestine

   Answer for Q 94 on page 356

95. The bacteria detected in localized aggressive periodontitis are:
   (a) *Borrelia vincenti*, medium size spirochetes
   (b) *Fusiformis, Tanerella forsythus*
   (c) *Actinobacillus actinomycetemcomitans, capnocytophaga Spp., Eikenella corrodens, campylobacter rectus, prevotella intermedia*
   (d) *Mycoplasma, capnocytophaga sputigena, spirocheles*
   (e) *Treponema denticola, fusobacterium nucleatum, rectus, Actinobacillus Actinomycetemcomitans*

   Answer for Q 95 on page 356

96. Acute periodontal abscess is treated by:
   (a) Gingivoplasty
   (b) Gingivectomy
   (c) Periodontal flap procedure
   (d) Antibiotics
   (e) Drainage through the gingival sulcus or by an external incision

   Answer for Q 96 on page 356

97. Tumor metastasizing to gingiva is/are:
   (a) Papilloma
   (b) Central giant cell carcinoma of the jaw
   (c) Fibroma
   (d) Lipoma
   (e) Adenocarcinoma of colon, renal cell carcinoma, hypernephroma, lung carcinoma

   Answer for Q 97 on page 356

98. Periodontal destruction is considered moderate when:
    - (a) 3–4 mm of clinical attachment loss has occurred in chronic periodontitis
    - (b) 1–2 mm of clinical attachment loss has occurred in chronic periodontitis
    - (c) 5 mm or more of clinical attachment loss has occurred in chronic periodontitis
    - (d) 0–1 mm of clinical attachment loss has occurred
    - (e) 0.5–0.9 mm of clinical attachment loss has occurred in chronic periodontitis

    Answer for Q 98 on page 356

99. Primary endodontic lesion requires:
    - (a) Minor periodontal treatment only
    - (b) Periodontal surgical treatment only
    - (c) A combined periodontal and endodontic treatment
    - (d) Endodontic treatment only
    - (e) A periodontal flap procedure

    Answer for Q 99 on page 356

100. False gingival enlargement is caused by:
    - (a) Underlying drug induced gingival enlargement
    - (b) Underlying inflammation of periodontal ligament
    - (c) Underlying dental and osseous structures
    - (d) By epulis
    - (e) Sarcoidosis

    Answer for Q 100 on page 356

101. Hypophosphatasia is characterized by:
    - (a) High level of serum alkaline phosphatase and phosphoethanolamine
    - (b) Low level of serum alkaline phosphatase and high level of phosphoehtanolamine
    - (c) Low level of serum alkaline phosphatase and low level of phosphoethanolamine
    - (d) High level of alkaline phosphatase and low level of phosphoethanolamine
    - (e) Low level of acid phosphatase and alkaline phosphatase

    Answer for Q 101 on page 356

102. Necrotising ulcerative periodontitis:
   (a) Is associated with deep periodontal pockets
   (b) Is associated with a crater like depression at the tip of interdental papilla and vesicle formation
   (c) Is associated with a crater like interdental bony depression
   (d) Is not responsive to any therapy
   (e) Leads to gingival recession because of faulty tooth brushing

   Answer for Q 102 on page 357

103. Subclinical gingivitis is:
   (a) Characterized by vascular proliferation
   (b) Characterized by predominantly lymphocytes microscopically
   (c) Characterized by predominantly plasma cells microscopically
   (d) Characterized by erythema, bleeding on probing
   (e) Characterized by increased crevicular fluid flow and infiltration of sulcular and junctional epithelium by polymorphonuclear leukocytes

   Answer for Q 103 on page 357

104. The amount of gingival crevicular fluid is:
   (a) Decreased when inflammation is present
   (b) Increase by trauma from occlusion
   (c) Decreased by mastication of coarse foods and smoking
   (d) Decreased by ovulation and hormonal contraceptives
   (e) Increased by tooth brushing and gingival massage

   Answer for Q 104 on page 357

105. Dentogingival unit:
   (a) Is sulcular epithelium and gingival fibers
   (b) Is junctional epithelium and gingival fibers
   (c) Is sulcular epithelium and periodontal fibers
   (d) Is junctional epithelium and periodontal fibers
   (e) Is oral epithelium and gingival fibers

   Answer for Q 105 on page 357

106. Transseptal fibers extend:

(a) Obliquely from the cementum just beneath the junctional epithelium to the alveolar crest

(b) From the cementum in a coronal direction obliquely to the bone

(c) From the cementum to cementum in the furcation areas of the multirooted teeth

(d) Interproximally over the alveolar crest and are embedded in cementum of adjacent teeth

(e) At right angles to the long axis of the tooth from cementum to the alveolar bone

Answer for Q 106 on page 357

107. The growth of *Porphyromonas gingivalis* is enhanced by metabolic by products:

(a) Succinate from *Campylobacter rectus*

(b) Protoheme from *Capnocytophaga*

(c) Protoheme from *Campylobacter rectus*

(d) Succinate from *Veillonella*

(e) Protoheme from *Fusobacterium*

Answer for Q 107 on page 357

108. Leukemic gingival enlargement:

(a) Occurs in edentulous areas

(b) Occurs in chronic leukemia

(c) Occurs by abnormal accumulation of leukemia cells in dermal and subcutaneous connective tissue

(d) Occurs by dense cellular accumulation in papillary layer of connective tissue

(e) Occurs by dense cellular accumulation in reticular layer of connective tissue

Answer for Q 108 on page 357

109. A linear (Burtonian line) steel gray gingival pigmentation associated with local inflammation occurs in:

(a) Bismuth intoxication

(b) Lead intoxication

(c) Mercury intoxication

(d) Arsenic intoxication

(e) Chromium intoxication

Answer for Q 109 on page 357

110. The initial colonizers in the dental plaque are:

(a) *Fusobacterium nucleatum, prevotella intermedia*

(b) *Capnocytophaga species, campylobacter rectus*

(c) *Tannerella forsythus, bacterionema maturochottii*

(d) *Streptococcus sanguis, actinomyces viscosus*

(e) *Eikehella corrodens, actinobacills actenomycetem comitans*

Answer for Q 110 on page 357

111. A forcibly embedded tooth brush bristle may be retained in the gingiva and cause:

(a) Gingival recession

(b) Periodontal pocket

(c) Attachment loss

(d) Bone loss

(e) Gingival abscess

Answer for Q 111 on page 357

112. Vitamin B deficiency results in:

(a) Deep periodontal pockets

(b) Hemorrhagic diathesis in the gingival

(c) Loss of lamina dura

(d) Glossitis, glossodynia, gingivitis, inflammation of entire oral mucosa

(e) Accelerated gingival wound healing

Answer for Q 112 on page 357

113. There is partial or complete loss of lamina dura in:

(a) Hypoparthyroidism

(b) Hyperparathyroidism

(c) Beri beri

(d) Pellgra

(e) Hypervitaminosis D

Answer for Q 113 on page 357

114. Mineralization of plaque may start intracellularly in:

   (a) *Streptococcus sanguis* and *actinomyces viscosus* species

   (b) *Porphyromonas gingivalis* and *prevotela* intermedia species

   (c) *Diptheroids, bacterionema, veillonella* species

   (d) *Borrelia vincenti* and *Actinobacillus Actinomycetemcomitans*

   (e) *Capnocytophaga* and *Campylobacter rectus* and *Tenneralla forsythus*

   Answer for Q 114 on page 357

115. Severe generalized periodontitis has been reported in:

   (a) Tetralogy of Fallot (ToF)

   (b) Tetralogy of Eisenmenger syndrome

   (c) Initial lesion

   (d) Early lesion

   (e) Vitamin A deficiency

   Answer for Q 115 on page 357

116. Mineral precipitation results from a local rise in the degree of saturation of calcium and phosphate ions because:

   (a) A decrease in the pH of the saliva cause precipitation of calcium and phosphate ions

   (b) An increase in the pH of the saliva cause precipitation of calcium and phosphate ions by lowering of precipitation constant

   (c) A decrease in pH of saliva lowers precipitation constant leading to precipitation of calcium and phosphate ion

   (d) An increase in the pH of saliva increases precipitation constant leading to precipitation of calcium and phosphate ions

   (e) An increase in the pH of saliva with no effect on precipitation constant

   Answer for Q 116 on page 357

117. The incidence of lingual recession and pocket formation and radiographic evidence of bone loss among subjects with a mean age of 22 years who wore lingual "barbells" for 2 years or more according to Campbell et al is:

   (a) 97%

   (b) 50%

   (c) 62%

   (d) 10%

   (e) 5%

Answer for Q 117 on page 357

118. Non eugenol periodontal dressing:
   (a) The retention is by chemically interlocking in the interdental areas
   (b) Contact allergy to eugenol has been reported
   (c) There is asbestos
   (d) Is placed for two weeks
   (e) Is placed for one week

Answer for Q 118 on page 358

119. Synthetic resorbable suturing materials in periodontal surgery is:
   (a) Polyglycolic
   (b) Expanded polytetra fluoroethylene
   (c) Nylon
   (d) Polyester
   (e) Chromic gut

Answer for Q 119 on page 358

120. Excisional new attachment procedure involves:
   (a) A periodontal flap
   (b) A free gingival graft
   (c) A regenerative osseous procedure
   (d) Root planning
   (e) Internal bevel incision from the margin of the free gingiva apically to point below bottom of pocket

Answer for Q 120 on page 358

121. Non bone graft materials used in periodontal surgery include:
   (a) Cartilage, cementum, xenograft
   (b) Dentin, plaster of Paris, allografts
   (c) Ceramics, coral derived material ls, autografts
   (d) Cartilage, sclera, dura, dentin, cementum
   (e) Xenografts, dentin

Answer for Q 121 on page 358

122. Papilla preservation flap:

(a) Is a conventional flap procedures?

(b) Is used when narrow interdental spaces are present

(c) Is used for teeth with wide interdental spaces

(d) Is a partial thickness flap

(e) Is a apically displaced flap

Answer for Q 122 on page 358

123. Guided tissue regeneration involves:

(a) Formation of cementum with recession of gingiva

(b) Epithelial migration on the cementum surface

(c) Biomend, a bovine achilles tendon collagen that resorbs in 4–18 weeks

(d) A resective osseous procedure

(e) Atrisorb a polyglycolic acid gel

Answer for Q 123 on page 358

124. Average human biologic width is:

(a) 3 mm

(b) 2 mm

(c) 4 mm

(d) 1 mm

(e) 0.5 mm

Answer for Q 124 on page 358

125. Löe et al found the rate of bone loss to average about:

(a) 0.2 mm a year for facial surfaces and about 0.3 mm a year for proximal surfaces

(b) 0.3 mm a year for facial surfaces and about 0. 2mm a year for proximal surfaces

(c) 0.5 mm a year for facial surfaces and about 0.05 mm a year for proximal surfaces

(d) 0.1 mm a year for facial surfaces and about 1.00 mm a year for proximal surfaces

(e) 0.5 mm a year for facial surfaces and about 1.5 mm a year for proximal surfaces

Answer for Q 125 on page 358

126. The distance between the apical extent of the calculus and alveolar crest in human periodontal pockets is:

(a) 0.2 mm

(b) 3 mm

(c) 1.97 mm (=33.16%)

(d) 4 mm

(e) 0.02 mm

Answer for Q 126 on page 358

127. Horizontal bone loss is present in:

(a) Localized aggressive periodontitis

(b) Generalized aggressive periodontitis

(c) Infrabony pockets

(d) Chronic periodontitis

(e) Acute necrotizing ulcerative gingivitis

Answer for Q 127 on page 358

128. Regional lymph node enlargement is present in:

(a) Acute pericoronitis [15]

(b) Lichen planus

(c) Pemphigoid

(d) Pemphigus vulgaris

(e) Chronic ulcerative stomatitis

Answer for Q 128 on page 358

129. Look carefully into the following diagram and select the correct label for the biological human width.

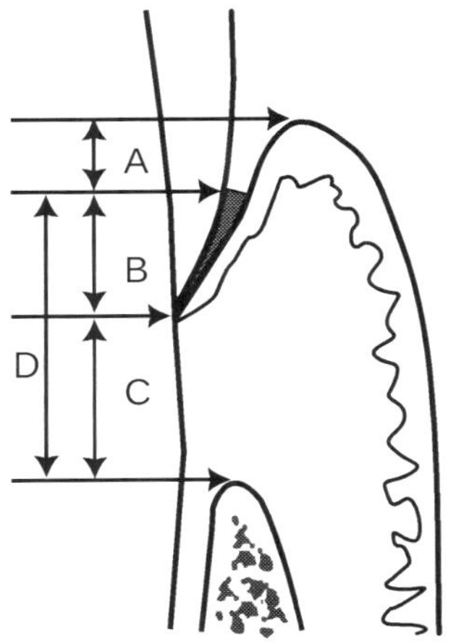

(a) Biological width is A

(b) Biological width is B

(c) Biological width is D

(d) Biological width is C

Answer for Q 129 on page 358

18.2 Answers with Comments:

1. The correct answer is **B** – Fixed or immovable joints between bones and teeth or bones and other bones through tough fibrous tissue. Gomphosis can allow a very tiny movements between parts.

   Back to Q 1 on page 321
2. The correct answer is **D** – The possible sources of exposure include lead contaminated water or paint and mercury or silver containing drugs.

   Back to Q 2 on page 321
3. The correct answer is **A** – No explanation is available for this answer.

   Back to Q 3 on page 322
4. The correct answer is **D** – Periodontal condition in which the marginal gingiva surrounding the tooth is enlarged in a form resembling a doughnut.

   Back to Q 4 on page 322
5. The correct answer is **D** – No explanation is available for this answer.

   Back to Q 5 on page 322
6. The correct answer is **A** – No explanation is available for this answer.

   Back to Q 6 on page 322
7. The correct answer is **B** – No explanation is available for this answer.

   Back to Q 7 on page 322
8. The correct answer is **B** – No explanation is available for this answer.

   Back to Q 8 on page 323
9. The correct answer is **A** – No explanation is available for this answer.

   Back to Q 9 on page 323
10. The correct answer is **A** – No explanation is available for this answer.

    Back to Q 10 on page 323
11. The correct answer is **B** – Poor oral hygiene is the most important factor contributing to gingivitis in children.

Back to Q 11 on page 323

12. The correct answer is **B** – No explanation is available for this answer.

Back to Q 12 on page 323

13. The correct answer is **C** – No explanation is available for this answer.

Back to Q 13 on page 324

14. The correct answer is **B** – No explanation is available for this answer.

Back to Q 14 on page 324

15. The correct answer is **C** – No explanation is available for this answer.

Back to Q 15 on page 324

16. The correct answer is **D** – Any chronic inflammation is characterized by infiltration with lymphocytes, plasma cells, and polymorph nuclear leukocytes.

Back to Q 16 on page 324

17. The correct answer is **A** – No explanation is available for this answer.

Back to Q 17 on page 324

18. The correct answer is **D** – No explanation is available for this answer.

Back to Q 18 on page 325

19. The correct answer is **D** – No explanation is available for this answer.

Back to Q 19 on page 325

20. The correct answer is **B** – No explanation is available for this answer.

Back to Q 20 on page 325

21. The correct answer is **B** – No explanation is available for this answer.

Back to Q 21 on page 325

22. The correct answer is **D** – No explanation is available for this answer.

Back to Q 22 on page 325

23. The correct answer is **B** – No explanation is available for this answer.

Back to Q 23 on page 326

24. The correct answer is **A** – Prognosis - A > B > C > D.

Back to Q 24 on page 326

25. The correct answer is **B** – No explanation is available for this answer.

Back to Q 25 on page 326

26. The correct answer is **C** – No explanation is available for this answer.

Back to Q 26 on page 326

27. The correct answer is **A** – No explanation is available for this answer.

Back to Q 27 on page 326

28. The correct answer is **D** – No explanation is available for this answer.

Back to Q 28 on page 327

29. The correct answer is **B** – No explanation is available for this answer.

Back to Q 29 on page 327

30. The correct answer is **A** – No explanation is available for this answer.

Back to Q 30 on page 327

31. The correct answer is **D** – No explanation is available for this answer.

Back to Q 31 on page 327

32. The correct answer is **D** – No explanation is available for this answer.

Back to Q 32 on page 327

33. The correct answer is **A** – No explanation is available for this answer.

Back to Q 33 on page 328

34. The correct answer is **D** – No explanation is available for this answer.

Back to Q 34 on page 328

35. The correct answer is **D** – No explanation is available for this answer.

Back to Q 35 on page 328

36. The correct answer is **A** – No explanation is available for this answer.

Back to Q 36 on page 328

37. The correct answer is **A** – No explanation is available for this answer.

Back to Q 37 on page 328

38. The correct answer is **C** – No explanation is available for this answer.

Back to Q 38 on page 329

39. The correct answer is **A** – Oral lesions may resemble actinomycosis, Dimorphic fungus is causing the disease,Associated with erythema multiforme.

Back to Q 39 on page 329

40. The correct answer is **D** – No explanation is available for this answer.

Back to Q 40 on page 329

41. The correct answer is **B** – No explanation is available for this answer.

Back to Q 41 on page 329

42. The correct answer is **A** – No explanation is available for this answer.

Back to Q 42 on page 329

43. The correct answer is **B** – No explanation is available for this answer.

Back to Q 43 on page 330

44. The correct answer is **D** – No explanation is available for this answer.

Back to Q 44 on page 330

45. The correct answer is **C** – No explanation is available for this answer.

Back to Q 45 on page 330

46. The correct answer is **D** – All of the mentioned bacteria in the list are responsible for adult periodontitis except *S. sonnei*, which is responsible for acute diarrhea.

Back to Q 46 on page 330

47. The correct answer is **B** – No explanation is available for this answer.

Back to Q 47 on page 330

48. The correct answer is **A** – No explanation is available for this answer.

Back to Q 48 on page 331

49. The correct answer is **A** – No explanation is available for this answer.

Back to Q 49 on page 331

50. The correct answer is **D** – No explanation is available for this answer.

Back to Q 50 on page 331

51. The correct answer is **A** – No explanation is available for this answer.

Back to Q 51 on page 331

52. The correct answer is **B** – No explanation is available for this answer.

Back to Q 52 on page 331

53. The correct answer is **A** – No explanation is available for this answer.

Back to Q 53 on page 332

54. The correct answer is **E** – ANUG is caused by Gram-negative aerobic bacteria, usually in the mandible, has a very distinctive smell (fetor oris) and is more common in smokers and those with poor oral hygiene.

Back to Q 54 on page 332

55. The correct answer is **D** – No explanation is available for this answer.

Back to Q 55 on page 332

56. The correct answer is **A** – No explanation is available for this answer.

Back to Q 56 on page 332

57. The correct answer is **E** – The bacterial is anaerobic and oxygen in hydrogen peroxide render the environment unsuitable for its growth. The most efficacious mouthwash is hydrogen peroxide, and the

bacterial component is treated with metronidazole. Amoxicillin and erythromycin would be ineffective in treatment of this condition.

Back to Q 57 on page 332

58. The correct answer is **B** – Tooth mobility is graded as shown in the table below:
    (a) Movement of the crown of a tooth in the horizontal plane is 0.2–1 mm
    (b) Movement of the crown of a tooth in the horizontal plane is greater than 1 mm
    (c) Movement of the crown of a tooth in the vertical plane

Back to Q 58 on page 333

59. The correct answer is **D** – No explanation is available for this answer.

Back to Q 59 on page 333

60. The correct answer is **C** – No explanation is available for this answer.

Back to Q 60 on page 333

61. The correct answer is **A** – No explanation is available for this answer.

Back to Q 61 on page 333

62. The correct answer is **B** – None of the others are relevant to periodontal disease.

Back to Q 62 on page 333

63. The correct answer is **B** – No explanation is available for this answer.

Back to Q 63 on page 334

64. The correct answer is **D** – No explanation is available for this answer.

Back to Q 64 on page 334

65. The correct answer is **C** – Hypophosphatasia, as well as Ehlers–Danlos syndrome are associated with abnormal collagen formation and periodontal disease. Papillon–Lefèvre syndrome is associated with abnormal neutrophil function, which contributes to the severity of periodontal disease.

Back to Q 65 on page 334

66. The correct answer is **C** – No explanation is available for this answer.

Back to Q 66 on page 334

67. The correct answer is **C** – No explanation is available for this answer.

Back to Q 67 on page 334

68. The correct answer is **D** – The probe shown is the Williams' probe, which has 1 mm increments for accurate measurement of the pocket depth.

Back to Q 68 on page 335

69. The correct answer is **A** – No explanation is available for this answer.

Back to Q 69 on page 335

70. The correct answer is **B** – No explanation is available for this answer.

Back to Q 70 on page 335

71. The correct answer is **C** – *A. actinomycetemcomitans* is a capnophilic, non-motile rod that possesses a potent leucotoxin, which causes lysis of polymorphonuclear leukocytes.

Back to Q 71 on page 335

72. The correct answer is **D** – No explanation is available for this answer.

Back to Q 72 on page 336

73. The correct answer is **A** – As these are the first teeth to erupt, they seem to be the teeth which are affected most by juvenile periodontitis.

Back to Q 73 on page 336

74. The correct answer is **E** – No explanation is available for this answer.

Back to Q 74 on page 336

75. The correct answer is **D** – No explanation is available for this answer.

Back to Q 75 on page 336

76. The correct answer is **B** – No explanation is available for this answer.

Back to Q 76 on page 336

77. The correct answer is **C** – No explanation is available for this answer.

Back to Q 77 on page 337

78. The correct answer is **D** – No explanation is available for this answer.

Back to Q 78 on page 337

79. The correct answer is **B** – A Gracey no 1 or no 2 is ideally shaped to facilitate scaling of all surfaces of anterior teeth.

Back to Q 79 on page 337

80. The correct answer is **B** – No explanation is available for this answer.

Back to Q 80 on page 337

81. The correct answer is **D** – No explanation is available for this answer.

Back to Q 81 on page 337

82. The correct answer is **D** – No explanation is available for this answer.

Back to Q 82 on page 338

83. The correct answer is **E** – No explanation is available for this answer.

Back to Q 83 on page 338

84. The correct answer is **E** – No explanation is available for this answer.

Back to Q 84 on page 338

85. The correct answer is **B** – No explanation is available for this answer.

Back to Q 85 on page 338

86. The correct answer is **E** – No explanation is available for this answer.

Back to Q 86 on page 339

87. The correct answer is **C** – No explanation is available for this answer.

Back to Q 87 on page 339

88. The correct answer is **E** – No explanation is available for this answer.

Back to Q 88 on page 339

89. The correct answer is **A** – No explanation is available for this answer.

Back to Q 89 on page 339

90. The correct answer is **A** – No explanation is available for this answer.

Back to Q 90 on page 340

91. The correct answer is **A** – No explanation is available for this answer.

Back to Q 91 on page 340

92. The correct answer is **C** – No explanation is available for this answer.

Back to Q 92 on page 340

93. The correct answer is **D** – No explanation is available for this answer.

Back to Q 93 on page 340

94. The correct answer is **B** – No explanation is available for this answer.

Back to Q 94 on page 341

95. The correct answer is **C** – No explanation is available for this answer.

Back to Q 95 on page 341

96. The correct answer is **E** – No explanation is available for this answer.

Back to Q 96 on page 341

97. The correct answer is **E** – No explanation is available for this answer.

Back to Q 97 on page 341

98. The correct answer is **A** – No explanation is available for this answer.

Back to Q 98 on page 342

99. The correct answer is **D** – No explanation is available for this answer.

Back to Q 99 on page 342

100. The correct answer is **C** – No explanation is available for this answer.

Back to Q 100 on page 342

101. The correct answer is **C** – No explanation is available for this answer.

Back to Q 101 on page 342

102. The correct answer is **C** – No explanation is available for this answer.

Back to Q 102 on page 343

103. The correct answer is **E** – No explanation is available for this answer.

Back to Q 103 on page 343

104. The correct answer is **E** – No explanation is available for this answer.

Back to Q 104 on page 343

105. The correct answer is **B** – No explanation is available for this answer.

Back to Q 105 on page 343

106. The correct answer is **D** – No explanation is available for this answer.

Back to Q 106 on page 344

107. The correct answer is **C** – No explanation is available for this answer.

Back to Q 107 on page 344

108. The correct answer is **E** – No explanation is available for this answer.

Back to Q 108 on page 344

109. The correct answer is **B** – No explanation is available for this answer.

Back to Q 109 on page 344

110. The correct answer is **D** – No explanation is available for this answer.

Back to Q 110 on page 345

111. The correct answer is **E** – No explanation is available for this answer.

Back to Q 111 on page 345

112. The correct answer is **D** – No explanation is available for this answer.

Back to Q 112 on page 345

113. The correct answer is **B** – No explanation is available for this answer.

Back to Q 113 on page 345

114. The correct answer is **C** – No explanation is available for this answer.

Back to Q 114 on page 346

115. The correct answer is **B** – No explanation is available for this answer.

Back to Q 115 on page 346

116. The correct answer is **B** – No explanation is available for this answer.

Back to Q 116 on page 346

117. The correct answer is **B** – No explanation is available for this answer.

Back to Q 117 on page 346

118. The correct answer is **E** – No explanation is available for this answer.

Back to Q 118 on page 347

119. The correct answer is **A** – No explanation is available for this answer.

Back to Q 119 on page 347

120. The correct answer is **E** – No explanation is available for this answer.

Back to Q 120 on page 347

121. The correct answer is **B** – No explanation is available for this answer.

Back to Q 121 on page 347

122. The correct answer is **C** – No explanation is available for this answer.

Back to Q 122 on page 348

123. The correct answer is **C** – No explanation is available for this answer.

Back to Q 123 on page 348

124. The correct answer is **B** – No explanation is available for this answer.

Back to Q 124 on page 348

125. The correct answer is **A** – No explanation is available for this answer.

Back to Q 125 on page 348

126. The correct answer is **C** – No explanation is available for this answer.

Back to Q 126 on page 349

127. The correct answer is **D** – No explanation is available for this answer.

Back to Q 127 on page 349

128. The correct answer is **A** – No explanation is available for this answer.

Back to Q 128 on page 349

129. The correct answer is **C** – The biological human width is the label D in the figure, it is the sum of B (epithelial attachment) and C (connective tissue attachment) i.e., from the base of the gingival sulcus to the crest of the alveolar bone.

Back to Q 129 on page 349

Chapter 19
Multi Span Questions

These are question that covers more than one chapter.

Choose **one or more** of the most appropriate answers. Some questions may have **more than one** correct answer. You have to choose all the correct answers as best as you can.

19.1 MCQs Questions

1. Collagen is a protein found in all of the following tissues **except**:
   (a) Bone
   (b) Dentin
   (c) Enamel
   (d) Cementum

   Answer for Q 1 on page 383
2. Black hairy tongue is characterized by excessive proliferation of:
   (a) Fungiform papillae
   (b) Filiform papillae
   (c) Cicumvallate papillae
   (d) Foliate papillae

   Answer for Q 2 on page 383
3. Langhans giant cell are usually found in:
   (a) Acute inflammation
   (b) Pyogenic granuloma
   (c) Rheumatic carditis
   (d) TB

   Answer for Q 3 on page 383

4. A benign tumor composed of a proliferation of capillaries is called a:
   (a) Schwannoma
   (b) Hemangioma
   (c) Lipoma
   (d) Osteoma

   Answer for Q 4 on page 383

5. Touton giant cells are usually found in:
   (a) Chronic inflammatory conditions
   (b) Multiple myeloma
   (c) Histiocytosis Y (verruciform xanthoma)
   (d) Tuberculosis

   Answer for Q 5 on page 384

6. In addition to testing the pulp vitality with either cold or an electric pulp tester, which of the following clinical tests or procedures would be the most appropriate to assist in making a diagnosis?
   (a) Orthopantomogram
   (b) Bite-wing radiograph
   (c) Percussion
   (d) Crack testing

   Answer for Q 6 on page 384

7. Dorothy Reed giant cell are usually found in:
   (a) Measles
   (b) Viral infection
   (c) Hodgkin's disease
   (d) Actinomycosis

   Answer for Q 7 on page 384

8. Which of the following would most clearly differentiate an acute periodontal abscess from an acute periapical abscess?
   (a) Pigmentation of the gingivae
   (b) Nature of the swelling
   (c) Degree of tooth mobility
   (d) Response to a test for vitality
   (e) Tenderness to percussion

   Answer for Q 8 on page 384

9. A 25-years-old male complained of many minute vesicles on the vermillion border of the upper lip. The vesicles were preceded by an "itching" sensation. The patient stated the vesicles develop "two or three times" a year. The most likely diagnosis is:
   (a) Impetigo
   (b) Herpes zoster
   (c) Recurrent herpes simplex infection
   (d) Primary herpetic stomatitis
   (e) Recurrent aphthous ulceration

   Answer for Q 9 on page 384

10. A patient presents with painless, bluish lump (10 mm in diameter) just inside the vermillion border of the lower lip. The most likely diagnosis is:
   (a) Smoker's keratosis
   (b) Squamous cell carcinoma
   (c) Mucocele
   (d) Fibroma
   (e) Fibro-epithelial polyp

   Answer for Q 10 on page 384

11. A patient develops unilateral facial paralysis within ten minutes after an attempted inferior alveolar nerve block on the same side. The most logical explanation is that the injection was made into the:
   (a) Parotid gland
   (b) Masseter muscle
   (c) Maxillary artery
   (d) Pterygomandibular ligament
   (e) Buccinator muscle

   Answer for Q 11 on page 384

12. ♣ Which of the following are correct with regard to dentinogenesis imperfecta?

    (a) It is caused by a defect in fibronectin formation

    (b) The defect is transmitted as an autosomal dominant condition, the gene for which is closely related to the one that causes amelogenesis imperfecta

    (c) Dentinogenesis imperfecta affects permanent teeth only with sparing of the deciduous ones

    (d) Enamel on teeth with dentinogenesis imperfecta is practically normal, but is weakly attached and hence chips away easily

    (e) Radiographs of teeth with dentinogenesis imperfecta show teeth with obliterated pulp chambers and short stunted roots.

    Answer for Q 12 on page 384

13. ♣ Which of the following are predisposing conditions for osteomyelitis?

    (a) Chronic malnutrition

    (b) Paget's disease

    (c) Sickle cell anemia

    (d) Diabetes insipidus

    (e) Chronic alcoholism

    Answer for Q 13 on page 384

14. Which of the following statements about cysts or cyst like lesions of the jaws are correct?

    (a) A radicular (periapical cyst) cysts have an epithelial lining composed of stratified squamous epithelium, and often contain hyaline bodies (Rushton's bodies)

    (b) Dentigerous cysts have cyst walls similar to radicular cysts, with inflammatory changes commonly seen in the wall

    (c) Aneurysmal bone cysts have an epithelial lining composed of columnar epithelium

    (d) Cholesterol clefts within a cyst wall are pathognomonic of a radicular cyst

    (e) Odontogenic keratocysts (keratocystic odontogenic tumors) have an epithelial lining of uniform thickness, with a flat lower border, and a thin fibrous wall

    Answer for Q 14 on page 384

15. A patient with a white patch in her mouth. She has had a biopsy performed and you have the report in front of you. Which of the following are appropriate actions to take depending on the diagnosis reported?
    (a) An excision of the lesion is required because the report states that it is a white sponge nevus
    (b) No further treatment is needed because the lesion is leukoedema
    (c) No further treatment is required because the lesion is sublingual keratosis
    (d) Referral to appropriate specialist for management is needed because the lesion is severely dysplastic
    (e) An excision of the lesion is required because it is frictional keratosis

    Answer for Q 15 on page 384

16. Which of the following statements regarding salivary lumps are correct?
    (a) A 1 cm lump in the upper lip is most likely to be mucocele
    (b) A 1 cm lump in the lower lip is most likely to be mucocele
    (c) About 75% of tumors in the submandibular gland are malignant
    (d) About 30% of all salivary gland tumors occur in the sublingual gland and the majority of these are malignant
    (e) Intraoral salivary glands account for about 10% of all salivary gland tumors with about half of these being benign

    Answer for Q 16 on page 385

17. Which of the following are types of Langerhans' cells histiocytosis?
    (a) Letterer–Siwe syndrome
    (b) Solitary eosinophilic granuloma
    (c) Hand–Schuller–Christian disease
    (d) Melkersson–Rosenthal syndrome
    (e) Solitary plasmacytoma

    Answer for Q 17 on page 385

18. Which of the following statements regarding biopsies are correct?
    (a) When choosing the site to biopsy in a large lesion the most important consideration is to place the biopsy in the site that is likely to heal with the least amount of discomfort to the patient
    (b) A suture need not be placed through the tissue to be biopsied if you are using non-toothed forceps, as these will not crush the tissue and will not leave marks on the specimen
    (c) Sloughing or necrotic areas of tissue should be avoided
    (d) A commonly used fixative is 20% formal saline
    (e) The specimen must not be processed until it has been in the fixative for at least 24 hours

    Answer for Q 18 on page 385

19. Which of the following are features of Gorlin–Goltz syndrome (basal cell carcinoma/jaw cyst syndrome)
    (a) Absence of clavicles
    (b) Early calcification of falx cerebri
    (c) Frontal and parietal bossing
    (d) Multiple dentigerous cysts
    (e) Multiple basal cell hemangiomas

    Answer for Q 19 on page 385

20. Which of the following are microscopic features of epithelial dysplasia?
    (a) Atypical mitosis
    (b) Hyperkeratinization
    (c) Loss of cellular polarity
    (d) Altered nuclear/cytoplasmic ratio
    (e) Loss or reduction of intercellular adherence

    Answer for Q 20 on page 385

21. Which of the following microscopic features are suggestive of the white lesion of lichen planus?
    (a) Saw tooth rete ridges
    (b) Hypokeratosis
    (c) Dense band of macrophages below the basement membrane
    (d) Basal cell liquefaction
    (e) Acantholysis

    Answer for Q 21 on page 385

22. Carcinoma of the lip:
    (a) Is commoner in the upper lip
    (b) Is often caused by chewing betel nut
    (c) Has a worse prognosis than intra-oral carcinoma
    (d) Is principally caused by alcohol consumption
    (e) Often occurs in patients with submucous fibrosis

    Answer for Q 22 on page 386

23. In anhidrotic ectodermal dysplasia:
    (a) There are often supernumerary teeth
    (b) Hair is usually scanty
    (c) A sex-linked recessive trait is usually the cause
    (d) Anhidrosis refers to the type of hair present
    (e) Teeth are often peg shaped

    Answer for Q 23 on page 386

24. Delayed eruption of teeth is a feature of which of the following conditions?
    (a) Cleidocranial dysostosis
    (b) Osteogenesis imperfecta
    (c) Rickets
    (d) Cherubism
    (e) Scurvy

    Answer for Q 24 on page 386

25. Regarding dental fluorosis:
    (a) It affects deciduous teeth and permanent teeth equally
    (b) It causes white or brownish mottling of teeth
    (c) Mottled teeth are less susceptible to caries than teeth not exposed to fluoride
    (d) It occurs in areas when the fluoride in drinking water exceeds 0.1 ppm
    (e) It occurs in areas when fluoride in the drinking water exceeds 2 ppm

    Answer for Q 25 on page 386

26. Regarding dental caries:

    (a) Lactobacilli are the bacteria that are the main cause of dental caries

    (b) Cariogenic bacteria produce acid

    (c) Glucose is more cariogenic than sucrose

    (d) Fructose is less cariogenic than sucrose

    (e) Sugar alcohols (polyols) are less cariogenic

    Answer for Q 26 on page 386

27. Acute osteomyelitis:

    (a) Affects the maxilla more commonly than the mandible

    (b) Always causes paresthesia in relation to the inferior dental nerve

    (c) Will not be apparent on radiographs until about 10 days

    (d) Usually causes sharp, shooting pain

    (e) May cause associated teeth to loosen

    Answer for Q 27 on page 386

28. Regarding actinomycosis:

    (a) It is a suppurative infection caused by a coccal bacterium, usually Actinomyces Israeli

    (b) It is more common in women than men

    (c) It usually affects middle-aged people

    (d) Multiple discharging sinuses are seen, and the pus contains "sulfur granules" (bacterial colonies)

    (e) It is treated with metronidazole

    Answer for Q 28 on page 386

29. Regarding radicular cysts:

    (a) The cyst capsule often contains cholesterol crystals

    (b) The cyst fluid often shimmers due to the keratin contained within

    (c) The cyst lining is formed of stratified squamous epithelium

    (d) Rushton's bodies in the cyst wall indicate that the cyst is actively growing

    (e) Radicular cysts are always associated with a non-vital pulp

    Answer for Q 29 on page 387

30. Keratocysts (keratocystic odontogenic tumors):
    (a) Are always multilocular
    (b) Are commoner in the mandible than the maxilla
    (c) Grow along the bone rather than expanding the jaw
    (d) Are always associated with a missing tooth
    (e) Commonly recur

    Answer for Q 30 on page 387

31. Patients with Gorlin–Goltz syndrome (or basal cell carcinoma/jaw cyst syndrome) have:
    (a) Precocious puberty
    (b) Palmar pits
    (c) Café au lait patches
    (d) Inherited as an autosomal dominant gene so that 25% of the affected person's children will also have the gene
    (e) Associated endocrine disease

    Answer for Q 31 on page 387

32. In syphilis:
    (a) A primary chancre in the oral cavity may appear about 3–4 weeks after infection
    (b) The primary chancre is also known as a snail track ulcer
    (c) The primary chancre often heals after 2 months with severe scarring
    (d) The secondary stage usually occurs 1–4 months after the primary infection
    (e) The tertiary stage involves the appearance of well-defined, rounded areas known as mucous patches

    Answer for Q 32 on page 387

33. Hairy leukoplakia:
    (a) Only ever occurs in human immunodeficiency virus (HIV)-positive patients
    (b) Is caused by candidal infection of the oral mucosa
    (c) Commonly affects the dorsum of the tongue
    (d) Is a premalignant condition
    (e) Has koilocyte-like cells in the prickle cell layer

    Answer for Q 33 on page 387

34. Regarding an oral dysplastic lesion:

(a) It should be managed with 6-monthly check-up at the dentist clinic

(b) Stop any habits that may be contributory, e.g., smoking, alcohol consumption

(c) Surgical removal of the whole dysplastic area

(d) Leukoplakias have a higher risk of malignant transformation than erythroplakia

(e) High-risk sites include the hard palate

Answer for Q 34 on page 388

35. Salivary calculi:

(a) Commonly cause dry mouth

(b) Occur most commonly in the sublingual gland

(c) Occur most commonly in the parotid gland

(d) Are always visible on radiographs

(e) May be asymptomatic

Answer for Q 35 on page 388

36. Regarding salivary gland tumors:

(a) About 75% of all salivary gland tumors occur in the parotid gland

(b) About 10% of all salivary gland tumors occur in the minor salivary glands

(c) A tumor in the parotid gland is more likely to be malignant than a tumor in the minor salivary glands

(d) Most tumors in the sublingual salivary gland are benign

(e) The commonest salivary gland tumor is a adenoid cystic carcinoma

Answer for Q 36 on page 388

37. Regarding salivary gland tumors:

(a) Pleomorphic adenomas usually undergo malignant change

(b) Pleomorphic adenomas may contain fibrous, myxoid and chondroid tissue

(c) Mucoepidermoid carcinomas have a characteristic "Swiss cheese" pattern

(d) Acinic cell carcinomas commonly spread along nerve sheaths

(e) Adenoid cystic carcinomas have a poor prognosis

Answer for Q 37 on page 388

38. Which of the following investigations are appropriate for the lesions?
    (a) Incisional biopsy for a suspected squamous cell carcinoma
    (b) Incisional biopsy for a suspected hemangioma
    (c) Excisional biopsy for a suspected Fibro-epithelial polyp
    (d) Excisional biopsy for a white patch of unknown origin
    (e) Incisional biopsy for a mucous extravasation cyst

    Answer for Q 38 on page 388

39. Regarding ameloblastoma:
    (a) It usually presents between the ages of 15 and 20 years
    (b) It is the commonest odontogenic neoplasm
    (c) Commonly presents as a monolocular cyst on radiographs
    (d) It is common in the posterior mandible
    (e) Follicular ameloblastoma is the commonest type

    Answer for Q 39 on page 388

40. With respect to fibrous dysplasia:
    (a) It is commoner in females
    (b) It typically affects the maxilla
    (c) It is painful
    (d) Histologically there is irregular resorption and deposition of bone
    (e) Commonly occurs in the fourth decade

    Answer for Q 40 on page 388

41. With respect to osteosarcoma:
    (a) It is a complication of Paget's disease of bone
    (b) It is commoner in the maxilla
    (c) Paresthesia may be the presenting feature
    (d) It is commoner in males
    (e) It is most commonly seen in children

    Answer for Q 41 on page 389

42. Regarding hyperparathyroidism:
   (a) Characterized by raised plasma calcium levels
   (b) It presents histologically with giant cell lesions
   (c) Jaw lesions are commonly present
   (d) Patients may present with enlargement of the skull
   (e) It is most commonly secondary to chronic renal failure (CRF)

   Answer for Q 42 on page 389

43. Which of the following are true of cherubism?
   (a) Autosomal dominant trait
   (b) It is commoner in males
   (c) The middle third of the face is usually hypoplastic
   (d) Presents with lesions also known as Brown's tumors
   (e) The lesion cease growth with caseation of skeletal growth

   Answer for Q 43 on page 389

44. Which of the following are potentially malignant oral lesions/conditions?
   (a) Speckled leukoplakia
   (b) Tertiary syphilis
   (c) Paterson–Kelly syndrome (Plummer-Vinson Syndrome)
   (d) Chronic candidiasis
   (e) Medium rhomboid glossitis

   Answer for Q 44 on page 389

45. Regarding Warthin's tumor (adenolymphoma):
   (a) It is commoner in males
   (b) Tall columnar eosinophilic cells covering masses of lymphoid tissue is the characteristic histological appearance
   (c) It is the commonest type of salivary tumor
   (d) Average age of presentation is 40 years
   (e) 10% are bilateral

   Answer for Q 45 on page 389

46. Which of the following features would raise suspicion of a malignant salivary tumor?

(a) Facial nerve palsy

(b) Soft rubbery consistency

(c) Sudden increase in size

(d) Lesion is in a minor salivary gland rather than in the parotid

(e) Skin ulceration

Answer for Q 46 on page 389

47. Which of the following are true of oral submucous fibrosis?

(a) It is associated with smoking

(b) It is at risk of malignant transformation

(c) It is managed by topical corticosteroids

(d) It characteristically affects the buccal mucosa

(e) It may present with trismus

Answer for Q 47 on page 389

48. Regarding odontomes:

(a) They are hamartomas

(b) They usually present around the age of 30 years

(c) They can undergo malignant transformation

(d) They most commonly present in the anterior maxilla

(e) The lesion is composed of cementum embedded in fibrous tissue and a surrounding capsule

Answer for Q 48 on page 389

49. Which of the following statements are true?

(a) Ameloblastic fibromas usually present around the age of 50 years

(b) Ghost and ameloblastic cells are characteristically seen in ameloblastic fibromas

(c) Calcifying epithelial odontogenic tumor is also known as Pindborg's tumor

(d) Calcifying epithelial odontogenic tumors are locally invasive

(e) Adenomatoid odontogenic tumors most commonly present in the anterior maxilla

Answer for Q 49 on page 390

50. The excessive formation of scar tissue is called:

(a) Fibroma

(b) Myxoma

(c) Keloid

(d) Myoma

(e) Carcinoma

Answer for Q 50 on page 390

51. Atrophy of the pharyngeal and gastric mucosa, koilonychias (spoon nails) and predisposition to oral carcinoma in postmenopausal women are features of:

(a) Iron deficiency anemia

(b) Pernicious anemia

(c) Sturge-Weber-Dimitri syndrome

(d) Plummer-Vinson syndrome

(e) Trisomy 21

Answer for Q 51 on page 390

52. A normal clot retraction time, which is independent of coagulation time, is indicative of a normal number of circulating:

(a) Platelets

(b) Lymphocytes

(c) Monocytes

(d) Red blood cells

(e) Neutrophils

Answer for Q 52 on page 390

53. The blood of a patient with an acute infectious process would be expected to demonstrate:

(a) Lymphocytosis

(b) Leukocytosis

(c) Monocytosis

(d) Leukopenia

(e) Erythrocytosis

Answer for Q 53 on page 390

54. A biopsy would be of value in the diagnosis or oral lesions of:
    (a) Amyloidosis
    (b) Carcinoma in situ
    (c) Tuberculosis
    (d) Lichen planus
    (e) All of above

    Answer for Q 54 on page 390

55. The irradiation to the head region does not cause:
    (a) Xerostomia
    (b) Osteoradionecrosis
    (c) Radiation caries
    (d) Interference with tooth development
    (e) Ramsay Hunt syndrome

    Answer for Q 55 on page 390

56. Vesicles or bullae of the mucous membrane or skin are seen in all the following **except**:
    (a) Herpes simplex
    (b) Herpes zoster
    (c) Agranulocytosis
    (d) Pemphigus
    (e) SLE

    Answer for Q 56 on page 390

57. White lesions of the oral mucosa are characteristic of the following **except**:
    (a) Hyperkeratosis
    (b) Leukoedema
    (c) Lichen planus
    (d) Medium rhomboid glossitis
    (e) Acanthosis

    Answer for Q 57 on page 390

58. The peak incidence of gingivitis in children occurs at ages:
    (a) Birth-6 months
    (b) 1-3 years
    (c) 5-7 years
    (d) 7-10 years
    (e) 10-13 years

    Answer for Q 58 on page 390

59. Oral cytological smears are of no value in the diagnosis of:
    (a) Oral cancer
    (b) Primary intraoral herpes simplex
    (c) Recurrent intraoral herpes simplex
    (d) Herpes zoster
    (e) Lipoma

    Answer for Q 59 on page 390

60. The so-called "split papule," an erosive lesion involving the commissure of the lips, is actually:
    (a) An aphthous ulcer
    (b) A traumatic ulcer
    (c) A mucous patch
    (d) A fever blisters
    (e) Koplik's spot

    Answer for Q 60 on page 390

61. A 38-year-old woman developed soreness of the tongue and was referred to a local otolaryngology unit. She is found to have iron-deficiency anemia and she says she has been experiencing difficulty in swallowing. Endoscopy and barium swallow reveal erythematous esophageal spots. What syndrome does this patient have?
    (a) Steven-Johnson syndrome
    (b) Plummer-Vinson (Patterson-Kelly-Brown syndrome)
    (c) Discoid Lupus Erythematosus
    (d) Psoriasis

    Answer for Q 61 on page 390

62. An 85-year-old man presented with a 2-month history of a numb lip on the left side. His dentist had suggested that he leave his lower denture out for 2 weeks but this made no difference. A radiograph revealed a diffuse radiolucent lesion in the region of the left mental foramen. He was referred to the

hospital where, on taking a full history, the patient admitted to hematuria and weight loss over the last 3 months. A lateral skull radiograph reveals multiple radiolucent lesions in the skull and jaws. What syndrome does this patient have?

(a) Squamous cell carcinoma
(b) Carcinoma in situ
(c) Multiple myeloma
(d) Osteomalacia

Answer for Q 62 on page 390

63. Which of the following is correct?

(a) Pyknosis – shrinkage of nucleus
(b) Karyolysis – Dissolution of nucleus
(c) Karyorrhexis – fragmentation of nucleus
(d) All of the above

Answer for Q 63 on page 390

64. A specimen for a biopsy should be taken from:

(a) Necrotic area
(b) Subdermal layer
(c) Border of an ulcerated area
(d) Center of an ulcerated area

Answer for Q 64 on page 390

65. Granulomas are lesions which consist of granulation tissue. They usually result from failure of the body to eradicate the infection. This failure may be attributed to:

(a) Peculiar characteristic of some organism
(b) Decreased body resistance
(c) Persistence of the irritant and failure of the body to totally eliminate.
(d) All of the above

Answer for Q 65 on page 391

66. One of the following is a granular cell lesion:

(a) Congenital epulis of newborn
(b) Squamous cell carcinoma
(c) Basal cell carcinoma
(d) Fibroma

Answer for Q 66 on page 391

67. The nature of the granules found in cells of oncocytoma (oxyphilic adenoma) is:

(a) Lysosomes

(b) Zymogen

(c) Mitochondria

(d) Fat globules

Answer for Q 67 on page 391

68. How are necrotizing ulcerative gingivitis and necrotizing ulcerative periodontitis different?

(a) By name

(b) By bacterial type

(c) By anatomical extension of necrosis

(d) By treatment

Answer for Q 68 on page 391

69. Mulberry Molars are typically encountered in which of the following?

(a) Primary syphilis

(b) Secondary syphilis

(c) Congenital syphilis

(d) Latent syphilis

Answer for Q 69 on page 391

70. Which of the following is the most recognized form of Candidiasis?

(a) Pseudomembranous candidiasis

(b) Angular chelitis

(c) Candidal leukoplakia

(d) Mucocutaneous candidiasis

Answer for Q 70 on page 391

71. Bald tongue (loss of filiform papilla) is related to which of the following conditions?

(a) Antibiotic sore mouth

(b) Burning mouth syndrome

(c) Sjogren's disease

(d) Denture stomatitis

Answer for Q 71 on page 391

72. A well-demarcated erythematous zone in the midline posterior dorsum of the tongue can usually be diagnosed as which of the following?
    (a) Median rhomboid glossitis
    (b) Exfoliative chelitis
    (c) Papillary hyperplasia
    (d) Chronic multifocal candidiasis
    Answer for Q 72 on page ??
73. What is the most common form of primary herpes simplex infection known as?
    (a) Herpetic whitlow
    (b) Herpetic paronychia
    (c) Acute herpetic gingivostomatitis
    (d) Herpes labialis
    Answer for Q 73 on page 391
74. Which of the following is the most common site for recurrent herpes infection?
    (a) Buccal mucosa
    (b) Vermilion border (Lips)
    (c) Finger
    (d) Tongue
    Answer for Q 74 on page 391
75. In Shingles the emphasis is on prevention, why?
    (a) To avoid scarring
    (b) Post herpetic neuralgia is difficult to treat
    (c) Hyperpigmentation is irreversible
    (d) It is contagious
    Answer for Q 75 on page 391
76. A 4-year-old patient came to the clinic where his mother gave a history of flu-like symptoms, vesicles in the anterior regions of the mouth and cutaneous lesions (fingers and toes). What is the most likely diagnosis?
    (a) Herpangina
    (b) Acute lymphonodular pharyngitis
    (c) Hand, foot and mouth disease
    (d) Infectious mononucleosis
    Answer for Q 76 on page 391

77. Which of the following conditions is strongly associated with HIV?
    (a) Mycobacterial infection
    (b) HIV associated salivary gland disease
    (c) Thrombocytopenia
    (d) Kaposi sarcoma

    Answer for Q 77 on page 391

78. What is the most important sign that indicate the lesion is malignant?
    (a) Invasion of the surrounding structure
    (b) Bone expansion
    (c) Root resorption of the adjacent teeth
    (d) Metastasis

    Answer for Q 78 on page 391

79. What is the most clinically significant odontogenic tumor of the following?
    (a) Ameloblastoma
    (b) Odontogenic myxoma
    (c) Odontoma
    (d) Ameloblastic fibroma

    Answer for Q 79 on page 391

80. The following is the most common type of ameloblastoma:
    (a) Multicystic ameloblastoma
    (b) Unicystic ameloblastoma
    (c) Peripheral ameloblastoma
    (d) Malignant ameloblastoma

    Answer for Q 80 on page 391

81. The unique feature in ameloblastic carcinoma is:
    (a) Cause sever bone expansion
    (b) Cause root resorption
    (c) Cause numbness of the jaw
    (d) Has extensive cytological atypia

    Answer for Q 81 on page 392

82. Rosette-like structures is a histological feature that present in the following tumor:
    (a) Clear cell odontogenic carcinoma
    (b) Adenomatoid odontogenic tumor
    (c) Calcifying epithelial odontogenic tumor
    (d) Squamous odontogenic tumor

Answer for Q 82 on page 392

83. Amyloid like structures is a histological feature that present in the following tumor:
    (a) Clear cell odontogenic carcinoma
    (b) Adenomatoid odontogenic tumor
    (c) Calcifying epithelial odontogenic tumor
    (d) Squamous odontogenic tumor

Answer for Q 83 on page 392

84. Liesegang ring calcification is a histological feature that present in the following tumor:
    (a) Clear cell odontogenic carcinoma
    (b) Adenomatoid odontogenic tumor
    (c) Calcifying epithelial odontogenic tumor
    (d) Squamous odontogenic tumor

Answer for Q 84 on page 392

85. The following tumor appear like multiple small teeth in the radiographic film:
    (a) Ameloblastic fibroma
    (b) Compound odontoma
    (c) Complex odontoma
    (d) Ameloblastic fibro-odontoma

Answer for Q 85 on page 392

86. One of the following tumors should be in the differential diagnosis of mixed tumors in the x-ray:
    (a) Ameloblastic fibroma
    (b) Compound odontoma
    (c) Complex odontoma
    (d) Ameloblastic fibro-odontoma

Answer for Q 86 on page 392

87. Tumor that has jelly like texture grossly is:

    (a) Odontogenic fibroma

    (b) Granular cell odontogenic tumor

    (c) Odontogenic myxoma

    (d) Cementoblastoma

    Answer for Q 87 on page 392

88. A 42-year-old man presented with a hard papule which is crater shaped on the skin side of the lower lip. Upon histological examination, keratin plugs were found. The most probable diagnosis is:

    (a) Keratoacanthoma

    (b) Traumatic ulcer

    (c) Melanoma

    (d) Lipoma

    Answer for Q 88 on page 392

89. Which of the following tumors may undergo spontaneous regression?

    (a) Rodent ulcer

    (b) Squamous cell carcinoma

    (c) Papilloma

    (d) Keratoacanthoma

    Answer for Q 89 on page 392

90. Cauliflower like appearance is characteristic feature of one of the following:

    (a) Papilloma

    (b) Physiological pigmentation

    (c) Capillary hemangioma

    (d) Aphthous ulcer

    Answer for Q 90 on page 392

91. The following lesion is very similar to squamous cell papilloma clinically and histologically:

    (a) Squamous cell carcinoma

    (b) Verruca vulgaris

    (c) Mucous retention cyst

    (d) Mucous extravasation cyst

    Answer for Q 91 on page 392

92. The most likely etiologic factor for verruca vulgaris is:
    (a) Ultraviolet rays of sun
    (b) Chronic mechanical irritation
    (c) Viral infection
    (d) Bacterial infection

    Answer for Q 92 on page 392

93. Multiple hemangiomas are a usual feature of **all** the following syndromes **except**:
    (a) Peutz-Jeghers syndrome
    (b) von-Hippel Lindau disease
    (c) Osler Weber-Rendu disease
    (d) Sturge-Weber syndrome

    Answer for Q 93 on page 392

94. Central hemangioma of the mandible usually appears in radiographs as:
    (a) Unilocular radiolucent area
    (b) Multilocular radiolucent area
    (c) Mixed radiolucency with radiopacities
    (d) Radiopaque lesion

    Answer for Q 94 on page 392

95. Pseudoepitheliomatous hyperplasia is a characteristic feature of one of the following tumors:
    (a) Keratoacanthoma
    (b) Fibroma
    (c) Lipoma
    (d) Squamous cell carcinoma

    Answer for Q 95 on page 392

96. Juvenile melanoma is a:
    (a) Malignant tumor
    (b) Histologically malignant but clinically benign
    (c) Locally malignant (locally invasive)
    (d) None of the above

    Answer for Q 96 on page 392

97. The type of nevi that results from melanocytes arrested deep in the dermis is termed:

    (a) Intradermal nevus

    (b) Blue nevus

    (c) Junctional nevus

    (d) Compound nevus

    Answer for Q 97 on page 392

98. ♣ Hair-on-end appearance is a characteristic radiographic feature of:

    (a) Thalassemia

    (b) Sickle cell anemia

    (c) Malaria

    (d) Lymphoma

    Answer for Q 98 on page 393

99. ♣ Foam cells are macrophages loaded with lipids usually found in:

    (a) Periapical granuloma

    (b) Radicular cysts

    (c) Verruciform xanthoma

    (d) Foreign body granuloma

    (e) Langerhans histiocytosis

    Answer for Q 99 on page 393

100. ♣ Tzanck cells are acantholytic cells appear free floating the in the epithelial clefts in cases of:

    (a) Herpes simplex

    (b) Varicella and herpes zoster

    (c) Pemphigus vulgaris

    (d) Herpangina

    (e) Cytomegalovirus

    Answer for Q 100 on page 393

101. ♣ Ghost cells are Greatly enlarged eosinophilic epithelial cells without visible nuclei that can be found in:

    (a) Calcifying odontogenic cyst (Gorlin cyst)

    (b) Ameloblastoma

    (c) Ameloblastic odontoma

    (d) Complex odontome

    (e) Ghost cell odontogenic carcinoma

Answer for Q 101 on page 393

102. ♣ Pathergy reaction may be found in:
   (a) Psoriasis
   (b) Behçet's disease
   (c) Pemphigus vulgaris
   (d) pyoderma gangrenosum

Answer for Q 102 on page 393

103. Immunoelectrophoresis test is used to measure the exact amount of:
   (a) Red blood cells
   (b) Bence Jones proteins in the urine
   (c) White blood cells
   (d) Platelets

Answer for Q 103 on page 393

104. Kveim test is used in:
   (a) Sarcoidosis
   (b) Syphilis
   (c) Actinomycosis
   (d) Tuberculosis

Answer for Q 104 on page 394

19.2 Answers with Comments:

1. The correct answer is **C** – Proteins of enamel are not collagen but mostly are ameloblastin, enamelin, tuftelin and amelogenin.

   Back to Q 1 on page 359

2. The correct answer is **B** – Black hairy tongue results form excessive proliferation of filiform papillae associated with increase in keratin production or a decrease in normal desquamation (shedding of surface epithelial cells).

   Back to Q 2 on page 359

3. The correct answer is **D** – Do not confuse Langhans giant cell with Langerhans cells, the latter are tissue-resident macrophages of the skin, and contain organelles called Birbeck granules.

   Back to Q 3 on page 359

4. The correct answer is **B** – No explanation is available for this answer.

Back to Q 4 on page 360

5. The correct answer is **C** – Touton giant cells are a type of multinucleated giant cell in which nuclei forms a ring in the cytoplasm. Usually seen in lesions with high lipid content such as fat necrosis, xanthoma, and xanthelasma and xanthogranulomas. They are also found in dermatofibroma.

Back to Q 5 on page 360

6. The correct answer is **C** – No explanation is available for this answer.

Back to Q 6 on page 360

7. The correct answer is **C** – No explanation is available for this answer.

Back to Q 7 on page 360

8. The correct answer is **D** – No explanation is available for this answer.

Back to Q 8 on page 360

9. The correct answer is **C** – No explanation is available for this answer.

Back to Q 9 on page 361

10. The correct answer is **C** – No explanation is available for this answer.

Back to Q 10 on page 361

11. The correct answer is **A** – No explanation is available for this answer.

Back to Q 11 on page 361

12. The correct answer is **DE** – Dentinogenesis imperfecta is due to a defect in collagen formation not fibronectin. It is inherited as an autosomal dominant condition and is closely related to osteogenesis imperfecta. It affects deciduous and permanent teeth, and in certain types of osteogenesis imperfecta deciduous teeth are affected. Enamel on teeth with dentinogenesis imperfecta is practically normal but is chipped away easily as the scalloping of the enamel dentin junction is lost.

Back to Q 12 on page 362

13. The correct answer is **ABCE** – Many chronic illnesses predispose patients to osteomyelitis. Poorly controlled diabetes mellitus, but not diabetes insipidus, is a predisposing factor.

Back to Q 13 on page 362

14. The correct answer is **AE** – Dentigerous cysts have cyst walls similar to radicular cysts but inflammatory changes are rare. Aneurysmal bone cysts are not proper cysts and do not have an epithelial lining. Cholesterol clefts within a cyst wall are indicative of inflammation, and not specific to a particular cyst type.

Back to Q 14 on page 362

15. The correct answer is **BD** – Both white sponge nevus and leukoedema are benign and do not need any active treatment; simple reassurance is all that is required. Friction keratosis is also benign, and removal of the irritant source will cause the patch to disappear. No active treatment of the keratotic

patch is needed. Sublingual keratosis is similar to leukoplakia in a sublingual position. There are differing reports of rates of malignant change in this lesion but it should still be managed as a leukoplakic lesion.

Back to Q 15 on page 363

16. The correct answer is **BE** – A small lump in the upper lip is most likely to be a salivary gland tumor, often a pleomorphic adenoma whereas a lump in the lower lip is most likely to be a mucocele. About a third of tumors in the submandibular gland are malignant. About 0.3% of all salivary gland tumors occur in the sublingual gland and the majority of these are malignant.

Back to Q 16 on page 363

17. The correct answer is **ABC** – Langerhans' cells are antigen-presenting cells present in the epithelium. If they give rise to bone tumors, three forms are recognized: Letterer–Siwe syndrome, solitary eosinophilic granuloma and multifocal eosinophilic granuloma, including Hand–Schuller–Christian disease. Melkersson Rosenthal syndrome is a condition in which patients have facial paralysis along with chronic granulomatous lesions similar to Crohn's disease. Plasmacytoma is a tumor of plasma cells, not Langerhans' cells.

Back to Q 17 on page 363

18. The correct answer is **C** – When choosing the site to biopsy in a large lesion the most important consideration is to select the most suspicious looking area(s). A suture should be placed through the tissue to be biopsied for several reasons: it can be used to orientate the biopsy, it can prevent it being aspirated and it will prevent crush marks that can be made with any type of instrument. A commonly used fixative is 10% formal saline, which is formaldehyde solution in normal saline. The length of time it takes a specimen to fix depends on its size. Smaller specimens will fix in less than 24 hours so could be processed sooner.

Back to Q 18 on page 364

19. The correct answer is **B** – Gorlin–Goltz (basal cell carcinoma/jaw cyst) syndrome has many features including calcified falx cerebri, multiple basal cell carcinomas, skeletal abnormalities and multiple odontogenic keratocysts (keratocystic odontogenic tumors). The clavicles are absent in cleidocranial dysostosis.

Back to Q 19 on page 364

20. The correct answer is **ACDE** – Dysplasia is a term used to describe histological abnormalities seen in both premalignant and malignant cells. Abnormal features include: abnormal mitoses and increased number of mitoses; loss of polarity; drop-shaped rete ridges; abnormal intercellular adherence; and abnormal nuclear/cytoplasmic ratio. Abnormal keratiniztion occurs in cells situated more basally than in the layers in which cells normally keratinize. Hyperkeratinization is not a feature of dysplasia.

Back to Q 20 on page 364

21. The correct answer is **AD** – The typical histological features of lichen planus include saw tooth rete ridges, hyperkeratosis or parakeratosis, a dense band of lymphocytes below the basement membrane and basal cell liquefaction.

    Back to Q 21 on page 364

22. The correct answer is – All statements are false. Carcinoma of the lip is commoner on the lower lip. It is often identified early because it is visible and hence has a better prognosis than intra-oral carcinoma. The main risk factor for carcinoma of the lip is exposure to sunlight, and it is not affected by alcohol consumption or betel nut chewing in the same way as intra-oral carcinoma. Intra-oral carcinoma commonly occurs in patients with submucous fibrosis.

    Back to Q 22 on page 365

23. The correct answer is **BCE** – Anhidrotic ectodermal dysplasia is usually a sex-linked recessive trait that results in hypodontia, hypotrichosis (scanty and wispy hair) and anhidrosis (inability to sweat). Any teeth present are often peg shaped or conical.

    Back to Q 23 on page 365

24. The correct answer is **ACD** – Delayed eruption of teeth usually occurs in cleidocranial dysostosis and rickets. In cherubism eruption may be delayed due to displacement by the giant cell lesions.

    Back to Q 24 on page 365

25. The correct answer is **BCE** – Excess fluoride ingestion causes dental fluorosis. Fluoride is usually present in drinking water and unwanted effects are seen when it exceeds 2ppm, however, mottling can occur at lower levels. Permanent teeth are usually affected, it rarely affects deciduous teeth, and mottling appears as white or brown areas on the teeth with varying degrees of pitting.

    Back to Q 25 on page 365

26. The correct answer is **BD** – Viridans streptococci are the most cariogenic bacteria and not lactobacilli, which tend to appear in bacterial plaque after caries has developed. All cariogenic bacteria produce acid. The most cariogenic sugar is sucrose – both glucose and fructose are less cariogenic than sucrose. Sugar alcohols are less cariogenic and so are used in "sugar-free" foods.

    Back to Q 26 on page 366

27. The correct answer is **CE** – Acute osteomyelitis commonly affects the mandible. Osteomyelitis of the maxilla is rare although it may occur in infants. Acute osteomyelitis is associated with severe, deep-seated, throbbing pain, the associated teeth become tender and loose, and pus may exude from the socket. Alteration in sensation in relation to the inferior dental nerve may occur, but not in all cases. Radiographic changes are not visible initially, only becoming apparent after about 10 days, when loss of trabeculae and areas of bone destruction are evident.

    Back to Q 27 on page 366

28. The correct answer is **CD** – Actinomycosis is a suppurative infection that is usually caused by Actinomyces israeli, a filamentous bacterium. It most commonly tends to affect men aged about 30–60 years. Multiple discharging sinuses are seen, and the pus contains granules known as "sulfur granules", which are colonies of Actinomyces species. Treatment involves drainage of the pus along with penicillin or tetracycline.

Back to Q 28 on page 366

29. The correct answer is **ACE** – Radicular cysts are formed following infection or inflammation of the pulp and are associated with non-vital roots. The cyst lining is formed of stratified squamous epithelium, which contains hyaline or Rushton's bodies, which indicate the odontogenic origin of the cyst. The cyst capsule contains cholesterol crystals and the cholesterol in the cyst fluid gives it a shimmering appearance.

Back to Q 29 on page 366

30. The correct answer is **BCE** – Keratocysts (keratocystic odontogenic tumors) are often unilocular when small and become multilocular as they enlarge. They are thought to be formed from the remnants of the dental lamina and so are not always associated with a missing tooth. They are commoner in the mandible than the maxilla. They commonly recur due to the difficulty of removing all of the friable lining.

Back to Q 30 on page 367

31. The correct answer is **BD** – The features of Gorlin–Goltz syndrome are multiple keratocysts (keratocystic odontogenic tumors), multiple basal cell carcinomas, intra-cranial abnormalities such as calcification of the falx cerebri, and frontal bossing and other skeletal abnormalities including bifid ribs. Gorlin's syndrome is an autosomal dominant condition so 50% of the affected person's children will also have the gene. They have pits on their palms and on the soles of their feet. Allbright's syndrome presents with precocious puberty, Café au lait patches, polyostotic fibrous dysplasia, and endocrine hyperfunction.

Back to Q 31 on page 367

32. The correct answer is **AD** – An oral chancre appears in primary syphilis about 3–4 weeks after infection. It often heals without scarring after a couple of months. In secondary syphilis the oral lesions consist of ulcers that are covered with a greyish slough known as snail track ulcers. When ulcers join together, larger areas are involved and these are known as mucous patches. The lesion in tertiary syphilis is the gumma.

Back to Q 32 on page 367

33. The correct answer is **E** – Hairy leukoplakia occurs most commonly in homosexual men infected with HIV. It also occurs in immunodeficient patients although it is not as common. It is often secondarily infected with Candida, and occurs most commonly on the lateral borders of the tongue. It is not a

premalignant condition. Histologically there is hyperkeratosis or parakeratosis. In the prickle cell layer are vacuolated and ballooned cells with dark nuclei surrounded by a clear halo – koilocyte-like cells.

Back to Q 33 on page 367

34. The correct answer is **B** – Dysplastic lesions should be reviewed 3 months after elimination of risk factors and regularly thereafter. Surgical excision of the lesion may be indicated if the lesion persists, depending on the degree of dysplasia, and site and extent of the lesion. Erythroplasia have a much higher risk of malignant transformation than homogeneous leukoplakias. The high-risk sites include the ventrolateral surfaces of the tongue, floor of the mouth and soft palate/fauces.

Back to Q 34 on page 368

35. The correct answer is **E** – Salivary calculi occur most commonly in the submandibular gland and may be asymptomatic. They are not always visible on radiographs and do not cause a dry mouth.

Back to Q 35 on page 368

36. The correct answer is **AB** – About three-quarters of all salivary gland tumors occur in the parotid gland, and about a tenth occur in the minor salivary glands. A tumor in a minor gland is more likely to be malignant as about a third are malignant, whereas in the parotid gland only about 15% are malignant. However, a tumor in the sublingual gland is most likely to be malignant as over 80% of tumors in this site are malignant. The commonest salivary gland tumor is the pleomorphic adenoma.

Back to Q 36 on page 368

37. The correct answer is **BE** – Only about 2–4% of pleomorphic adenomas undergoes malignant change. They may contain a wide variety of tissue types including fibrous, myxoid and elastic. The characteristic "Swiss cheese" appearance and spread along nerve sheaths is seen in adenoid cystic carcinomas. Adenoid cystic carcinomas grow slowly, metastasize late, and have a poor prognosis.

Back to Q 37 on page 368

38. The correct answer is **AC** – Incisional biopsies should be done on squamous cell carcinomas and white patches of unknown origin. An excisional biopsy is appropriate for a fibroepithelial polyp and a mucous extravasation cyst. Biopsy should not be attempted on a suspected hemangioma.

Back to Q 38 on page 369

39. The correct answer is **BDE** – Ameloblastoma usually presents between the ages of 30 and 50 years, and it presents as a multilocular cyst. The other types of ameloblastoma are: plexiform, acanthomatous, basal cell and granular cell. Unicystic ameloblastomas are considered as a distinct entity to the solid variants of ameloblastoma.

Back to Q 39 on page 369

40. The correct answer is **AB** – In fibrous dysplasia normal bone is replaced by fibrous tissue. It usually affects the maxilla and people below the age of 20. It is not often painful. Irregular resorption and deposition of bone is seen in Paget's disease.

Back to Q 40 on page 369

41. The correct answer is **ACD** – Osteosarcoma is rare and more common in the mandible. It is most commonly seen between the ages of 30 and 40 years and in males. It occurs as a complication of Paget's disease, although it is not common.

Back to Q 41 on page 369

42. The correct answer is **ABE** – Skull enlargement occurs with Paget's disease. Osteolytic lesions in bone are more commonly the result of secondary hyperparathyroidism (eg CRF) than primary (hyperplasia or adenoma of parathyroids).

Back to Q 42 on page 370

43. The correct answer is **ABE** – Cherubism is inherited as an autosomal dominant trait. It presents with expansion of the maxilla. The lesion cease growth with caseation of skeletal growth. Brown tumors are seen secondary to hyperparathyroidism.

Back to Q 43 on page 370

44. The correct answer is **ABCD** – Various potentially malignant conditions occur in the oral cavity including erythroplakia, dysplastic and speckled leukoplakia, oral submucous fibrosis, tertiary syphilis, chronic candidiasis and lichen planus. There is also high incidence of oral and esophageal cancer in Paterson–Kelly syndrome. Median rhomboid glossitis is not a potentially malignant lesion.

Back to Q 44 on page 370

45. The correct answer is **ABE** – The male to female ratio of occurrence of Warthin's tumor is 7:1. It is a benign tumor, making up 7–8% of salivary tumors. The average age of presentation is 70 years; 40 years is the average age for presentation of pleomorphic adenomas.

Back to Q 45 on page 370

46. The correct answer is **ACDE** – A mass of hard consistency is more likely to be malignant. Sudden increase in size of a salivary mass, even if it has been present for many years, should alert the clinician to a risk of malignant mass. Pain, nerve involvement and nodal metastases are also signs of malignant growth.

Back to Q 46 on page 371

47. The correct answer is **BDE** – Oral submucous fibrosis is associated with betel quid chewing (smokeless tobacco). Intra-lesional injections of steroids have been tried, but the benefit is limited. The risk of malignant transformation is reported to be around 5–8%.

Back to Q 47 on page 371

48. The correct answer is **AD** – Odontomes usually present between the ages of 10 and 20 years, and are benign lesions. They most commonly present in the anterior maxilla and posterior mandible. The lesion is composed of pulp, dentin, enamel and cementum.

Back to Q 48 on page 371

49. The correct answer is **CDE** – Ameloblastic fibromas usually present in children or young adults. Ghost and ameloblastic cells are seen in calcifying odontogenic cysts.

    Back to Q 49 on page 371

50. The correct answer is **C** – No explanation is available for this answer.

    Back to Q 50 on page 372

51. The correct answer is **D** – No explanation is available for this answer.

    Back to Q 51 on page 372

52. The correct answer is **A** – No explanation is available for this answer.

    Back to Q 52 on page 372

53. The correct answer is **B** – No explanation is available for this answer.

    Back to Q 53 on page 372

54. The correct answer is **E** – No explanation is available for this answer.

    Back to Q 54 on page 373

55. The correct answer is **E** – No explanation is available for this answer.

    Back to Q 55 on page 373

56. The correct answer is **C** – No explanation is available for this answer.

    Back to Q 56 on page 373

57. The correct answer is **D** – No explanation is available for this answer.

    Back to Q 57 on page 373

58. The correct answer is **E** – No explanation is available for this answer.

    Back to Q 58 on page 374

59. The correct answer is **E** – No explanation is available for this answer.

    Back to Q 59 on page 374

60. The correct answer is **C** – No explanation is available for this answer.

    Back to Q 60 on page 374

61. The correct answer is **B** – No explanation is available for this answer.

    Back to Q 61 on page 374

62. The correct answer is **C** – No explanation is available for this answer.

    Back to Q 62 on page 374

63. The correct answer is **D** – No explanation is available for this answer.

    Back to Q 63 on page 375

64. The correct answer is **C** – No explanation is available for this answer.

Back to Q 64 on page 375

65. The correct answer is **D** – No explanation is available for this answer.

Back to Q 65 on page 375

66. The correct answer is **A** – No explanation is available for this answer.

Back to Q 66 on page 375

67. The correct answer is **C** – No explanation is available for this answer.

Back to Q 67 on page 376

68. The correct answer is **C** – No explanation is available for this answer.

Back to Q 68 on page 376

69. The correct answer is **C** – No explanation is available for this answer.

Back to Q 69 on page 376

70. The correct answer is **A** – No explanation is available for this answer.

Back to Q 70 on page 376

71. The correct answer is **A** – No explanation is available for this answer.

Back to Q 71 on page 376

72. The correct answer is **A** – No explanation is available for this answer.

Back to Q 70 on page 376

73. The correct answer is **C** – No explanation is available for this answer.

Back to Q 73 on page 377

74. The correct answer is **B** – No explanation is available for this answer.

Back to Q 74 on page 377

75. The correct answer is **B** – No explanation is available for this answer.

Back to Q 75 on page 377

76. The correct answer is **C** – No explanation is available for this answer.

Back to Q 76 on page 377

77. The correct answer is **D** – No explanation is available for this answer.

Back to Q 77 on page 378

78. The correct answer is **D** – No explanation is available for this answer.

Back to Q 78 on page 378

79. The correct answer is **A** – No explanation is available for this answer.

Back to Q 79 on page 378

80. The correct answer is **A** – No explanation is available for this answer.

Back to Q 80 on page 378

81. The correct answer is **D** – No explanation is available for this answer.

Back to Q 81 on page 378

82. The correct answer is **B** – No explanation is available for this answer.

Back to Q 82 on page 379

83. The correct answer is **C** – No explanation is available for this answer.

Back to Q 83 on page 379

84. The correct answer is **C** – No explanation is available for this answer.

Back to Q 84 on page 379

85. The correct answer is **B** – No explanation is available for this answer.

Back to Q 85 on page 379

86. The correct answer is **D** – No explanation is available for this answer.

Back to Q 86 on page 379

87. The correct answer is **C** – No explanation is available for this answer.

Back to Q 87 on page 380

88. The correct answer is **A** – No explanation is available for this answer.

Back to Q 88 on page 380

89. The correct answer is **D** – No explanation is available for this answer.

Back to Q 89 on page 380

90. The correct answer is **A** – No explanation is available for this answer.

Back to Q 90 on page 380

91. The correct answer is **B** – No explanation is available for this answer.

Back to Q 91 on page 380

92. The correct answer is **C** – No explanation is available for this answer.

Back to Q 92 on page 381

93. The correct answer is **A** – No explanation is available for this answer.

Back to Q 93 on page 381

94. The correct answer is **B** – No explanation is available for this answer.

Back to Q 94 on page 381

95. The correct answer is **A** – No explanation is available for this answer.

Back to Q 95 on page 381

96. The correct answer is **B** – No explanation is available for this answer.

Back to Q 96 on page 381

97. The correct answer is **B** – No explanation is available for this answer.

Back to Q 97 on page 382

98. The correct answer is **AB** – When the diploic space of the skull vault expands, the trabeculae become thicker, giving the diploic space a hair-on-end appearance on radiographs. These perpendicular trabeculae are scattered throughout the skull vault and radiolucent marrow hyperplasia. It is classically described in plain skull radiographs although can also be appreciated on CT or MRI 3. Causes include: Thalassemia; sickle cell anemia; hereditary spherocytosis and iron deficiency anemia.

Back to Q 98 on page 382

99. The correct answer is **ABCE** – Foam cells are macrophages loaded with lipids, usually cholesterol. The lipid dissolves in xylol during the preparation of the microscopic slides, leaving spaces similar to foam. Foam cells are found surrounding cholesterol clefts in periapical granulomas and radicular cysts. They are also found in some tumors, such as verruciform xanthoma and Langerhans histiocytosis. Also, foam cells may be found lining the coronaries, and it is assumed that they contribute to the plaque formation with subsequent atherosclerosis and coronary heart disease.

Back to Q 99 on page 382

100. The correct answer is **ABCE** – Tzanck cells are acantholytic cells appear free floating the in the epithelial clefts in cases of pemphigus vulgaris and some other vesiculobullous lesions. They loss intercellular bridges (desmosomes) and thus become rounded with pyknotic nuclei.

Back to Q 100 on page 382

101. The correct answer is **AE** – Ghost cells are greatly enlarged eosinophilic epithelial cells without visible nuclei, referred to as "ghost cells" are present within the stellate reticulum-like cells (nature uncertain, may represent keratin). Recently, ghost cells were found to be amelogenin positive suggesting the ameloblastic differentiation of ghost cells. The cells are found in *calcifying odontogenic cyst* (also termed as Gorlin cyst, Ghost cell tumors) and also in *ghost cell odontogenic carcinoma.*

Back to Q 101 on page 382

102. The correct answer is **BD** – Pathergy is a skin condition in which a minor trauma, hapten or antigen leads to the development of skin lesions or ulcers that may be resistant to healing.

Pathergy is seen with both Behçet's disease and pyoderma gangrenosum[1]. A highly similar phenomenon known as the ***Koebner phenomenon*** occurs in autoimmune diseases such as psoriasis, and systemic lupus erythematosus.

Pathergy may be helpful in the diagnosis of Behçet's disease by attempting to induce a pathergy reaction with a test known as a "Skin Prick Test".

Back to Q 102 on page 383

[1] Pyoderma gangrenosum is a rare, non-infectious inflammatory skin disease where painful pustules or nodules become ulcers that progressively enlarge.

103. The correct answer is **B** – Immunoelectrophoresis is a general term for a number of biochemical methods for separation and characterization of proteins based on electrophoresis.

In medical practice it is used to measure the exact amount of Bence Jones proteins in the urine, a technique which is helpful in the diagnosis of myeloma.

Back to Q 103 on page 383

104. The correct answer is **A** – Kveim test is an intradermal test for ***sarcoidosis*** in which an antigen prepared from the lymph nodes or spleen of human sarcoidosis patients is injected intracutaneously. The test is positive when an infiltrated area, papule, nodule, or superficial necrosis appears around the site of injection. If the patient has been on treatment (e.g. glucocorticoids), the test may be false negative.

Back to Q 104 on page 383

Chapter 20
Oral Pathology and Medicine for Saudi Board Quiz (Examples)

Choose **one or more** of the most appropriate answers. Some questions may have **more than one** correct answer. You have to choose all the correct answers as best as you can.

20.1 MCQs Questions

1. Osteogenesis Imperfecta occur due to:
   (a) Improper osteoblastic activity
   (b) Collagen I maturation defect
   (c) Osteoclastic cells malfunction
   (d) Poorly differentiated osteocytes
   Answer for Q 1 on page 444
2. The drug most commonly used to treat trigeminal neuralgia is:
   (a) Diazepam (Valium)
   (b) Carbamazepine (Tegretol)
   (c) Ergotamine
   (d) Phenytoin (Dilantin)
   (e) Metronidazole (Flagyl)
   Answer for Q 2 on page 444
3. In osteopetrosis:
   (a) The number of osteoclasts increase
   (b) The number of osteoclasts decrease
   (c) There is no change in osteoclasts number
   (d) Osteoblast cells increase
   Answer for Q 3 on page 444

4. Aphthous ulcer, compared with herpes ulcer is:
   (a) More characteristic in histology
   (b) Leaves scar
   (c) Less response to stress
   (d) Occur in lining mucosa.

   Answer for Q 4 on page 444
5. All of the following are signs of Paget's disease **except**:
   (a) Cotton wool appearance in the X-Ray
   (b) Decrease blood level of alkaline phosphatase
   (c) Increase urinary hydroxyproline
   (d) Bone pain

   Answer for Q 5 on page 444
6. Syphilis first appearance:
   (a) Multiple vesicle
   (b) Erythematous reaction
   (c) Ulcer
   (d) Bullae

   Answer for Q 6 on page 444
7. Child with vesicle on the hard palate with history of malaise for 3 days what is the possible diagnosis:
   (a) Herpes simplex
   (b) Erythema multiform
   (c) Herpes zoster
   (d) Herpangina

   Answer for Q 7 on page 444
8. The disease that has large number of unerupted supernumerary teeth is:
   (a) Paget's disease
   (b) Cleidocranial dysplasia
   (c) Osteogenesis imperfecta
   (d) Down syndrome

   Answer for Q 8 on page 444

9. Which virus is present in the patient's mouth all his Life?
   (a) Herpes Simplex
   (b) Herpes zoster
   (c) Varicella Virus
   (d) None of the above

   Answer for Q 9 on page 445

10. Calcium channel blockers cause increased salivary secretion:
    (a) True
    (b) False
    (c) Note sure

    Answer for Q 10 on page 445

11. In Maccune-Albright syndrome cell mutation occur:
    (a) Early embryonic life
    (b) Late embryonic life
    (c) In postnatal life
    (d) In childhood

    Answer for Q 11 on page 445

12. The most common type of biopsy used in oral cavity is:
    (a) Excisional biopsy
    (b) Incisional biopsy
    (c) Aspiration through needle
    (d) Punch biopsy

    Answer for Q 12 on page 445

13. 10-years old child present with bilateral swelling of submandibular area, what could be the disease:
    (a) Facial fibrous dysplasia
    (b) Pleomorphic adenoma
    (c) Cherubism
    (d) Paget's disease of bone

    Answer for Q 13 on page 445

14. In osteosarcoma there is elevation in the periosteum in:
    (a) Parosteal osteosarcoma
    (b) Periosteal osteosarcoma
    (c) Endosteal osteosarcoma
    (d) None of the above

    Answer for Q 14 on page 445

15. The scientific evidence in dictating that oral Lichen planus is a "premalignant Lesion" is:
    (a) Very strong
    (b) Non-existent
    (c) Moderately strong
    (d) Weak

    Answer for Q 15 on page 445

16. One of the differential diagnoses of focal cemento-osseous dysplasia is:
    (a) Condensing osteitis
    (b) Paget's disease
    (c) Osteosarcoma
    (d) None of the above

    Answer for Q 16 on page 446

17. Oral lesions of lichen planus usually appear as:
    (a) White striae
    (b) Red plaque
    (c) Shallow ulcers
    (d) Papillary projections

    Answer for Q 17 on page 446

18. Oral lesions of lichen planus:
    (a) Are usually painful
    (b) Rarely appear before lesion elsewhere on the body
    (c) May be part of a syndrome in which lesions also appear on the skin, conjunctiva and genitalia
    (d) Often appear in nervous, high-strung individuals

    Answer for Q 18 on page 446

19. All of the following are oral features of acquired immunodeficiency syndrome (AIDS) **except**:
    (a) Candidiasis.
    (b) Erythema multiform
    (c) Hairy leukoplakia
    (d) Rapidly progressing periodontitis
    Answer for Q 19 on page 446
20. Van der Woude syndrome has all of the following **except**:
    (a) Cleft lip
    (b) Paramedian pit
    (c) Cleft palate
    (d) Tongue tie
    Answer for Q 20 on page 446
21. ♣ A patient presents to your clinic complaining of a dry mouth. Which of the following would be suitable initial investigations to carry out to help determine the primary cause of the condition?
    (a) CT scan of the major salivary glands
    (b) Labial gland biopsy
    (c) Blood tests to determine anti-Lo and anti-Ra antibodies
    (d) Salivary flow rate
    (e) Ultrasound of the salivary glands
    Answer for Q 21 on page 446
22. ♣ You wish to provide symptomatic relief for a patient with a dry mouth. Which of the following drugs could be used?
    (a) Saliva Orthana
    (b) Glandosane
    (c) Pilocarpine
    (d) Hyoscine
    Answer for Q 22 on page 446
23. Complex hemihyperplasia is called when:
    (a) One whole side of the body is affected
    (b) Both side of the body are affected
    (c) Single limb is affected with complication
    (d) Single limb is affected without complication
    Answer for Q 23 on page 446

24. ♣ Which of the following drugs can result in tooth discoloration?
    (a) Chlorhexidine
    (b) Fluorides
    (c) Iron
    (d) Tetracyclines
    (e) Minocycline

    Answer for Q 24 on page 446

25. Metastatic tumor that results in radiopaque mass in the jaw is:
    (a) Renal cancer
    (b) Lung cancer
    (c) Prostate cancer
    (d) Thyroid cancer

    Answer for Q 25 on page 447

26. ♣ Causes of halitosis include:
    (a) Starvation
    (b) Alcohol
    (c) Cytotoxic drugs
    (d) Renal failure
    (e) Hepatic failure

    Answer for Q 26 on page 447

27. ♣ Which of the following statements about infections are correct?
    (a) Mumps is a common bacterial infection that causes bilateral enlargement of the parotid glands
    (b) Foot and mouth disease is caused by Coxsackie A virus and is characterized by a viral rash and oral ulceration
    (c) The Epstein–Barr virus causes infectious mononucleosis, in which petechiae of the palate and ulceration of the fauces are seen
    (d) Primary herpetic stomatitis is caused by the herpes zoster virus, usually type 1 and is a condition in which intra-oral vesicles occur, which rapidly break down to form ulcerated areas
    (e) A patient with a facial palsy and vesicles of herpes zoster in the external auditory meatus is likely to have Ramsay–Hunt syndrome

    Answer for Q 27 on page 447

28. ♣ Which of the following statements are correct with respect to the salivary glands and calculi?
    (a) Meal time syndrome only occurs if a patient has a blockage in salivary flow due to a salivary calculus
    (b) Salivary calculi form more commonly in the parotid gland than the submandibular gland
    (c) Encouraging salivary flow by chewing may help small salivary calculi to pass out through the salivary duct
    (d) Salivary calculi are more common in males than in females
    (e) Salivary calculi are always radiopaque due to calcium deposits, and hence are visible on radiographs

    Answer for Q 28 on page 447

29. A patient present with tender swelling in the palatal area. Associated teeth were normal. Radiographic examination of the area shows radiolucent area with honeycomb appearance. Excessive bleeding was encountered upon entering into the lesion. Most probable diagnosis of the lesion is:
    (a) Radicular cyst
    (b) Aneurysmal bone cyst
    (c) Hemorrhagic bone cyst
    (d) Mid-palatal cyst

    Answer for Q 29 on page 447

30. ♣ Which of the following are well-known effects of chewing betel nut/paan[1]?
    (a) Oral submucous fibrosis
    (b) Oral dysplasia
    (c) Oral candidiasis
    (d) Cervical caries
    (e) Fissured depapillated tongue

    Answer for Q 30 on page 448

31. A cyst occurring under the tongue, caused by obstruction of salivary gland duct, is called:
    (a) Dentigerous cyst
    (b) Dermoid cyst
    (c) Ranula
    (d) Periodontal cyst

    Answer for Q 31 on page 448

[1] Paan is a preparation of betel leaf with areca nut widely consumed throughout Asia, Indian subcontinent and East Asia (mainly Taiwan). It is chewed for its stimulant effects. After chewing, it is either spat out or swallowed.

32. ♣ Which of the following factors predispose a patient to oral and oropharyngeal squamous cell carcinoma?
   (a) Smokeless tobacco use
   (b) Sunlight
   (c) Viral infection
   (d) Vitamin C deficiency
   (e) Vitamin K deficiency

   Answer for Q 32 on page 448

33. ♣ Which of the following statements are correct regarding medications used to treat various types of pain in the orofacial region?
   (a) Idiopathic facial pain or atypical facial pain may be treated effectively with tricyclic antidepressants
   (b) Temporal arteritis may be treated effectively with clonazepam
   (c) Trigeminal neuralgia may be treated effectively with carbamazepine
   (d) Trigeminal neuralgia may be treated effectively with gabapentin
   (e) Post-herpetic neuralgia may be treated effectively with aciclovir

   Answer for Q 33 on page 448

34. All the following cysts present as radiolucent lesions **except**:
   (a) Nasopalatine
   (b) Globulomaxillary
   (c) Dermoid cyst
   (d) Periapical cyst

   Answer for Q 34 on page 448

35. ♣ Which of the following descriptions of the types of facial pain are correct?
   (a) Myofascial pain is often poorly localized
   (b) Pain from internal derangement of the temporomandibular joint is usually poorly localized
   (c) Periodic migrainous neuralgia (cluster headache) is often associated with facial flushing on the affected side of the face
   (d) If a young patient is diagnosed with migrainous neuralgia (cluster headache), it may well be due to multiple sclerosis
   (e) Atypical facial pain (idiopathic facial pain) is often poorly localized and may occur in the absence of organic signs

   Answer for Q 35 on page 448

36. ♣ Which of the following conditions are associated with a known increased risk of malignant change?
    (a) Geographic tongue
    (b) Hairy leukoplakia
    (c) Sublingual keratosis
    (d) Denture stomatitis
    (e) Erosive lichen planus

    Answer for Q 36 on page 448

37. ♣ A patient presents with a sore mouth. Which hematological tests would you request?
    (a) Full blood count (FBC)
    (b) Serum ferritin
    (c) Alkaline phosphatase levels
    (d) Urea and electrolytes (U&Es)
    (e) Mean corpuscular volume (MCV)

    Answer for Q 37 on page 448

38. ♣ Which of the following are common signs of primary herpetic gingivostomatitis?
    (a) Dry mouth
    (b) Intra-oral vesicles
    (c) Circumoral vesicles
    (d) Intra-oral ulcers

    Answer for Q 38 on page 449

39. The most commonly involved tooth with dentigerous cyst is the:
    (a) Maxillary first premolar
    (b) Maxillary canine
    (c) Mandibular canine
    (d) Mandibular third molar

    Answer for Q 39 on page 449

40. ♣ Which of the following are used to treat patients with primary herpetic gingivostomatitis?
    (a) A broad-spectrum antibiotic
    (b) Analgesics
    (c) An antifungal medication
    (d) Fluids
    (e) Aciclovir

    Answer for Q 40 on page 449

41. The following statements are true for latent bone cyst **except**:

   (a) It is developmental lingual mandibular salivary gland depression

   (b) It is a salivary gland aberrancy

   (c) Located between the lower border of the mandible and the inferior alveolar canal

   (d) Located above the inferior alveolar canal

   Answer for Q 41 on page 449

42. ♣ Which of the following are features of secondary Sjögren's syndrome?

   (a) Dry mouth (xerostomia)

   (b) Insomnia (loss of smell)

   (c) Connective tissue disease

   (d) Dry eyes (xerophthalmia)

   (e) Increased incidence of oral squamous cell carcinoma (SCC)

   Answer for Q 42 on page 449

43. ♣ Which of the following describes the pain of trigeminal neuralgia?

   (a) Dull ache

   (b) Electric shock-like

   (c) Activated by touching a trigger zone

   (d) Usually prevents patients' sleeping

   (e) Lasts for hours

   Answer for Q 43 on page 449

44. ♣ Which of the following can be used to treat trigeminal neuralgia?

   (a) Jaw exercises in retruded position

   (b) Carbamazepine

   (c) Baclofen

   (d) Phenytoin

   (e) Flumazenil

   Answer for Q 44 on page 449

45. Which of the following is not a true cyst?

   (a) Gingival cyst

   (b) Calcifying odontogenic cyst

   (c) Dentigerous cyst

   (d) Aneurysmal bone cyst

   Answer for Q 45 on page 450

46. ♣ Which of the following drugs has gingival hyperplasia as a side effect?

(a) Phenytoin

(b) Carbamazepine

(c) Nifedipine

(d) Cisplatin

(e) Ciclosporin

Answer for Q 46 on page 450

47. ♣ Which of the following conditions are strongly associated with human immunodeficiency virus (HIV) infection?

(a) Kaposi's carcinoma

(b) Hairy leukoplakia

(c) Candidiasis

(d) Lichen planus

(e) Narcotizing ulcerative gingivitis

Answer for Q 47 on page 450

48. ♣ Which of the following drugs commonly cause lichenoid reactions?

(a) Gold

(b) Non-steroidal anti-inflammatory drugs (NSAIDs)

(c) β-Blockers

(d) Carbamazepine

(e) Oral hypoglycaemics

Answer for Q 48 on page 450

49. ♣ Which of the following are types of lichen planus?

(a) Reticular

(b) Erosive

(c) Pseudomembranous

(d) Bullous

(e) Hyperplastic

Answer for Q 49 on page 450

50. Odontogenic keratocyst develops:
    (a) In place of a missing tooth
    (b) On the fully formed crown
    (c) As result of obstruction of salivary flow by a keratin plug
    (d) From dental lamina remnants in the mandible and maxilla

    Answer for Q 50 on page 450

51. ♣ Which of the following are treatments options for lichen planus?
    (a) No treatment
    (b) Fluconazole
    (c) Betnesol (betamethasone)
    (d) Azathioprine
    (e) Pilocarpine

    Answer for Q 51 on page 450

52. The cyst that shows scallops between the roots of the teeth in its X-ray picture is:
    (a) Aneurysmal bone cyst
    (b) Staphne bone cyst
    (c) Simple bone cyst
    (d) Gorlin cyst

    Answer for Q 52 on page 450

53. ♣ Which of the following conditions are associated with bullous lesions?
    (a) Epidermolysis bullosa
    (b) Linear Ig A disease
    (c) Erythema multiforme
    (d) Pemphigus
    (e) Bulimia

    Answer for Q 53 on page 450

54. An epithelial lining is typically found in:
    (1) Traumatic bone cyst
    (2) Keratocyst
    (3) Mucous extravasation cyst

(4) Dentigerous cyst

(a) 1, 2 and 4 are correct

(b) 2 and 4 correct

(c) 2 and 3 correct

(d) 1, 2 and 3 correct

Answer for Q 54 on page 450

55. ♣ Which of the following statements are true?

(a) Lichen planus is characterized by mononuclear inflammatory infiltrate in the lamina propria

(b) The rate of malignant transformation with lichen planus is in the order of 10%

(c) Patients with systemic lupus erythematosus (SLE) may present with a malar rash

(d) Pemphigus is more common in children

(e) Behçet's syndrome may present with conjunctivitis and uveitis

Answer for Q 55 on page 450

56. ♣ Which of the following are true regarding Sjögren's syndrome?

(a) It is more common in females

(b) Primary Sjögren's may be associated with rheumatoid arthritis

(c) Autoantibodies against ribonucleotides are found: SS-A or Ro and SS-B or La

(d) May lead to B-cell lymphoma (MALTOMA)

(e) Tricyclic antidepressants may be helpful

Answer for Q 56 on page 451

57. Regarding aphthous ulcers:

(a) They are more common in males

(b) The herpetiform-type are more common in males

(c) Hematinic deficiencies are detected in approximately 50% of cases

(d) They can be associated with cessation of smoking

(e) They are often helped by the used of antidepressants

Answer for Q 57 on page 451

58. Features of glandular odontogenic cyst **do not** include:

(a) Commonly seen in the mandible

(b) Exhibits a non-aggressive clinical course

(c) The cyst is lining might contain cuboidal and goblet cells

(d) Recurrence is expected

Answer for Q 58 on page 451

59. ♣ Which of the following lesions/conditions are caused by viruses?

 (a) Koplik's spots
 (b) Herpetiform ulcers
 (c) Herpes labialis
 (d) Ramsay–Hunt syndrome
 (e) Lyme disease

Answer for Q 59 on page 451

60. ♣ Patients with which of the following conditions are more likely to get oral candidal infections than those without?

 (a) Patients undergoing chemotherapy
 (b) Sjögren's syndrome
 (c) Diabetes mellitus
 (d) Anemia
 (e) Undernutrition

Answer for Q 60 on page 451

61. ♣ Which of the following conditions can be associated with oral mucosal disease?

 (a) Crohn's disease
 (b) Irritable bowel syndrome (IBS)
 (c) Ulcerative colitis
 (d) Peutz–Jeghers syndrome
 (e) Bowen's disease

Answer for Q 61 on page 451

62. ♣ Which of the following are treatments for dry mouth?

 (a) Pilocarpine
 (b) Salivary substitutes based on carboxymethylcellulose
 (c) Mucin-based salivary substitutes
 (d) Atropine
 (e) Hyoscine

Answer for Q 62 on page 451

63. Which of the following pathological lesions usually has an empty lumen:
   (a) Radicular cyst
   (b) Mucocele
   (c) Dermoid cyst
   (d) Traumatic bone cyst

   Answer for Q 63 on page 452

64. ♣ Angular cheilitis can be:
   (a) Caused by candidal infection of the commissures
   (b) Caused by Staphylococcus aureus infection of the commissures
   (c) Caused by an increase in occlusal vertical dimension in patients wearing dentures
   (d) Treated with aciclovir cream
   (e) Treated with miconazole cream

   Answer for Q 64 on page 452

65. The microscopic appearance of translucent, dark, body of the lesion and surface zones represents the carious lesion of:
   (a) Deep dentin caries
   (b) Destructive cementum caries
   (c) Early dentin caries
   (d) Early enamel caries

   Answer for Q 65 on page 452

66. ♣ Although the etiology of recurrent aphthous ulceration is unknown, which of the following are thought to be associated with aphthous ulceration?
   (a) Smoking
   (b) Hematinic deficiencies
   (c) Stress
   (d) Family history
   (e) HIV

   Answer for Q 66 on page 452

67. ♣ Which of the following oral lesions are known to be related to candidal infections?

    (a) Antibiotic sore mouth

    (b) Denture stomatitis

    (c) Median rhomboid glossitis

    (d) Geographical tongue (erythema migrans)

    (e) Hairy leukoplakia

    Answer for Q 67 on page 452

68. ♣ Dry mouth may be caused by:

    (a) Hyperbaric oxygen treatment of osteoradionecrosis

    (b) Sjögren's syndrome

    (c) Sarcoidosis

    (d) Bell's palsy

    (e) Parkinson's disease

    Answer for Q 68 on page 452

69. Liquefaction foci and transverse clefts are structures see in:

    (a) Dentin caries

    (b) Deep enamel caries

    (c) Early enamel caries

    (d) Superficial cementum caries

    Answer for Q 69 on page 452

70. ♣ Regarding oral cancer:

    (a) It accounts for approximately 10% of cancers in the UK

    (b) It is commoner in men

    (c) Smoking and heavy alcohol intake are synergistic risk factors

    (d) Chewed tobacco (betel nut) is safer than smoked tobacco

    (e) It may arise in white patches

    Answer for Q 70 on page 452

71. The location of smooth surface caries includes:

    (a) Buccal surface of the upper second molar

    (b) Lingual surface of the upper central incisor

    (c) Mesial surface of the lower first molar

    (d) Occlusal surface of the upper second molar

    Answer for Q 71 on page 453

72. ♣ Which of the following are potentially malignant oral lesions?
    (a) Oral submucous fibrosis
    (b) Speckled leukoplakia
    (c) Actinic cheilitis
    (d) Erythema multiforme

    Answer for Q 72 on page 453

73. Increased radiodensity around sites of chronic dental infection is suggestive of:
    (a) Suppurative osteomyelitis.
    (b) Sclerosing osteomyelitis
    (c) Stafne bone defect.
    (d) Dry socket

    Answer for Q 73 on page 453

74. ♣ Regarding mucous membrane pemphigoid:
    (a) It is commoner in men
    (b) The onset is in the third to fourth decade
    (c) It is characterized by deposits of immunoglobulins and complement components in the basement membrane
    (d) It is characterized by loss of intercellular adherence of supra-basal spinous cells
    (e) Ocular involvement may lead to blindness

    Answer for Q 74 on page 453

75. ♣ Desquamative gingivitis is seen in which of the following conditions?
    (a) Lichen planus
    (b) Pemphigus vulgaris
    (c) Erythema multiforme
    (d) Erythema migrans
    (e) Mucous membrane pemphigoid

    Answer for Q 75 on page 453

76. The commonly affected age group with Garre's osteomyelitis is the:
    (a) Childhood and adolescence
    (b) Newborn
    (c) Old age
    (d) Middle age

    Answer for Q 76 on page 453

77. ♣ Regarding Bell's palsy:

(a) It is an upper motor neurone lesion

(b) It causes a unilateral paralysis of all the muscles of facial expression

(c) It is thought to be due to compression of the facial nerve in the pterygomaxillary fissure

(d) Loss of taste may also be associated

(e) It is usually treated with low-dose steroids

Answer for Q 77 on page 453

78. ♣ Regarding herpes infections of the trigeminal area:

(a) Reactivation of the herpes simplex virus usually causes cold sores on the lips

(b) Herpetic whitlow can be caught only from patients with primary herpes infections

(c) Post-herpetic neuralgia follows a herpes simplex infection

(d) Post-herpetic neuralgia usually responds well to treatment with carbamazepine

(e) Post-herpetic neuralgia usually occurs in young patients

Answer for Q 78 on page 454

79. ♣ Petechial hemorrhage is characteristic of which of the following condition?

(a) Agranulocytosis

(b) Neutropenia

(c) Pernicious anemia

(d) Thrombocytopenic purpura

Answer for Q 79 on page 454

80. ♣ Bacteria found in gingivitis are localized in:

(a) Connective tissue fibers

(b) Gingival Sulcus

(c) Alveolar bone

(d) Periodontal ligament

Answer for Q 80 on page 454

81. Epimyoepithelial islands are common histological feature of:

(a) Pleomorphic adenoma

(b) Adenocystic carcinoma

(c) Sicca syndrome

(d) Epidemic parotitis

Answer for Q 81 on page 454

82. ♣ Histological examination of the tissues in desquamative gingivitis reveals:
   (a) Hyperkeratosis
   (b) Elongation of the rete pegs
   (c) Aggregations of giant cells
   (d) Local loss of the basement membrane

   Answer for Q 82 on page 454

83. One of the following malignant tumors tend to spread through perineural lymphatics:
   (a) Kaposi's sarcoma
   (b) Mucoepidermoid carcinoma
   (c) Adenocystic carcinoma
   (d) Osteogenic sarcoma

   Answer for Q 83 on page 454

84. ♣ One of the earlier signs of cavernous sinus thrombosis is due to deficit in the function of:
   (a) Trochlear nerve
   (b) Abducens nerve
   (c) Oculomotor nerve
   (d) Ophthalmic division of trigeminal nerve

   Answer for Q 84 on page 454

85. ♣ Exfoliative cytology is mainly used in the definitive diagnosis of the:
   (a) Oral cancer
   (b) Fungal infection
   (c) Vesiculobullous diseases
   (d) Viral infection

   Answer for Q 85 on page 454

86. ♣ Of the following locations, the one in which the prognosis of epidermoid carcinoma is least favorable is:
   (a) Lower lip
   (b) Hard palate
   (c) Buccal mucosa
   (d) Posterior lateral border of tongue

   Answer for Q 86 on page 454

87. The most common development disorder affecting the tongue is:
    (a) Median rhomboid glossitis
    (b) Fissured tongue
    (c) White spongy nevus
    (d) Black hairy tongue
    Answer for Q 87 on page 455

88. Mumps is caused by:
    (a) Orthomyxovirus
    (b) Paramyxovirus
    (c) Rhabdovirus
    (d) Retrovirus
    Answer for Q 88 on page 455

89. A flat, circumscribed discoloration of skin or mucosa that may vary in size and shape is referred to as:
    (a) Epulis
    (b) Macule
    (c) Nodule
    (d) Papule
    Answer for Q 89 on page 455

90. One of the following tumors can affect parotid gland bilaterally:
    (a) Basal cell adenoma
    (b) Canalicular adenoma
    (c) Papillary cystadenoma
    (d) Papillary cystadenoma lymphomatosum
    Answer for Q 90 on page 455

91. A twenty-year-old woman complains that regular, gentle brushing of her teeth is painful besides causing profuse bleeding. Oral examination reveals the loss of epithelium from the attached gingiva of both arches. Which of the following dermatological problems is this patient most likely to have?
    (a) Benign mucous membrane pemphigoid
    (b) Chronic discoid lupus erythematosus
    (c) Pemphigus
    (d) Psoriasis
    Answer for Q 91 on page 455

92. Which of the following is also known as "mixed" tumor?

    (a) Warthin's tumor

    (b) Oncocytoma

    (c) canalicular adenoma

    (d) Pleomorphic adenoma

    Answer for Q 92 on page 455

93. Which of the following is an oral manifestation of lichen planus?

    (a) Dentinogenesis imperfecta

    (b) Fordyce spots

    (c) White, chalky enamel surface

    (d) White radiating lines on the buccal mucosa

    Answer for Q 93 on page 455

94. Among the following, which is the most common site of occurrence of pleomorphic adenoma?

    (a) Hard palate

    (b) Soft palate

    (c) Parotid gland

    (d) Submandibular gland

    Answer for Q 94 on page 455

95. Which of the following tumors occurs almost **exclusively** in parotid gland?

    (a) Oncocytoma

    (b) Myoepithelioma

    (c) Pleomorphic adenoma

    (d) Papillary cystadenoma lymphomatosum

    Answer for Q 95 on page 455

96. Antinuclear antibodies are seen in:

    (a) SLE

    (b) Systemic sclerosis

    (c) Morphea[2]

    (d) All of the above

    Answer for Q 96 on page 455

[2] Morphea is a localized scleroderma that involves patches of hardened and discolored skin on the face, hands, and feet, or anywhere else on the body.

97. Which of the following is **not** a growth pattern for adenoid cystic carcinoma?
    (a) Solid
    (b) Cribriform
    (c) Follicular
    (d) Tubular
    (e) Plexiform

    Answer for Q 97 on page 455

98. Which of the following diseases of the skin is the most likely to be associated with partial or total anodontia?
    (a) Erythema multiforme
    (b) Hereditary ectodermal dysplasia
    (c) Keratosis follicularis
    (d) Treacher Collins syndrome
    (e) Franceschetti's syndrome

    Answer for Q 98 on page 455

99. Which of the following is **absent** in CREST syndrome?
    (a) Calcinosis cutis
    (b) Raynaud's phenomenon
    (c) Telangiectasia
    (d) Endocrine disorders
    (e) Sclerodactyly

    Answer for Q 99 on page 456

100. Nikolsky's sign is positive in:
    (a) Bullous pemphigus
    (b) Epidermolysis bullosa
    (c) Herpes simplex
    (d) Erythema multiforme
    (e) Steven Johnson syndrome

    Answer for Q 100 on page 456

101. Look in the following picture and guess the most probable diagnosis

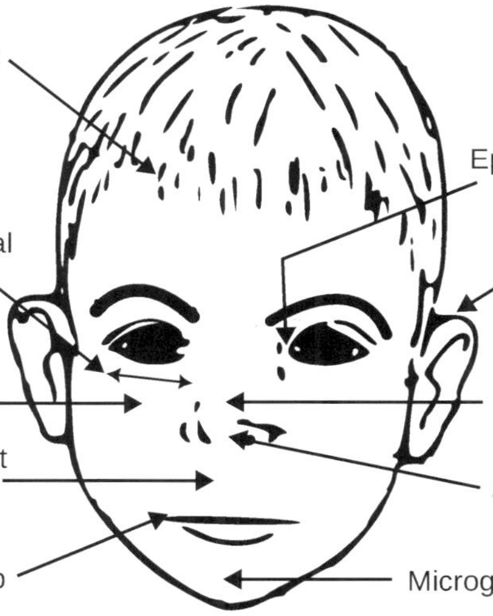

(a) Achondroplasia

(b) Cleidocranial dysplasia

(c) Fetal alcohol syndrome

(d) Pierre Robin sequence

(e) Treacher Collins syndrome

Answer for Q 101 on page 456

102. Monro's microabscess are seen in:

(a) Pemphigus

(b) Lichen planus

(c) Leukoplakia

(d) Psoriasis

Answer for Q 102 on page 456

103. In lichen planus the basal cells which are shrunken with an eosinophilic cytoplasm and with a pyknotic and fragmented nuclei are called:

(a) Tzanck cells

(b) Civatte bodies

(c) Donovan bodies

(d) Rushton bodies

Answer for Q 103 on page 456

104. Mumps (epidemic parotitis):
   (a) Is caused by an adenovirus
   (b) Is transmitted by droplet spread from infected saliva
   (c) Complications are more common in children rather than adults
   (d) Recurrent attacks are not uncommon
   Answer for Q 104 on page 456

105. Grinspan's syndrome is associated with:
   (a) Hypertension, diabetes, lichen planus
   (b) Oral, ocular, genital lesions
   (c) Hypertension with oral lesions
   (d) Pemphigus, CHF, diabetes
   Answer for Q 105 on page 456

106. Regarding fetal alcohol syndrome:
   (a) invasive dental procedures are contraindicated if the patient displays behavioral signs/symptoms that pose a risk to himself or the dental team during procedures
   (b) invasive dental procedures should be postponed for getting medical consultation if the patient has any cardiac condition
   (c) Antibiotic prophylaxis required
   (d) All of the above
   Answer for Q 106 on page 456

107. The most common form of inheritance of ectodermal dysplasia is:
   (a) Autosomal recessive
   (b) Autosomal dominant
   (c) X-linked dominant
   (d) X-linked recessive
   Answer for Q 107 on page 456

108. In Sjogren's syndrome:
   (a) Proliferation of the acini
   (b) Occurs early in childhood
   (c) Common in males than females
   (d) Increased incidence of malignant lymphoma
   Answer for Q 108 on page 456

109. Which sites are characteristically affected in Stevens–Johnson syndrome?
   (a) Conjunctiva, genitalia, oral mucosa
   (b) Liver, spleen, pancreas
   (c) Oral mucosa, lacrimal apparatus, ears
   (d) Parotid gland, palate, conjunctiva

   Answer for Q 109 on page 456

110. Which one of the following is **NOT** a lichenoid reaction?
   (a) Graft versus Host disease
   (b) Fixed drug eruption
   (c) Secondary syphilis
   (d) Pemphigus vulgaris

   Answer for Q 110 on page 456

111. Squamous cell papilloma is similar histologically and clinically to:
   (a) Verruca vulgaris
   (b) Keratoacanthoma
   (c) Squamous cell carcinoma
   (d) Congenital epulis of newborn

   Answer for Q 111 on page 456

112. Oral diagnostic features of scleroderma include all of the following, **except**:
   (a) Pseudoankylosis of the T.M. Joint
   (b) Widening of the oral aperture
   (c) A hard and a rigid tongue
   (d) Difficulty in swallowing

   Answer for Q 112 on page 456

113. The most important difference between verruca vulgaris and squamous cell papilloma is:
   (a) Presence of intranuclear inclusion bodies
   (b) Presence of hyperkeratosis
   (c) Presence of acanthosis
   (d) More longer rete pegs

   Answer for Q 113 on page 457

114. A typical example of an immunologically mediated collagen vascular/connective tissue disorder is:

(a) Lichen planus

(b) Pemphigus vulgaris

(c) Lupus erythematosus

(d) Epidermolysis bullosa

Answer for Q 114 on page 457

115. Pseudoepitheliomatous hyperplasia is a characteristic feature of:

(a) Keratoacanthoma

(b) Squamous cell papilloma

(c) Verruca vulgaris

(d) Pyogenic granuloma

Answer for Q 115 on page 457

116. Fine needle aspiration biopsy is indicated to diagnose:

(a) Necrotic pulp

(b) Pemphigus

(c) Traumatic ulcer

(d) Chronic gingivitis

Answer for Q 116 on page 457

117. Juvenile melanomas are clinically benign, although they are histologically malignant:

(a) Both statements are correct

(b) Both statements are incorrect

(c) The first statement is only correct

(d) The second statement is only correct

Answer for Q 117 on page 457

118. Subepithelial vesicles are characteristic all of the following **except**:

(a) Bullous pemphigoid

(b) Pemphigus

(c) Epidermolysis bullosa acquisita

(d) Cicatrical pemphigoid

Answer for Q 118 on page 457

119. In blue nevus the nevus cells are:
   (a) Spindle shaped
   (b) Rounded
   (c) Epithelioid
   (d) Polyhydral

   Answer for Q 119 on page 457

120. An independent, uncoordinated new growth of tissue which is potentially capable of unlimited growth and does not regress after removal of stimulus is:
   (a) Tumor
   (b) Neoplasm
   (c) Swelling
   (d) All of the above

   Answer for Q 120 on page 457

121. Which is a degeneration disorder characterized by atrophic changes of the deeper structures (e.g., fat, muscle, cartilage & bone) involving one side of the face:
   (a) Miescheris syndrome
   (b) Peutz-Jeghers syndrome
   (c) Parry Romberg syndrome
   (d) Scleroderma

   Answer for Q 121 on page 457

122. In cicatricial pemphigoid, which antigen is bound by IgG on the epidermal side of the salt split skin technique:
   (a) Laminin 5
   (b) XVII collagen
   (c) Epitigrin
   (d) BP antigen 1 & 2

   Answer for Q 122 on page 457

123. L.E. Cell phenomenon in peripheral blood is seen in:
   (a) Systemic Lupus Erythematosus
   (b) Ischemic heart disease
   (c) Infective endocarditis
   (d) Rheumatic heart disease

   Answer for Q 123 on page 457

124. "Self-healing carcinoma" is term usually applied to one of the following:

(a) Acanthoma

(b) Papilloma

(c) Keratoacanthoma

(d) Verrucous carcinoma

Answer for Q 124 on page 457

125. Which of the followings is the most common lesion of the skin?

(a) Intradermal nevus

(b) Junctional nevus

(c) Compound nevus

(d) Spindle cell nevus

Answer for Q 125 on page 457

126. Erosive lichen planus resembles which of the following:

(a) Monilial gingivitis

(b) Acute ulcerative gingivitis

(c) Desquamative gingivitis

(d) Herpetic gingivitis

Answer for Q 126 on page 457

127. Origin of peripheral giant cell granuloma is:

(a) Gingiva

(b) Interdental papilla

(c) Mucoperiosteum

(d) Tongue

Answer for Q 127 on page 457

128. Grinspan's syndrome is associated with:

(a) Lichen planus

(b) Aphthous ulcer

(c) Leukoplakia

(d) Oral submucous fibrosis

Answer for Q 128 on page 457

129. Which of the followings represent a hamartomatous malformation rather than a true neoplasm?

(a) Hemangioma

(b) Lymphangioma

(c) Blue nevus

(d) All of the above

Answer for Q 129 on page 458

130. Desmoplakin is the target antigen in:

(a) Pemphigus foliaceous

(b) Pemphigus Vulgaris

(c) Drug-induced pemphigus

(d) Paraneoplastic pemphigus

Answer for Q 130 on page 458

131. One of the following lesions might be related to vitamin B12 deficiency:

(a) Frictional keratosis

(b) Lichen planus

(c) Oral submucous fibrosis

(d) Keratoacanthoma

Answer for Q 131 on page 458

132. Top to bottom epithelial dysplasia usually refers to:

(a) Severe epithelial dysplasia

(b) Moderate epithelial dysplasia

(c) Mild epithelial dysplasia

(d) None of the above

Answer for Q 132 on page 458

133. Unusual extensibility of the tongue is a characteristic feature of:

(a) Syphilis

(b) Darier-White disease

(c) Ehlers-Danlos syndrome

(d) Epidermolysis bullosa

Answer for Q 133 on page 458

134. 60-year-old diabetic female presented with burning sensation to spicy food, Intraoral examination revealed multiple periodontal abscess and keratotic area in a lace pattern with occasional erosive areas inside the lace pattern. Syndrome associated with this disease is:

(a) Peutz Jeghers syndrome

(b) Sjogren's syndrome

(c) Down's syndrome

(d) Grinspan syndrome

Answer for Q 134 on page 458

135. En coup de sabre is most likely to be associated with which type of scleroderma?

(a) Linear

(b) Radicular

(c) Vertical

(d) Ovoid

Answer for Q 135 on page 458

136. Histopathologic study of lichen planus shows:

(a) Antiepithelial antibodies

(b) Scattered infiltrate with ill-defined lower border

(c) Mixed cellular inflammatory infiltrate

(d) Presence of T-lymphocytes predominantly

Answer for Q 136 on page 458

137. Cafe au lait macules are seen in:

(a) Albright's syndrome and Bloom's syndrome

(b) Von Reklinghausen's neurofibromatosis

(c) None of them

(d) All of the above

Answer for Q 137 on page 458

138. About hairy leukoplakia, only one statement is **not** correct:

(a) Commonly affect immunodeficient patients

(b) Characterized histologically by ballooning cells

(c) Caused by human papilloma virus

(d) Found on lateral borders of the tongue

Answer for Q 138 on page 458

139. Psoriasis is associated with:
   (a) Lupus erythematosus
   (b) Lupus vulgaris
   (c) Benign median rhomboid glossitis
   (d) Geographic tongue

   Answer for Q 139 on page 458

140. Mumps (epidemic parotitis):
   (a) Is caused by an adenovirus
   (b) Is transmitted by droplets spread from infected saliva
   (c) Complications are more common in children rather than adults
   (d) Recurrent attacks are not uncommon

   Answer for Q 140 on page 458

141. White radiating lines can be observed in case of lesions of:
   (a) Erythema multiforme
   (b) Lichen planus
   (c) Pemphigus
   (d) Leukoplakia

   Answer for Q 141 on page 458

142. Pemphigus is characterized by:
   (a) Hyperparakeratosis
   (b) Hyperorthokeratosis
   (c) Acantholysis
   (d) Acanthosis

   Answer for Q 142 on page 458

143. A 60-year-old diabetic female presented with burning sensation to spicy food. Intraoral examination revealed multiple periodontal abscess and keratotic area in a lace pattern with occasional erosive areas inside the lace pattern. Histological feature will be:
   (a) Saw tooth rete ridges
   (b) Bulbous rete ridges
   (c) Elongated rete ridges
   (d) Flattened rete ridges

   Answer for Q 143 on page 458

144. One of the following conditions is considered as an undifferentiated variant of squamous cell carcinoma:

(a) Spindle cell carcinoma

(b) Verrucous carcinoma

(c) Krompecker's carcinoma

(d) None of the above

Answer for Q 144 on page 458

145. Mucocutaneous lesion associated with neoplasia:

(a) Paraneoplastic pemphigus

(b) Parapemphigus

(c) Pemphigus vegetans

(d) Familial benign pemphigus

Answer for Q 145 on page 458

146. One of the following features is related to stage 2 of TNM system:

(a) Palpable but not fixed unilateral lymph nodes

(b) Palpable but not fixed ipsilateral lymph nodes

(c) Non palpable lymph nodes

(d) Evidence of distant metastasis

Answer for Q 146 on page 459

147. ALL the following are inherited disorders of connective tissue **except**:

(a) Marfan syndrome

(b) McArdle's disease

(c) Ehlers-Danlos syndrome

(d) Alport syndrome

Answer for Q 147 on page 459

148. Cicatricial pemphigoid is the synonym for:

(a) pemphigus vulgaris

(b) mucous membrane pemphigoid

(c) paraneoplastic pemphigus

(d) Hailey-Hailey disease

Answer for Q 148 on page 459

149. Pathologic calcification is seen in:
   (a) Scleroderma
   (b) Lupus erythematosus
   (c) Dystrophic epidermolysis bullosa
   (d) Lichen planus

   Answer for Q 149 on page 459

150. A 3-year-old patient has extensive vesicles on their lips, tongue, and oral mucous membrane. After 2–4 days, vesicles rupture, forming painful ulcers. The patient has a mild fever. What will be the diagnosis?
   (a) Steven-Johnson syndrome
   (b) Primary herpetic gingivostomatitis
   (c) Acute ulcerative necrotizing gingivitis
   (d) Erythema multiforme

   Answer for Q 150 on page 459

151. Evidence of distant metastasis is related to one of the following stages of TNM system:
   (a) Stage 1
   (b) Stage 2
   (c) Stage 3
   (d) Stage 4

   Answer for Q 151 on page 459

152. Oral, ocular and genital lesions are seen in:
   (a) Erythema multiforme
   (b) SLE
   (c) Stevens-Johnson syndrome
   (d) None of them

   Answer for Q 152 on page 459

153. Tzanck smear test is used in the diagnosis of:
   (a) Pemphigus
   (b) ANUG
   (c) Lichen planus
   (d) Aphthous disease

   Answer for Q 153 on page 459

154. Parakeratin lining the clefts and parakeratin plugging is a hallmark of:

(a) Basal cell carcinoma

(b) Epidermoid carcinoma

(c) Transitional cell carcinoma

(d) Verrucous carcinoma

Answer for Q 154 on page 459

155. Multiple pulp stones are seen in:

(a) Down's syndrome

(b) Ehler's Danlos syndrome

(c) Apert's syndrome

(d) Marfan Syndrome

Answer for Q 155 on page 459

156. Erythema multiforme is:

(a) Bacterial infection

(b) An acute self-limiting disease, of skin and oral mucous membrane

(c) Painless vesicular self-limiting disease

(d) A viral disease

Answer for Q 156 on page 459

157. Which of the following viruses might be implicated as the causative factor of nasopharyngeal carcinoma?

(a) Human papilloma virus

(b) Human immunodeficiency virus

(c) Epstein Barr virus

(d) Cytomegalovirus

Answer for Q 157 on page 459

158. Target Lesions are observed in case of:

(a) Erythema multiforme

(b) Psoriasis

(c) Lichen planus

(d) Pemphigus vulgaris

Answer for Q 158 on page 459

159. Lupus erythematosus is:
   (a) Autoimmune disorder
   (b) Neoplastic condition
   (c) Degenerative condition
   (d) Reactive Lesion

   Answer for Q 159 on page 459

160. Oral Lesions are not seen in:
   (a) Psoriasis
   (b) Pemphigoid
   (c) Candidiasis
   (d) Stevens-Johnson syndrome

   Answer for Q 160 on page 459

161. False about mucous membrane pemphigoid:
   (a) Twice in female
   (b) Disease associated antigen are most frequently present in lamina densa
   (c) Oral mucosa is most frequently involved
   (d) Autoantibodies towards basement membrane protein

   Answer for Q 161 on page 459

162. The swollen degenerating epithelial cell due to acantholysis is:
   (a) Tzanck cell
   (b) Prickle cell
   (c) Anitschow cell
   (d) Ghost cell

   Answer for Q 162 on page 460

163. Primary lesion in lichen planus is:
   (a) Bulla
   (b) Vesicle
   (c) Papule
   (d) Macule

   Answer for Q 163 on page 460

164. Koebner's phenomenon is seen with:

(a) Psoriasis

(b) Erythema multiforme

(c) Impetigo

(d) Pemphigoid

Answer for Q 164 on page 460

165. Which of the following is inherited as an autosomal dominant trait?

(a) Bullous pemphigoid

(b) White sponge nevus

(c) Lichen planus

(d) Pemphigus vulgaris

Answer for Q 165 on page 460

166. Wickham's striae are seen in:

(a) Leukoedema

(b) Erythema multiforme

(c) Lichen planus

(d) Leukoplakia

Answer for Q 166 on page 460

167. In ectodermal dysplasia all of the following structures are affected **except**:

(a) Teeth

(b) Salivary glands

(c) Nails

(d) Hair

Answer for Q 167 on page 460

168. Ehlers Danlos syndrome is?

(a) X-Linked recessive

(b) X-Linked Dominant

(c) Autosomal recessive

(d) Autosomal Dominant

Answer for Q 168 on page 460

169. Butterfly rash is typically seen in:
   (a) Systemic lupus erythematosus
   (b) Herpes simplex
   (c) Scleroderma
   (d) None of them

   Answer for Q 169 on page 460

170. Joint erosions are not a feature of:
   (a) Rheumatoid arthritis
   (b) Multicentric reticulo-histiocytosis
   (c) Systemic Lupus erythematosus
   (d) Psoriasis

   Answer for Q 170 on page 460

171. Xeroderma pigmentosum is characterized by:
   (a) Autosomal dominant inheritance
   (b) Inability to repair sunlight induced damage to DNA
   (c) Acanthosis of epithelium with elongation of rete ridges
   (d) Irregular accumulation of melanin in the basal cell layer

   Answer for Q 171 on page 460

172. All are diseases of skin **except**:
   (a) Keratosis follicularis
   (b) Erythema multiforme
   (c) Psoriasis form lesion
   (d) Erythema migrans

   Answer for Q 172 on page 460

173. Intraepithelial vacuolation with formation of vesicle or bulla intraepithelially above the basal layer is characteristically seen in:
   (a) Pemphigus
   (b) Lichen planus
   (c) Bullous pemphigoid
   (d) Candida albicans

   Answer for Q 173 on page 460

174. Darier's disease is associated with:

(a) Vitamin A deficiency and involvement of oral epithelium and skin
(b) Diffuse tender ulceration on the palate predominantly
(c) Pernicious anemia
(d) Rickets with involvement of teeth and bones

Answer for Q 174 on page 460

175. Which of the following individual show susceptibility to dental caries?

(a) Down syndrome
(b) Pierre robin syndrome
(c) Epidermolysis bullosa
(d) Hereditary fructose intolerance

Answer for Q 175 on page 460

176. Which of the following is not a type of lichen planus?

(a) Hypertrophic
(b) Atrophic
(c) Verrucous
(d) Erosive

Answer for Q 176 on page 460

177. Autoantibodies Anti Ro and Anti La are completely absent in:

(a) Sjogren's syndrome
(b) Diffuse Scleroderma
(c) Rheumatoid arthritis
(d) Systemic lupus erythematosus

Answer for Q 177 on page 460

178. Immunofluorescence is seen at basement membrane as patchy distribution in:

(a) Lichen Planus
(b) Pemphigus
(c) Pemphigoid
(d) Lupus erythematosus

Answer for Q 178 on page 460

179. Histological clefts in lichen planus are:

(a) Auspitz's sign

(b) Civatte bodies

(c) Wickham's Striae

(d) Max - Joseph spaces

Answer for Q 179 on page 461

180. The most common lesion in Mucous membrane pemphigoid is:

(a) Esophageal ulcer

(b) Ulcer of Soft palate

(c) Symblepharon

(d) Desquamative gingivitis

Answer for Q 180 on page 461

181. Which of the following are seen in ectodermal dysplasia?

(a) Defective or absence of sweat glands

(b) Hyperpyrexia

(c) Protuberant lips and frontal bossing

(d) Any of them

Answer for Q 181 on page 461

182. In which of the following disorders a circulating antibody directed to intercellular cementing substance of stratified squamous epithelium is observed:

(a) Pemphigus vulgaris

(b) Bullous pemphigoid

(c) Verrucous vulgaris

(d) Lichen planus

Answer for Q 182 on page 461

183. Fish Net pattern in pemphigus vulgaris is seen in which of the following tests?

(a) Tzanck smear

(b) Histopathology

(c) Direct immunofluorescence

(d) FNAC

Answer for Q 183 on page 461

184. Intraepithelial bullae are found in:

   (a) Pemphigoid

   (b) Pemphigus

   (c) Bullous pemphigoid

   (d) Bullous lichen planus

   Answer for Q 184 on page 461

185. A 60-year-old has got severe bulla and target lesion which erythema around halo and genital Lesions:

   (a) Herpes zoster

   (b) Stevens Johnson syndrome

   (c) Herpes simplex

   (d) Herpangina

   Answer for Q 185 on page 461

186. Bullae formation after striking an intact skin/mucosal surface is known as:

   (a) Chovstek's sign

   (b) Tinel's sign

   (c) Babinski's sign

   (d) Nikolsky's sign

   Answer for Q 186 on page 461

187. Hydropic degeneration of the basal cell of the stratum germinativum is a feature of?

   (a) Leukoplakia

   (b) Lichen Planus

   (c) Pemphigus

   (d) Syphilis

   Answer for Q 187 on page 461

188. Steven-Johnson syndrome involves:

   (a) Type I hypersensitivity reaction

   (b) Type IV hypersensitivity reaction

   (c) Type II hypersensitivity reaction

   (d) Type III hypersensitivity reaction

   Answer for Q 188 on page 461

189. Lichen planus:
   (a) Must be excised
   (b) Treated only by medication
   (c) Can undergo malignant change
   (d) Is an idiosyncrasy reaction

Answer for Q 189 on page 461

190. Oral lesion associated with ulcerative colitis:
   (a) Pyostomatitis Vegetans
   (b) Sarcoidosis
   (c) Lichen planus
   (d) Dermatitis herpetiformis

Answer for Q 190 on page 461

191. Immunofluorescence test is positive in:
   (a) Psoriasis
   (b) Lupus erythematosus
   (c) Scleroderma
   (d) Myxoedema

Answer for Q 191 on page 461

192. Formation of multiple pinpoint bleeding spots on scratching the skin is characteristic of:
   (a) Pemphigus vulgaris
   (b) Lupus erythematosus
   (c) Psoriasis
   (d) Herpangina

Answer for Q 192 on page 461

193. Lichenoid reactions are mainly due to:
   (a) Intake of alcohol
   (b) Cigarette smoking
   (c) Betel nut chewing
   (d) Intake of certain drugs

Answer for Q 193 on page 461

194. A 45-years-old patient came to your clinic complaining of loose teeth with prolonged gingival bleeding. Recently, he lost his job and has been drinking heavily for the last three months. Currently he is

homeless. Based on the patient's history, social status and prolonged gingival bleeding, the function of which organ is compromised?

(a) Kidney
(b) Pancreas
(c) Liver
(d) Spleen

Answer for Q 194 on page 461

195. Surgical procedures involving the parotid gland may impose the greatest risk of damage to the:

(a) Facial vein
(b) Facial artery
(c) Internal carotid artery
(d) Retromandibular vein

Answer for Q 195 on page 462

196. Which layer of the epidermis contains stem cells undergoing mitosis?

(a) Basal cell layer
(b) Stratum corneum
(c) Stratum granulosum
(d) Stratum spinosum

Answer for Q 196 on page 462

197. Which one of the inflammatory cells would predominate in chronic sialadenitis if a biopsy is examined?

(a) Eosinophils
(b) Lymphocytes
(c) Macrophages
(d) Neutrophils

Answer for Q 197 on page 462

198. Which type of bone cells possess the capability to secrete collagenase?

(a) Osteoblasts
(b) Osteochondral progenitor cells
(c) Osteoclasts
(d) Osteocytes

Answer for Q 198 on page 462

199. Which type of bone cells possess the capability to secrete acid phosphatase?
   (a) Osteoblasts
   (b) Chondroblast
   (c) Osteoclasts
   (d) Osteocytes

Answer for Q 199 on page 462

200. Which type of bone cells possess the capability to secrete alkaline phosphatase?
   (a) Osteoblasts
   (b) Chondroblasts
   (c) Osteoclasts
   (d) Osteocytes

Answer for Q 200 on page 462

201. Addison's disease is characterized by:
   (a) Excess adrenal androgen production
   (b) Hyperfunction of the adrenal cortex
   (c) Hypofunction of the adrenal cortex
   (d) Increased glycolysis

Answer for Q 201 on page 462

202. A 3-Years-old-age child came with his mother. The chief Complaint "My daughter's teeth are loose and falling out." There is no history of facial injury. Radiographically, normal root morphology for lost anterior tooth. What is the most likely diagnosis?
   (a) Amelogenesis imperfecta
   (b) Dentinogenesis imperfecta
   (c) Hypophosphatasia
   (d) Cleidocranial dysplasia

Answer for Q 202 on page 462

203. The offspring of a genotypically normal mother and a father with an X-linked recessive disease will produce:
   (a) 50% affected sons
   (b) 100% affected sons
   (c) 100% affected daughters
   (d) 100% carrier daughters

Answer for Q 203 on page 462

204. Clear cells are commonly seen in which of the following lesions?

(a) Pleomorphic

(b) Warthin's tumor

(c) Pindborg tumor

(d) Adenomatoid odontogenic tumor

Answer for Q 204 on page 462

205. A-16-years old female attends your dental practice for an appointment. She is fit and healthy but has a phobia of dental injections. During administration of an inferior dental nerve block she becomes unwell and faints. What do you think is the most likely cause?

(a) Addisonian crisis

(b) Cerebrovascular accident

(c) Hypoglycemic shock

(d) Myocardial infarction

(e) Vasovagal attack

Answer for Q 205 on page 462

206. A 60-Year-old male with a history of Insulin-dependent Diabetes Mellitus loses consciousness during the course of dental treatment. What do you think is the most likely cause?

(a) Addisonian crisis

(b) Anaphylaxis

(c) Hyperglycemia

(d) Hypoglycemia

(e) Ketoacidosis

Answer for Q 206 on page 462

207. A 45-Year-old female develops acute anaphylaxis following administration of amoxicillin. Which one of the following drugs would be the most appropriate first line therapy?

(a) Adrenaline

(b) Chlorpheniramine

(c) Diazepam

(d) Hydrocortisone

(e) Salbutamol

Answer for Q 207 on page 462

208. A 4-year-old, child presents with fever, gingival bleeding and extensive oral ulceration in his mouth. His medical history is unremarkable. What would be your most likely diagnosis?

   (a) Candidal infection
   (b) Herpes Simplex infection
   (c) Herpes Zoster infection
   (d) Paramyxovirus infection
   (e) Recurrent Aphthous ulceration

   Answer for Q 208 on page 462

209. A 60-year-old male presents with unilateral facial paralysis, cutaneous lesions of external auditory meatus hearing defects, and vertigo. What would be your most likely diagnosis?

   (a) Bell's palsy
   (b) Melkersson Rosenthal syndrome
   (c) Moebius syndrome
   (d) Ramsay Hunt syndrome
   (e) Trigeminal neuralgia

   Answer for Q 209 on page 462

210. A-60-year old female presents with recurrent oral and corneal ulceration. Her biopsy specimen reveals subepithelial bullae. What is your most likely diagnosis?

   (a) Candidal infection
   (b) Lichen Planus
   (c) Mucous membrane pemphigoid
   (d) Pemphigus vulgaris
   (e) Squamous cell carcinoma

   Answer for Q 210 on page 462

211. A 55-Years-old female presents with severe, electrical and shocking pain in her right cheek triggered by light touch. Clinical examination does not reveal any local cause. Which drug is most likely to be effective for her?

   (a) Baclofen
   (b) Carbamazepine
   (c) Ergotamine
   (d) Paracetamol
   (e) Sumatriptan

   Answer for Q 211 on page 462

212. Which one of the following is the least likely indication for antibiotic prophylaxis to prevent bacterial endocarditis?

(a) Congenital heart disease
(b) Diabetes mellitus
(c) Previous history of endocarditis
(d) Rheumatic fever
(e) Valvular heart disease

Answer for Q 212 on page 463

213. A-55-year old edentulous female presents with an erythematous patch on her palate. She wears complete dentures and has a history of Insulin Dependent Diabetes Mellitus. You make a diagnosis of Denture stomatitis. Which drug is most likely to be effective for her?

(a) Augmentin
(b) Hydrocortisone
(c) Ibuprofen
(d) Miconazole
(e) Phenytoin

Answer for Q 213 on page 463

214. A-35-year old female presents with clicking in her right temporomandibular joint for the last six months. She does not have any pain or limitation of her mouth opening. Clinical examination does not reveal odontogenic cause. What does this condition most likely represent?

(a) Ankylosis of temporomandibular joint
(b) Fracture of the mandibular condyle
(c) Internal derangement of temporomandibular joint
(d) Myofascial pain
(e) Rheumatoid arthritis

Answer for Q 214 on page 463

215. Which one of the following conditions is least likely to be associated with immunosuppression?

(a) Acromegaly
(b) Agammaglobulinemia
(c) Anemia
(d) Diabetes mellitus
(e) Leukemia

Answer for Q 215 on page 463

216. Bone pain, renal calcinosis, and giant cell jaw lesions are most likely to be seen in which one of the following disorders?
   (a) Acromegaly
   (b) Fibrous dysplasia
   (c) Hyperparathyroidism
   (d) Hyperthyroidism
   (e) Paget's disease

   Answer for Q 216 on page 463

217. A-55-Y old female presents with a non-healing ulcer on the lateral border of her tongue. The ulcer has not responded to local measures. You suspect a squamous cell carcinoma. Which type of investigation would you perform for her?
   (a) Excisional biopsy
   (b) Exfoliative cytology
   (c) Immunoflourescence
   (d) Incisional biopsy
   (e) Needle aspiration

   Answer for Q 217 on page 463

218. Which one of the following statements regarding cluster headaches is least likely to be true?
   (a) Affects midface & circumorbital areas
   (b) Causes nasal stuffiness & facial flushing
   (c) May mimic anterior maxillary tooth ache
   (d) Mostly affects elderly females
   (e) Pain usually lasts for 15–30 minutes

   Answer for Q 218 on page 463

219. A-45-year old female presents with a 6 months history of recurrent mealtime swelling and pain in her right submandibular region. Clinical examination does not reveal any dental abnormality. What is the most likely cause for her symptoms?
   (a) Lymphadenitis
   (b) Sialolithiasis
   (c) Sialometaplasia
   (d) Sialorrhea
   (e) Xerostomia

   Answer for Q 219 on page 463

220. Which one of the following terms is most appropriate to describe pain occurring at the site of nerve injury?

(a) Analgesia

(b) Anesthesia

(c) Causalgia

(d) Hypesthesia

(e) Paresthesia

Answer for Q 220 on page 463

221. A-40-year old gentleman with a 6 months history of trauma to his face and complains of slight burning in his temporal area accompanied by increased sweating. What is the most likely diagnosis?

(a) Bell's palsy

(b) Cluster headache

(c) Frey's syndrome

(d) Postherpetic neuralgia

(e) Trigeminal neuralgia

Answer for Q 221 on page 463

222. A-55-year old male presents with hemorrhagic crusting of his lips following a course of antibiotic therapy. He does not have any systemic manifestations. What would be your most likely diagnosis?

(a) Anaphylaxis

(b) Bechet's syndrome

(c) Erythema multiforme

(d) Lichen Planus

(e) Pemphigus vulgaris

Answer for Q 222 on page 463

223. A-25-year old female with a history of betel quid chewing presents severe limitation of mouth opening. Clinical examination reveals palpable white fibrotic bands in her buccal mucosa bilaterally. What would be your most likely diagnosis?

(a) Oral submucous fibrosis

(b) Lichen planus

(c) Temporomandibular joint ankylosis

(d) Scleroderma

(e) Verrucous carcinoma

Answer for Q 223 on page 463

224. Which one of the following conditions is least likely to be associated with an increased risk of oral cancer?
    (a) Actinic cheilosis
    (b) Erythroplakia
    (c) Leukoedema
    (d) Leukoplakia
    (e) Plummer-Vinson syndrome

Answer for Q 224 on page 463

225. Perioral melanin pigmentation and intestinal polyps are most likely to be seen in which one of the following conditions?
    (a) ACTH therapy
    (b) Addison disease
    (c) Gorlin-Goltz Syndrome
    (d) Neurofibromatosis
    (e) Peutz–Jeghers syndrome

Answer for Q 225 on page 463

226. A neoplasm of enamel organ that **does not** undergo differentiation to the point of enamel or dentin formation is:
    (a) Odontome
    (b) Ameloblastoma
    (c) Calcifying epithelial odontogenic tumor
    (d) Adenomatoid odontogenic tumor

Answer for Q 226 on page 463

227. The most common malignancy in the oral cavity is:
    (a) Squamous cell carcinoma
    (b) Burkitt's lymphoma
    (c) Basal cell carcinoma
    (d) Adenocarcinoma

Answer for Q 227 on page 463

228. Extra-osseous ameloblastoma commonly occurs in:

(a) Gingiva

(b) Long bones

(c) Limbs

(d) Neck

Answer for Q 228 on page 464

20.2 Answers with Comments:

1. The correct answer is **B** – The underlying mechanism is usually a problem with connective tissue due to poorly formed type I collagen. In more than 90% of cases, OI occurs due to mutations in the COL1A1 or COL1A2 genes.

   Back to Q 1 on page 395

2. The correct answer is **B** – Carbamazepine (Tegretol, Carbatrol, and others) are used for the treatment of trigeminal neuralgia, and it's been shown to be effective in treating the condition.

   Back to Q 2 on page 395

3. The correct answer is **B** – In osteopetrosis, the main defect is the reduced osteoclastic activity.

   Back to Q 3 on page 395

4. The correct answer is **D** – Aphthous ulcers occurs mainly in the non-keratinized lining mucosa.

   Back to Q 4 on page 396

5. The correct answer is **B** – Urinary hydroxyproline levels are elevated in Paget's disease of bone, as a reflection of increased osteoclastic activity and bone resorption. Hydroxyproline is a product of collagen breakdown. Approximately 20-30% of total hydroxyproline levels are from bone resorption.

   Back to Q 5 on page 396

6. The correct answer is **C** – Chancre is the primary syphilis infection and appears as an indurated painless papule which soon ulcerates.

   Back to Q 6 on page 396

7. The correct answer is **A** – Primary herpetic gingivostomatitis is distributed in the whole oral cavity including keratinized and non-keratinized mucosa, while herpes zoster is always unilateral and herpangina is usually restricted to the soft palate and oropharynx.

   Back to Q 7 on page 396

8. The correct answer is **B** – Cleidocranial dysplasia is characterized by presence of many unerupted supernumerary and supplemental teeth.

Back to Q 8 on page 396

9. The correct answer is **A** – The virus remains latent in the oral epithelial cells or in the sensory ganglia. Thus, the virus is not completely eliminated from the oral cavity [9], [16]. Note that in the original exam, the correct answer was **D**, which we think is not the appropriate answer.

   The human herpesvirus (**HHV**) family (Herpetoviridae) are double-stranded DNA viruses, which includes mainly:

   (a) Herpes simplex virus (HSV), which includes HSV type 1 (HSV-1 or HHV-1 or herpes virus labialis) and HSV type 2 (HSV-2 or HHV-2 or herpes virus genitalis)

   (b) Varicella-zoster virus (VZV or HHV-3)

   (c) Epstein-Barr virus (EBV or HHV-4)

   (d) Cytomegalovirus (CMV or HHV-5)

   (e) HHV-6, and HHV-7 are closely related and thought to be responsible for symptomatic primary infection—termed **roseola** (**exanthema subitum**, **sixth disease**) – most often is caused by HHV-6 but also may be caused by HHV-7. Both viruses may replicate in salivary glands and establish latency in CD4+ T lymphocytes or other cell types. Reactivation occurs most frequently in immunocompromised patients and can result in widespread multi-organ infection, such as encephalitis, pneumonitis, bone-marrow suppression, and hepatitis.

   (f) HHV-8, involved in the pathogenesis of Kaposi sarcoma (KS)

   Humans are the only natural reservoir for these viruses, which are endemic worldwide.

   Back to Q 9 on page 397

10. The correct answer is **B** – False, because calcium channel blockers have no effects on salivary flow.

    Back to Q 10 on page 397

11. The correct answer is **A** – Maccune-Albright syndrome is a form of polystotic fibrous dysplasia in which mutation occurs in early embryonic life thus affecting multi-system of the body.

    Back to Q 11 on page 397

12. The correct answer is **A** – As the most common biopsy in the oral cavity is the excisional one.

    Back to Q 12 on page 397

13. The correct answer is **C** – Cherubism occurs bilaterally at young age.

    Back to Q 13 on page 397

14. The correct answer is **B** – New bone formation by the tumor under the periosteum will result in its elevation.

    Back to Q 14 on page 398

15. The correct answer is **C** – Patients with OLP were 4.8 times more likely to have OSCC than the matched referents. It is concluded that patients with OLP, and particularly the **erosive type** of OLP, should be

monitored closely for OSCC development, see reference [17]. Note that the original answer was **D**, which is in disagreement with the recent studies.

Back to Q 15 on page 398

16. The correct answer is **A** – Condensing osteitis is a localized lesion similar to cemento-osseous dysplasia.

    Back to Q 16 on page 398

17. The correct answer is **A** – The characteristic clinical feature of oral lichen planus is Wickham's stria which appears as white streaks.

    Back to Q 17 on page 398

18. The correct answer is **C** – Around 36% of cases of oral lichen planus are associated with skin lesions and around 46% of cases of lichen planus occur without oral lesions [18].

    Back to Q 18 on page 398

19. The correct answer is **B** – Till now, there is no reported cases of erythema multiforme occurring in association with AIDS.

    Back to Q 19 on page 399

20. The correct answer is **D** – Tongue tie is not a feature of Van der Woude syndrome.

    Back to Q 20 on page 399

21. The correct answer is **BDE** – In the absence of other signs and symptoms, CT scans of the major salivary glands are not normally carried out as part of the investigations for a dry mouth. A scan may be carried out if there is an enlargement of a salivary gland. Ultrasound is becoming more popular as a non-invasive investigation for salivary gland disease, and is often used when patients have dry mouths. Salivary flow rate is normally recorded as well. Blood tests are usually performed and include an antibody screen to test for anti-Ro and anti-La antibodies, which help in the diagnosis of Sjögren's syndrome, and also a labial gland biopsy.

    Back to Q 21 on page 399

22. The correct answer is **ABC** – Saliva Orthana and Glandosane are artificial saliva substitutes; Glandosane is acidic, whereas Saliva Orthana is non-acidic and contains fluoride. Pilocarpine is a non-selective muscarinic agonist that stimulates glandular secretions. It can be used to stimulate salivary flow but may have side effects such as sweating, gastrointestinal symptoms, and flushing of the face. Atropine and hyoscine are both anti-muscarinic drugs that are used to dry salivary secretions.

    Back to Q 22 on page 399

23. The correct answer is **A** – One whole side of the body is affected in cases of complex hemihyperplasia.

    Back to Q 23 on page 399

24. The correct answer is **ABCD** – Minocycline can lead to brown pigmentation of gingivae and mucosa but not of teeth. Chlorhexidine causes extrinsic staining of teeth. Tetracyclines and excessive fluoride cause intrinsic staining of teeth. Iron can cause extrinsic staining in infant teeth.

Back to Q 24 on page 400

25. The correct answer is **C** – Prostate cancer stimulates new bone formation hence, appear as a radiopaque mass.

Back to Q 25 on page 400

26. The correct answer is **ABCDE** – Halitosis or oral malodor is common and there are many causes including:

- Oral infections, sepsis in sinus and other part of respiratory tract
- Tumors
- GORD (gastro-oesophageal reflex disease)
- Volatile food stuffs, e.g., garlic, onions, curry
- Certain medical conditions, e.g., diabetic ketoacidosis and renal failure, which are associated with characteristic odor.
- Halitosis may also be psychogenic.

Back to Q 26 on page 400

27. The correct answer is **CE** – Mumps is caused by paramyxovirus and hence is a viral infection. It does cause painful enlargement of the parotid glands, but it may affect other glands as well. Hand, foot, and mouth disease is caused by Coxsackie A virus and is characterized by a viral rash and oral ulceration, whereas foot and mouth disease is a disease of cattle caused by a rhinovirus. Other signs and symptoms of infectious mononucleosis are cervical lymphadenopathy, sore throat, tonsillar exudates, and pyrexia. Primary herpetic stomatitis is usually caused by the type 1 herpes simplex virus. It does cause vesicular stomatitis, which may be accompanied by malaise, tiredness, and a sore throat. Herpes zoster infection in the geniculate ganglion causes Ramsay-Hunt syndrome. This causes facial weakness and vesicles of zoster to form in the ear and throat.

Back to Q 27 on page 400

28. The correct answer is **CD** – Meal time syndrome occurs if a patient has any type of blockage in salivary flow (e.g., calculus, stricture, mucus plug, etc.) from a major gland. 80 per cent of salivary calculi form in the submandibular gland, and it could be due to the composition of the saliva and the position and length of the duct. Salivary calculi occur most commonly in adult males. Not all salivary calculi are radiopaque, and sometimes they are only visualized on further imaging, e.g., a sialogram.

Back to Q 28 on page 401

29. The correct answer is **B** – Exploring or surgical intervention of aneurysmal bone cyst results in excessive bleeding.

    Back to Q 29 on page 401

30. The correct answer is **AB** – Chewing betel nut/paan is known to be a risk factor for oral submucous fibrosis, oral dysplasia and squamous cell carcinoma. Oral candidiasis, cervical caries and a fissured depapillated tongue are often caused by a dry mouth.

    Back to Q 30 on page 401

31. The correct answer is **C** – Ranula is the cyst resulting from obstruction of salivary glands under the tongue.

    Back to Q 31 on page 401

32. The correct answer is **ABC** – The etiology of oral squamous cell carcinoma is multifactorial and it is generally thought that the numerous risk factors include all kinds of tobacco usage, excessive alcohol usage, betel nut chewing, immunodeficiency, vitamin A deficiency, chronic infections such as candidal and syphilitic infections, and oral mucosal diseases including submucous fibrosis and lichen planus. Infection with the human papilloma virus (especially HPV-16) increases the risk of oropharyngeal cancer. Sunlight is also thought to play a role in lip cancer.

    Back to Q 32 on page 402

33. The correct answer is **ACD** – Temporal arteritis may be treated effectively with steroids. Post-herpetic neuralgia may be treated effectively with gabapentin or antidepressants. The initial viral infection may be effectively treated with aciclovir, but not the resultant neuralgic pain.

    Back to Q 33 on page 402

34. The correct answer is **C** – Dermoid cyst is a soft tissue cyst, hence it is negative in x-ray.

    Back to Q 34 on page 402

35. The correct answer is **ACE** – Pain due to internal derangement of the temporomandibular joint is usually well localized as opposed to myofascial pain, which is often poorly localized. Periodic migrainous neuralgia (cluster headache) is often associated with facial flushing, as well as a watery eye and a runny nose on the affected side. Young patients with symptoms of trigeminal neuralgia may have multiple sclerosis.

    Back to Q 35 on page 402

36. The correct answer is **CE** – Sublingual keratosis has a higher rate of malignant transformation than normal mucosa, as does erosive lichen planus. All the other conditions do not have a higher rate of malignant change.

    Back to Q 36 on page 403

37. The correct answer is **ABE** – A sore mouth may be due to hematological deficiency and hence blood tests are indicated when a patient complains of a sore mouth. FBC is indicated to determine if the patient is anemic. The anemic may be secondary to iron, folate or vitamin B12 deficiency. MCV is indicated to determine if the anemia is microcytic (eg iron deficiency) or macrocytic (B12 or folate deficiency).

    Back to Q 37 on page 403

38. The correct answer is **BD** – Primary herpetic gingivostomatitis is a viral infection caused by the herpes simplex virus. It is usually a subclinical infection. Patients have vesicles that may occur on any part of the oral mucosa, which burst leaving ulcers. Dry mouth and low hemoglobin are not usually seen in this condition. Labial vesicles are seen in recurrent herpes simplex infections and occasionally seen in primary herpetic gingivostomatitis.

    Back to Q 38 on page 403

39. The correct answer is **D** – Mandibular third molar is the most common site of dentigerous cyst. Maxillary canine is the second most common site.

    Back to Q 39 on page 403

40. The correct answer is **BDE** – Primary herpetic gingivostomatitis is a viral infection. Therefore, it is not treated with antibiotics or anti-fungals. Aciclovir can be used in severe cases and when there is widespread infection, but it needs to be given early. In milder cases bed rest, analgesics and fluids are usually sufficient

    Back to Q 40 on page 403

41. The correct answer is **D** – Latent bone cyst is located below the inferior alveolar canal.

    Back to Q 41 on page 404

42. The correct answer is **ACD** – In secondary Sjögren's syndrome, either xerostomia (dry mouth) or xerophthalmia (dry eyes) occurs in association with an autoimmune connective tissue disorder. Patients do not lose their sense of smell (anosmior have a higher incidence of oral SCC.

    Back to Q 42 on page 404

43. The correct answer is **BC** – Trigeminal neuralgia is an intense, excruciating, paroxysmal pain, often described as a shooting or electric shock-like pain. It lasts seconds and usually occurs when a trigger zone is touched. It does not usually keep patients awake at night.

    Back to Q 43 on page 404

44. The correct answer is **BCD** – Retruded jaw exercises are helpful in the management of temporomandibular joint dysfunction. Flumazenil is a benzodiazepine antagonist used for the reversal of the central sedative effects of benzodiazepines. Carbamazepine, baclofen and phenytoin may all be used for the treatment of trigeminal neuralgia.

    Back to Q 44 on page 404

45. The correct answer is **D** – Aneurysmal bone cyst is not lined by epithelium thus it is not a true cyst.

    Back to Q 45 on page 404

46. The correct answer is **ACE** – Gingival hyperplasia is a common side effect of calcium-channel blockers such as nifedipine and diltiazem. It also occurs with phenytoin and ciclosporin.

    Back to Q 46 on page 405

47. The correct answer is **BCE** – Kaposi's sarcoma is commonly associated with HIV infection. Hairy leukoplakia is strongly associated with HIV; non-HIV cases do occur but usually in immunocompromised patients. Candidal infections are extremely common in HIV-infected patients as is periodontal disease including acute necrotizing ulcerative gingivitis.

    Back to Q 47 on page 405

48. The correct answer is **ABCE** – Many drugs have been found to cause lichenoid reactions including anti-malarials, NSAIDs, gold, some tricyclic antidepressants, oral hypoglycemics, methyldopa, penicillamine and β-blockers.

    Back to Q 48 on page 405

49. The correct answer is **ABD** – Six types of lichen planus have been described: reticular, papular, plaque-like, atrophic (desquamative gingivitis), erosive/ulcerative and bullous. Pseudomembranous and hyperplastic are types of candidiasis.

    Back to Q 49 on page 405

50. The correct answer is **D** – Odontogenic keratocyst develops From dental lamina remnants in the jaws.

    Back to Q 50 on page 406

51. The correct answer is **ACD** – Treatment is not always required for lichen planus, and depends on the severity. Active treatment ranges from topical to systemic corticosteroids. In severe cases immunosuppressants, e.g., azathioprine and ciclosporin, may be necessary. Fluconazole is an anti-fungal used for the treatment of candidiasis. Pilocarpine is a parasympathomimetic used in the treatment of dry mouth.

    Back to Q 51 on page 406

52. The correct answer is **C** – Simple bone cyst (traumatic, solitary bone cyst) frequently extend between the roots of the associated teeth to produce a scalloped appearance that is characteristic of this lesion.

    Back to Q 52 on page 406

53. The correct answer is **ABD** – Epidermolysis bullosa and pemphigus may present with bullous lesions, as may linear IgA disease. Bulimia presents with tooth erosion, and erythema multiforme presents with ulcers and blood-stained, crusted lips.

54. The correct answer is **B** – Keratocysts and dentigerous cysts are true cysts lined by epithelium.

55. The correct answer is **ACE** – The rate of malignant transformation with lichen planus is in the order of 1%. Pemphigus is found mainly in middle-aged and older patients. SLE patients present with the classic malar 'butterfly' rash.

56. The correct answer is **ACD** – Secondary Sjögren's syndrome comprises dry eyes or dry mouth together with a connective tissue or autoimmune disease – not primary Sjögren's syndrome. Dry mouth is a side effect of tricyclic antidepressants.

    Back to Q 56 on page 407

57. The correct answer is **D** – Aphthous ulcers are slightly commoner in females than males. Hematinic deficiencies are detected in up to 20% of patients, and the ulcers can sometimes be associated with smoking cessation. The main treatment after correction of hematinic deficiencies is topical corticosteroids.

    Back to Q 57 on page 407

58. The correct answer is **B** – Glandular odontogenic cyst is an aggressive cyst.

    Back to Q 58 on page 407

59. The correct answer is **ACD** – Koplik's spots are seen in the buccal mucosa in patients with measles, which is an infection caused by paramyxovirus. Herpes labialis is caused by the herpes simplex virus and Ramsay–Hunt syndrome is due to herpes zoster of the geniculate ganglion. Herpetiform ulcers are a type of aphthous ulcer and are not caused by a virus. Lyme disease is caused by Borrelia burgdorferi, a spirochaetal bacterium, and is spread via ticks.

    Back to Q 59 on page 408

60. The correct answer is **ABCDE** – Candidal infections are commoner in patients with other underlying disease processes. Hence patients with anemia, diabetes mellitus and those who are malnourished or undergoing chemotherapy are more at risk of candidal infections. Patients with Sjögren's syndrome suffer from dry mouth, which puts them at greater risk of candidal infections.

    Back to Q 60 on page 408

61. The correct answer is **ACD** – Bowen's disease is carcinoma in situ of the skin. Crohn's disease may affect any part of the gastrointestinal tract and hence the oral cavity may be involved. Lesions seen are cobblestoning of the buccal mucosa, glossitis, mucosal tags and swelling of the lips. In Peutz–Jeghers syndrome pigmented macules are seen around the perioral region. In ulcerative colitis, aphthous ulcers may be seen possibly due to the malabsorption which accompanies the condition. IBS is not usually associated with oral lesions.

    Back to Q 61 on page 408

62. The correct answer is **ABC** – Pilocarpine stimulates muscarinic receptors in the salivary glands and hence increases the production of saliva. It is used for patients who have some residual salivary gland function following radiotherapy. Artificial saliva may be used for symptomatic relief of dry mouth and

can be based on carboxymethylcellulose or mucin. Atropine and hyoscine are anti-muscarinic drugs that dry up secretions.

Back to Q 62 on page 408

63. The correct answer is **D** – Traumatic bone cyst (simple bone cyst) is a hollow cavity that may be lined by a thin layer of granulation tissue.

Back to Q 63 on page 409

64. The correct answer is **ABE** – Angular cheilitis is a combined staphylococcal and fungal infection that occurs at the angles of the mouth. It has been previously attributed to a decreased occlusal vertical dimension in denture wearers, but increasing the vertical dimension alone will not treat the infection. Treatment can involve fusidic acid cream and an antifungal, e.g., miconazole. Aciclovir is an anti-viral medication and hence not indicated for angular cheilitis.

Back to Q 64 on page 409

65. The correct answer is **D** – The translucent, dark, body of the lesion and surface zones represents the carious lesion of enamel.

Back to Q 65 on page 409

66. The correct answer is **BCDE** – The cause of recurrent aphthous ulceration is unknown, but several associations have been made. Stress, hematinic deficiencies and a family history all predispose a patient to getting aphthae. The ulcers also occur in HIV infections, being more severe in the more immunocompromised cases. Smoking is not associated with aphthae, in fact patients who do not smoke or who have recently stopped smoking are more likely to suffer from aphthae.

Back to Q 66 on page 409

67. The correct answer is **ABC** – Antibiotic sore mouth and denture stomatitis are caused by candidal infection. Previously median rhomboid glossitis was thought to be a developmental condition, but it is now thought to be due to chronic atrophic candidal infection on the tongue. The cause of geographic tongue is unknown. Hairy leukoplakia occurs in HIV-infected patients and immunocompromised individuals. The lesion may be secondarily infected with Candida, but it is not the cause of the lesion.

Back to Q 67 on page 410

68. The correct answer is **BC** – Bell's palsy and Parkinson's disease are commonly associated with hypersalivation (ptyalism). Hyperbaric oxygen treatment does not cause a dry mouth although the patients may have a dry mouth following the radiotherapy. Both Sjögren's syndrome and sarcoidosis may cause a dry mouth.

Back to Q 68 on page 410

69. The correct answer is **A** – Liquefaction foci and transverse clefts are structures see in dentin caries.

Back to Q 69 on page 410

70. The correct answer is **BCE** – Oral cancer accounts for approximately 2% of cancers in the UK, and traditionally it was a disease of older men. However, the incidence is increasing in younger patients and women. Smoking and alcohol consumption are risk factors and are thought to act synergistically. Chewing betel nut is also a risk factor and important in the Indian subcontinent where it is commonly practiced. White patches in the mouth have a potential for malignant change.

Back to Q 70 on page 410

71. The correct answer is **A** – The location of smooth surface caries includes buccal surface of the upper second molar.

Back to Q 71 on page 410

72. The correct answer is **ABC** – Various potentially malignant conditions occur in the oral cavity. The lesion with the highest rate of malignant transformation is erythroplakia. Speckled leukoplakia and leukoplakia also have the potential to turn malignant. Oral submucous fibrosis, lichen planus, actinic cheilitis, chronic hyperplastic candidosis and lupus erythematosus are all potentially malignant lesions.

Back to Q 72 on page 411

73. The correct answer is **B** – Radiopacities are always associated with sclerosing osteomyelitis.

Back to Q 73 on page 411

74. The correct answer is **CE** – Loss of intercellular adherence of suprabasal spinous cells is characteristic of pemphigus vulgaris; in pemphigoid the split occurs at the level of the basement membrane. Mucous membrane pemphigoid is twice as common in women and usually affects people in their fifth to sixth decades. One complication of the disease is ocular involvement, which may lead to scarring and blindness.

Back to Q 74 on page 411

75. The correct answer is **ABE** - In desquamative gingivitis, the gingivae are red, inflamed and atrophic. It occurs in lichen planus, pemphigus vulgaris and mucous membrane pemphigoid.

Back to Q 75 on page 411

76. The correct answer is **A** – Garre's osteomyelitis occurs in young age.

Back to Q 76 on page 411

77. The correct answer is **BD** - Bell's palsy is a lower motor neural lesion of the facial nerve, and as such it causes unilateral paralysis of all the muscles of facial expression. Upper motor neurone lesions affecting the facial nerve do not cause paralysis of the forehead as there is some cross-over in innervation. The palsy is thought to be due to compression of the facial nerve in the stylomastoid canal. Loss of taste occurs due to the chorda tympani being affected. Treatment is usually with high-dose steroids initially, which are then tailed off.

Back to Q 77 on page 412

78. The correct answer is **A** - Reactivation of the herpes simplex virus does cause herpes labialis, which takes the form of cold sores on the lips. Herpetic whitlow can be caught from patients with primary or secondary herpetic infections. Post-herpetic neuralgia follows herpes zoster infection, and usually occurs in older people. The response to carbamazepine is often poor.

Back to Q 78 on page 412

79. The correct answer is **D** – Thrombocytopenic purpura. Petechial purpura is minor bleeding into the dermis that is flat and non-blanching. Petechiae are typically found in patients with thrombocytopenia or platelet dysfunction. Palpable purpura occurs in vasculitis. Ecchymosis, or bruising, is more extensive bleeding into deeper layers of the skin. The lesions are initially dark red or purple but become yellow as hemoglobin is degraded [19].

Back to Q 79 on page 412

80. The correct answer is **B** – Gingival sulcus. The pathologic changes of gingivitis are associated with the presence of oral microorganisms attached to the tooth and perhaps in or near the gingival sulcus [15].

Back to Q 80 on page 412

81. The correct answer is **C** – Epimyoepithelial islands are common histological feature of sicca (Sjögren syndrome)

Back to Q 81 on page 412

82. The correct answer is **A** – Hyperkeratosis. Hyperkeratosis is seen in many conditions that may present clinically as desquamative gingivitis e.g.: lichen planus, chronic ulcerative stomatitis, systemic lupus erythematosus, chronic cutaneous erythematosus, etc [15].

Back to Q 82 on page 413

83. The correct answer is **C** – Adenocystic carcinoma tends to spread along perineural lymphatics.

Back to Q 83 on page 413

84. The correct answer is **B** – Abducens nerve. Because the abducens nerve (cranial nerve VI) is usually the first nerve to become involved due to its location in the lateral wall of the cavernous sinus, an early sign may be an internal strabismus [20].

Back to Q 84 on page 413

85. The correct answer is **C** – Vesiculobullous diseases. It has been recognized that the exfoliative oral cytologic smear is also of value in the diagnosis of diseases other than carcinoma, particularly diseases which are characterized by the presence of certain specific cells. Thus, cytologic smears have been useful in the diagnosis of lesions of herpes simplex infection, herpes zoster, pemphigus vulgaris, benign familial pemphigus, keratosis follicularis, hereditary benign intraepithelial dyskeratosis, white sponge nevus, and pernicious and sickle cell anemia [11]

Back to Q 85 on page 413

86. The correct answer is **D** – Posterior lateral border of tongue. The epidermoid carcinoma/squamous cell carcinoma is the most common malignant neoplasm of the oral cavity. Although it may occur at any intraoral site, certain sites are more frequently involved than others. Because of the differences in clinical appearance, the nature of the lesion and particularly the prognosis, it is well to describe the tumors individually, as they may arise in these various areas. Of the areas of the oral cavity, the mortality rate is lowest for lip cancer (0.04 per 100,000) and highest for the tongue (0.7 per 100,000) [11].

Back to Q 86 on page 413

87. The correct answer is **B** – Fissured tongue is a condition frequently seen in the general population and it is characterized by grooves that vary in depth and are noted along the dorsal and lateral aspects of the tongue. Although a definitive etiology is unknown, a polygenic mode of inheritance is suspected because the condition is seen clustering in families who are affected. Patients are usually asymptomatic, and the condition is initially noted on routine intraoral examination as an incidental finding. The condition is relatively common, with an estimated prevalence of 6.8%–11% [4].

Back to Q 87 on page 414

88. The correct answer is **B** – No explanation is available for this answer.

Back to Q 88 on page 414

89. The correct answer is **B** – No explanation is available for this answer.

Back to Q 89 on page 414

90. The correct answer is **D** – No explanation is available for this answer.

Back to Q 90 on page 414

91. The correct answer is **A** – No explanation is available for this answer.

Back to Q 91 on page 414

92. The correct answer is **D** – No explanation is available for this answer.

Back to Q 92 on page 415

93. The correct answer is **D** – No explanation is available for this answer.

Back to Q 93 on page 415

94. The correct answer is **C** – No explanation is available for this answer.

Back to Q 94 on page 415

95. The correct answer is **D** – No explanation is available for this answer.

Back to Q 95 on page 415

96. The correct answer is **A** – No explanation is available for this answer.

Back to Q 96 on page 415

97. The correct answer is **C** – No explanation is available for this answer.

Back to Q 97 on page 416

98. The correct answer is **B** – No explanation is available for this answer.

Back to Q 98 on page 416

99. The correct answer is **D** – No explanation is available for this answer.

Back to Q 99 on page 416

100. The correct answer is **A** – No explanation is available for this answer.

Back to Q 100 on page 416

101. The correct answer is **C** – Fetal alcohol syndrome resulting from excess consumption of alcohol by pregnant women. Its main facial feature are flat indistinct philtrum, thin upper lip, and shortened distance between inner and outer corners of the eye and epicanthal folds. Other orofacial abnormalities in FAS may include: microdontia with defective enamel; cleft lip; cleft palate; malocclusion; and poor tongue thrusting. Mouth breathing resulting from orofacial deformities can lead to dry mouth.

Back to Q 101 on page 416

102. The correct answer is **D** – No explanation is available for this answer.

Back to Q 102 on page 417

103. The correct answer is **B** – No explanation is available for this answer.

Back to Q 103 on page 417

104. The correct answer is **B** – No explanation is available for this answer.

Back to Q 104 on page 418

105. The correct answer is **A** – No explanation is available for this answer.

Back to Q 105 on page 418

106. The correct answer is **D** – No explanation is available for this answer.

Back to Q 106 on page 418

107. The correct answer is **D** – No explanation is available for this answer.

Back to Q 107 on page 418

108. The correct answer is **D** – No explanation is available for this answer.

Back to Q 108 on page 418

109. The correct answer is **A** – No explanation is available for this answer.

Back to Q 109 on page 419

110. The correct answer is **D** – No explanation is available for this answer.

Back to Q 110 on page 419

111. The correct answer is **A** – No explanation is available for this answer.

Back to Q 111 on page 419

112. The correct answer is **B** – No explanation is available for this answer.

Back to Q 112 on page 419

113. The correct answer is **A** – No explanation is available for this answer.

Back to Q 113 on page 419

114. The correct answer is **C** – No explanation is available for this answer.

Back to Q 114 on page 420

115. The correct answer is **A** – No explanation is available for this answer.

Back to Q 115 on page 420

116. The correct answer is **B** – No explanation is available for this answer.

Back to Q 116 on page 420

117. The correct answer is **A** – No explanation is available for this answer.

Back to Q 117 on page 420

118. The correct answer is **B** – No explanation is available for this answer.

Back to Q 118 on page 420

119. The correct answer is **A** – No explanation is available for this answer.

Back to Q 119 on page 421

120. The correct answer is **B** – No explanation is available for this answer.

Back to Q 120 on page 421

121. The correct answer is **C** – No explanation is available for this answer.

Back to Q 121 on page 421

122. The correct answer is **B** – No explanation is available for this answer.

Back to Q 122 on page 421

123. The correct answer is **A** – No explanation is available for this answer.

Back to Q 123 on page 421

124. The correct answer is **C** – No explanation is available for this answer.

Back to Q 124 on page 422

125. The correct answer is **A** – No explanation is available for this answer.

Back to Q 125 on page 422

126. The correct answer is **C** – No explanation is available for this answer.

Back to Q 126 on page 422

127. The correct answer is **C** – No explanation is available for this answer.

Back to Q 127 on page 422

128. The correct answer is **A** – No explanation is available for this answer.

Back to Q 128 on page 422

129. The correct answer is **D** – No explanation is available for this answer.

Back to Q 129 on page 423

130. The correct answer is **D** – No explanation is available for this answer.

Back to Q 130 on page 423

131. The correct answer is **C** – No explanation is available for this answer.

Back to Q 131 on page 423

132. The correct answer is **A** – No explanation is available for this answer.

Back to Q 132 on page 423

133. The correct answer is **C** – No explanation is available for this answer.

Back to Q 133 on page 423

134. The correct answer is **D** – No explanation is available for this answer.

Back to Q 134 on page 424

135. The correct answer is **A** – No explanation is available for this answer.

Back to Q 135 on page 424

136. The correct answer is **D** – No explanation is available for this answer.

Back to Q 136 on page 424

137. The correct answer is **D** – No explanation is available for this answer.

Back to Q 137 on page 424

138. The correct answer is **C** – No explanation is available for this answer.

Back to Q 138 on page 424

139. The correct answer is **D** – No explanation is available for this answer.

Back to Q 139 on page 425

140. The correct answer is **B** – No explanation is available for this answer.

Back to Q 140 on page 425

141. The correct answer is **B** – No explanation is available for this answer.

Back to Q 141 on page 425

142. The correct answer is **C** – No explanation is available for this answer.

Back to Q 142 on page 425

143. The correct answer is **A** – No explanation is available for this answer.

Back to Q 143 on page 425

144. The correct answer is **A** – No explanation is available for this answer.

Back to Q 144 on page 426

145. The correct answer is **A** – No explanation is available for this answer.

Back to Q 145 on page 426

146. The correct answer is **B** – No explanation is available for this answer.

Back to Q 146 on page 426

147. The correct answer is **B** – No explanation is available for this answer.

Back to Q 147 on page 426

148. The correct answer is **B** – No explanation is available for this answer.

Back to Q 148 on page 426

149. The correct answer is **A** – No explanation is available for this answer.

Back to Q 149 on page 427

150. The correct answer is **B** – No explanation is available for this answer.

Back to Q 150 on page 427

151. The correct answer is **D** – No explanation is available for this answer.

Back to Q 151 on page 427

152. The correct answer is **C** – No explanation is available for this answer.

Back to Q 152 on page 427

153. The correct answer is **A** – No explanation is available for this answer.

Back to Q 153 on page 427

154. The correct answer is **D** – No explanation is available for this answer.

Back to Q 154 on page 428

155. The correct answer is **B** – No explanation is available for this answer.

Back to Q 155 on page 428

156. The correct answer is **B** – No explanation is available for this answer.

Back to Q 156 on page 428

157. The correct answer is **C** – No explanation is available for this answer.

Back to Q 157 on page 428

158. The correct answer is **A** – No explanation is available for this answer.

Back to Q 158 on page 428

159. The correct answer is **A** – No explanation is available for this answer.

Back to Q 159 on page 429

160. The correct answer is **A** – No explanation is available for this answer.

Back to Q 160 on page 429

161. The correct answer is **B** – No explanation is available for this answer.

Back to Q 161 on page 429

162. The correct answer is **A** – No explanation is available for this answer.

Back to Q 162 on page 429

163. The correct answer is **C** – No explanation is available for this answer.

Back to Q 163 on page 429

164. The correct answer is **A** – No explanation is available for this answer.

Back to Q 164 on page 430

165. The correct answer is **B** – No explanation is available for this answer.

Back to Q 165 on page 430

166. The correct answer is **C** – No explanation is available for this answer.

Back to Q 166 on page 430

167. The correct answer is **B** – No explanation is available for this answer.

Back to Q 167 on page 430

168. The correct answer is **D** – No explanation is available for this answer.

Back to Q 168 on page 430

169. The correct answer is **A** – No explanation is available for this answer.

Back to Q 169 on page 431

170. The correct answer is **C** – No explanation is available for this answer.

Back to Q 170 on page 431

171. The correct answer is **B** – No explanation is available for this answer.

Back to Q 171 on page 431

172. The correct answer is **D** – No explanation is available for this answer.

Back to Q 172 on page 431

173. The correct answer is **A** – No explanation is available for this answer.

Back to Q 173 on page 431

174. The correct answer is **A** – No explanation is available for this answer.

Back to Q 174 on page 432

175. The correct answer is **C** – No explanation is available for this answer.

Back to Q 175 on page 432

176. The correct answer is **C** – No explanation is available for this answer.

Back to Q 176 on page 432

177. The correct answer is **C** – No explanation is available for this answer.

Back to Q 177 on page 432

178. The correct answer is **A** – No explanation is available for this answer.

Back to Q 178 on page 432

179. The correct answer is **D** – No explanation is available for this answer.

Back to Q 179 on page 433

180. The correct answer is **D** – No explanation is available for this answer.

Back to Q 180 on page 433

181. The correct answer is **D** – No explanation is available for this answer.

Back to Q 181 on page 433

182. The correct answer is **A** – No explanation is available for this answer.

Back to Q 182 on page 433

183. The correct answer is **C** – No explanation is available for this answer.

Back to Q 183 on page 433

184. The correct answer is **B** – No explanation is available for this answer.

Back to Q 184 on page 434

185. The correct answer is **B** – No explanation is available for this answer.

Back to Q 185 on page 434

186. The correct answer is **D** – No explanation is available for this answer.

Back to Q 186 on page 434

187. The correct answer is **B** – No explanation is available for this answer.

Back to Q 187 on page 434

188. The correct answer is **D** – No explanation is available for this answer.

Back to Q 188 on page 434

189. The correct answer is **C** – No explanation is available for this answer.

Back to Q 189 on page 435

190. The correct answer is **B** – No explanation is available for this answer.

Back to Q 190 on page 435

191. The correct answer is **B** – No explanation is available for this answer.

Back to Q 191 on page 435

192. The correct answer is **C** – No explanation is available for this answer.

Back to Q 192 on page 435

193. The correct answer is **D** – No explanation is available for this answer.

Back to Q 193 on page 435

194. The correct answer is **C** – No explanation is available for this answer.

Back to Q 194 on page 435

195. The correct answer is **D** – No explanation is available for this answer.

Back to Q 195 on page 436

196. The correct answer is **A** – No explanation is available for this answer.

Back to Q 196 on page 436

197. The correct answer is **B** – No explanation is available for this answer.

Back to Q 197 on page 436

198. The correct answer is **B** – No explanation is available for this answer.

Back to Q 198 on page 436

199. The correct answer is **C** – No explanation is available for this answer.

Back to Q 199 on page 437

200. The correct answer is **A** – No explanation is available for this answer.

Back to Q 200 on page 437

201. The correct answer is **C** – No explanation is available for this answer.

Back to Q 201 on page 437

202. The correct answer is **C** – No explanation is available for this answer.

Back to Q 202 on page 437

203. The correct answer is **D** – No explanation is available for this answer.

Back to Q 203 on page 437

204. The correct answer is **C** – No explanation is available for this answer.

Back to Q 204 on page 438

205. The correct answer is **E** – No explanation is available for this answer.

Back to Q 205 on page 438

206. The correct answer is **D** – No explanation is available for this answer.

Back to Q 206 on page 438

207. The correct answer is **A** – No explanation is available for this answer.

Back to Q 207 on page 438

208. The correct answer is **B** – No explanation is available for this answer.

Back to Q 208 on page 439

209. The correct answer is **D** – No explanation is available for this answer.

Back to Q 209 on page 439

210. The correct answer is **C** – Benign mucous membrane pemphigoid (cicatricial pemphigoid) is characterized histologically by subepithelial bullae.

Back to Q 210 on page 439

211. The correct answer is **B** – No explanation is available for this answer.

Back to Q 211 on page 439

212. The correct answer is **B** – No explanation is available for this answer.

Back to Q 212 on page 440

213. The correct answer is **D** – No explanation is available for this answer.

Back to Q 213 on page 440

214. The correct answer is **C** – No explanation is available for this answer.

Back to Q 214 on page 440

215. The correct answer is **A** – No explanation is available for this answer.

Back to Q 215 on page 440

216. The correct answer is **C** – No explanation is available for this answer.

Back to Q 216 on page 441

217. The correct answer is **D** – No explanation is available for this answer.

Back to Q 217 on page 441

218. The correct answer is **D** – No explanation is available for this answer.

Back to Q 218 on page 441

219. The correct answer is **B** – No explanation is available for this answer.

Back to Q 219 on page 441

220. The correct answer is **C** – No explanation is available for this answer.

Back to Q 220 on page 442

221. The correct answer is **C** – No explanation is available for this answer.

Back to Q 221 on page 442

222. The correct answer is **C** – No explanation is available for this answer.

Back to Q 222 on page 442

223. The correct answer is **A** – No explanation is available for this answer.

Back to Q 223 on page 442

224. The correct answer is **C** – No explanation is available for this answer.

Back to Q 224 on page 443

225. The correct answer is **E** – No explanation is available for this answer.

Back to Q 225 on page 443

226. The correct answer is **B** – Ameloblastoma and ameloblastic fibroma do not have the capacity to produce enamel, dentin, cementum or calcification except on very rare occasions.

Back to Q 226 on page 443

227. The correct answer is **A** – No explanation is available for this answer.

Back to Q 227 on page 443

228. The correct answer is **A** – No explanation is available for this answer.

Back to Q 228 on page 444

References

[1] Miko I. Phenotype variability: penetrance and expressivity. Nature Education. 2008;1(1):137.

[2] Su Jm, Zeng Sj, Ye Xw, Wu Zf, Huang Xw, Pathak JL. Three years of follow-up of otodental syndrome in 3-year-old Chinese boy: a rare case report. BMC oral health. 2019;19(1):1-7. Available from: https://bmcoralhealth.biomedcentral.com/articles/10.1186/s12903-019-0860-z#citeas.

[3] Sánchez AR, Rogers III RS, Sheridan PJ. Tetracycline and other tetracycline-derivative staining of the teeth and oral cavity. International journal of dermatology. 2004;43(10):709-15.

[4] Rabiei M, Mohtashame Amiri Z, Masoodi Rad H, Niazi M, Niazi H. Frequency of tongue anomalies in primary school of Lahidjan. Journal of Guilan University of Medical Sciences. 2003;12(45):36-42.

[5] Jayam C, Choudhary P, Venkataraghavan K, Trivedi K, Shah S, Bandlapalli A. Linear Enamel Hypoplasia: Case Report. Journal of Advanced Oral Research. 2013 sep;4(3):12-5.

[6] El-Naggar AK, Chan JK, Grandis JR, Takata T, Slootweg PJ. WHO classification of head and neck tumours. International Agency for Research on Cancer; 2017.

[7] Ulrich M, Roewert-Huber J, González S, Rius-Diaz F, Stockfleth E, Kanitakis J. Peritumoral clefting in basal cell carcinoma: correlation of in vivo reflectance confocal microscopy and routine histology. Journal of Cutaneous Pathology. 2010 oct;38(2):190-5.

[8] Jewett FC, and Nelson BL . Dentinogenic ghost cell tumor;. Available from: https://www.pathologyoutlines.com/topic/mandiblemaxilladentinogenicghost.html.

[9] Neville BW, Damm DD, Chi AC, Allen CM. Oral and maxillofacial pathology. Fourth edition ed. Elsevier Health Sciences; 2015.

[10] Iorgulescu G. Saliva between normal and pathological. Important factors in determining systemic and oral health. Journal of medicine and life;2:303-7. Available from: https://www.ncbi.nlm.nih.gov/pmc/articles/PMC5052503/.

[11] Sivapathasundharam, B. Shafer's Textbook of Oral Pathology. 7th ed. Elsevier Health Sciences; 2016. Available from: https://www.amazon.com/Shafers-Textbook-Pathology-Rajendran-Sivapathasundharam/dp/813123097X.

[12] Abdel-Azim A M and Abdel-Azim A A. Oral and Maxillofacial Pathology: Tips and Tricks. theWay; 2020. Available from: https://www.amazon.com/dp/1734188219/ref=sr_1_1?keywords=tips+and+tricks+adel&qid=1576620609&sr=8-1.

[13] Mufadhal AA, Aldawla MA, Madfa AA. External and Internal Anatomy of Maxillary Permanent First Molars. In: Human Teeth - Key Skills and Clinical Illustrations. IntechOpen; 2020. .

[14] Luna LG. Manual of histologic staining methods of the Armed Forces Institute of Pathology. 3rd ed. New York, Blakiston Division, McGraw-Hill; 1968.

[15] Newman MG, Takei H, Klokkevold PR, Carranza FA. Newman and Carranza's clinical periodontology. Elsevier Health Sciences; 2018.

[16] Abdel-Azim A M and Abdel-Azim A A. Oral and Maxillofacial Pathology: A Study Guide. theWay; 2019. Available from: https://www.amazon.com/Oral-Maxillofacial-Pathology-Study-Guide/dp/1734188200/ref=olp_product_details?_encoding=UTF8&me=&qid=1572885040&sr=8-2.

[17] Laniosz V, Torgerson RR, Ramos-Rodriguez AJ, Ma JE, Mara KC, Weaver AL, et al. Incidence of squamous cell carcinoma in oral lichen planus: a 25-year population-based study. International journal of dermatology. 2019 Mar;58:296-301.

[18] Cassol-Spanemberg J, Blanco-Carrión A, Rodríguez-de Rivera-Campillo ME, Estrugo-Devesa A, Jané-Salas E, López-López J. Cutaneous, genital and oral lichen planus: A descriptive study of 274 patients. Medicina oral, patologia oral y cirugia bucal. 2019 Jan;24:e1-7.

[19] Ralston SH, Penman ID, Strachan MW, Hobson R. Davidson's Principles and Practice of Medicine E-Book. 23rd ed. Elsevier Health Sciences; 2018. Available from: https://books.google.com.eg/books/about/Davidson_s_Principles_and_Practice_of_Me.html?id=sTwGnwEACAAJ&redir_esc=y.

[20] Marx, R E and Stern, D . Oral and Maxillofacial Pathology: A Rationale for Diagnosis and Treatment. 2nd ed. Quintessence Publishing Company; 2012. Available from: http://books.google.com.sa/books?id=mCk5ywAACAAJ.

[21] Cawson R. Cawson's Essentials of Oral Pathology and Oral Medicine. Philadelphia: Churchill Livingstone, Elsevier; 2008.

[22] DeLong L, Burkhart N. General and oral pathology for the dental hygienist. LWW; 2013.

[23] El-Khoury J, Kibbi A, Abbas O. Mucocutaneous pseudoepitheliomatous hyperplasia: a review. Am J Dermatopathol. 2012 Apr;34(2):165-75. Available from: http://dx.doi.org/10.1097/DAD.0b013e31821816ab.

[24] Eversole L. Contemporary Oral and Maxillofacial Pathology. St. Louis: Mosby; 2004.

[25] Eversole L. Clinical outline of oral pathology: diagnosis and treatment. Pmph Bc Decker; 2002.

[26] Ibsen O. Oral Pathology for the Dental Hygienist. Philadelphia: Saunders; 2008.

[27] Langlais R. Color Atlas of Common Oral Diseases. Hagerstwon: Lippincott Williams & Wilkins; 2009.

[28] Langland OE, Langlais RP, Preece JW. Principles of dental imaging. Lippincott Williams & Wilkins; 2002.

[29] Levison D, Reid R. Muir's Textbook of Pathology. 14th ed. Levison D, Reid R, Fleming S, Harrison D, Burt A, editors. Hodder Arnold Publication; 2008.

[30] López de Blanc S, Sambuelli R, Femopase F, Luna N, Gravotta M, David D, et al. Bacillary angiomatosis affecting the oral cavity. Report of two cases and review. J Oral Pathol Med. 2000 Feb;29(2):91-6.

[31] MacDonald-Jankowski DS. Fibro-osseous lesions of the face and jaws. Clin Radiol. 2004 Jan;59(1):11-25.

[32] Pogrel A. The diagnosis and management of giant cell lesions of the jaws. Annals of Maxillofacial Surgery. 2012;2(2):102-6. Available from: http://www.amsjournal.com/article.asp?issn=2231-0746;year=2012;volume=2;issue=2;spage=102;epage=106;aulast=Pogrel;t=6.

[33] Regezi J. Oral Pathology. Philadelphia: Saunders; 2007.

[34] Scully C. Oral Medicine and Pathology at a Glance. Wiley-Blackwell; 2010.

[35] Shear M, Speight P. Cysts of the oral and maxillofacial regions. Wiley-Blackwell; 2008.

[36] Southam JV, Soames JC. Oral Pathology. Oxford shire: Oxford University Press; 2005.

[37] Zayour M, Lazova R. Pseudoepitheliomatous hyperplasia: a review. Am J Dermatopathol. 2011 Apr;33(2):112-22; quiz 123-6. Available from: http://dx.doi.org/10.1097/DAD.0b013e3181fcfb47.

[38] Malik S, Singh V, Singh G, Dahiya N. Central Giant Cell Granuloma of the Mandible: A Rare Presentation. IJHNS, Jaypee. 2014. Available from: http://www.jaypeejournals.com/eJournals/ShowText.aspx?ID=3993&Type=FREE&TYP=TOP&IN=_eJournals/images/JPLOGO.gif&IID=313&isPDF=YES.

[39] Powers-Fletcher M. A review of the biology and the laboratory diagnosis of Treponema pallidum. Journal of Continuing Education Topics & Issues. 2011;13(3). Available from: `http://www.freepatentsonline.com/article/Journal-Continuing-Education-Topics-Issues/268477987.html`.

[40] Shah A, Latoo S, Ahmad I. Multiple Myeloma and Dentistry - An Overview. MULTIPLE MYELOMA–AN OVERVIEW. 2011:207. Available from: `http://cdn.intechopen.com/pdfs-wm/26509.pdf`.

[41] Sharma NK, Singh AK, Pandey A, Verma V. Solitary plasmacytoma of the mandible: A rare case report. Natl J Maxillofac Surg. 2015;6(1):76-9. Available from: `http://dx.doi.org/10.4103/0975-5950.168214`.

[42] Witkop C. Amelogenesis imperfecta, dentinogenesis imperfecta and dentin dysplasia revisited: problems in classification. Journal of Oral Pathology & Medicine. 1988;17(9-10):547-53.

[43] Chaubal R, Tavri O, Sawant A, Singh C. Infantile Hemangioendothelioma of the Parotid Gland. Journal of clinical imaging science. 2017;7:5.

[44] Kotrashetti V, Sonawane V, Bainade K, Agarwal R. Infantile Hemangioendothelioma of the Parotid Gland. International Journal of Clinical Pediatrics. 2015;4(4). Available from: `http://www.theijcp.org/index.php/ijcp/article/view/227`.

[45] Tandon A, Jain B, Tandon R, Grover C, Pandhi D, Bhatt S. Infantile Hemangioendothelioma of the Parotid Gland: A Sonographic Diagnosis. Journal of Diagnostic Medical Sonography. 2011;27(3):131-4.

[46] Horie Y, Kato M. Juvenile hemangioma (infantile hemangioendothelioma) of the parotid gland associated with cytomegalovirus infection. Pathology international. 1999 Jul;49:668-71.

[47] Ayadi L, Khabir A, Boudawara T, Kharrat M, Makni S, Jlidi R. Cellular hemangioma of the parotid gland associated with an infection by cytomegalovirus. Revue de stomatologie et de chirurgie maxillo-faciale. 2003 Oct;104:290-3.

[48] Chatura K, Iqbal M. Parotid gland hemiangioma with cytomegalovirus infection. J Adv Clin Res Insights. 2015;2:31-2.

[49] Nagao K, Matsuzaki O, Shigematsu H, Kaneko T, Katoh T, Kitamura T. Histopathologic studies of benign infantile hemangioendothelioma of the parotid gland. Cancer. 1980 Nov;46:2250-6.

[50] Darrow DH, Greene AK, Mancini AJ, Nopper AJ. Diagnosis and Management of Infantile Hemangioma. Pediatrics. 2015 Oct;136:e1060-104.

[51] Routray S, Mohanty N, Panda S, Sahoo SR. Hemangiopericytoma / solitary fibrous tumor of mandible: A rare entity. Journal of oral and maxillofacial pathology: JOMFP. 2015;19:260-2.

[52] Makhasana JAS, Kulkarni MA, Vaze S, Shroff AS. Juvenile nasopharyngeal angiofibroma. Journal of oral and maxillofacial pathology: JOMFP. 2016;20:330.

[53] Ibsen OA, Phelan JA. Oral Pathology for the Dental Hygienist. Sixth ed. Elsevier Health Sciences; 2014.

[54] Bloch-Zupan A, Sedano H, Scully C. Dento/oro/craniofacial anomalies and genetics. 1st ed. Elsevier; 2012.

[55] Dakubo D Gabriel, editor. Mitochondrial genetics and cancer. Springer Science & Business Media; 2010.

[56] Roversi G, editor. Cancer prone diseases; 2018. Available from: `http://atlasgeneticsoncology.org/Kprones/Kproneliste.html`.

[57] Kumar V, Abbas AK, Aster JC. Robbins basic pathology. Tenth edition ed. Elsevier Health Sciences; 2017.

[58] Aggarwal A, Daniel MJ, Shetty RS, Kumar BN, Sumalatha CH, Srikanth E, et al. Oral Myiasis Caused by Chrysomya bezziana in Anterior Maxilla. Case reports in dentistry. 2014;2014:518427. Available from: `http://cdn.intechopen.com/pdfs-wm/26509.pdf`.

[59] Sharma A, Hedge A. Primary oral myiasis due to Chrysomya bezziana treated with Ivermectin. A case report. The Journal of clinical pediatric dentistry. 2010;34:259-61.

[60] Sankari LS, Ramakrishnan K. Oral myiasis caused by Chrysomya bezziana. Journal of oral and maxillofacial pathology : JOMFP. 2010 Jan;14:16-8.

[61] Han HS, Sharma R, Jeffery J, Noli C. Chrysomya bezziana (Diptera: Calliphoridae) infestation: case report of three dogs in Malaysia treated with spinosad/milbemycin. Veterinary dermatology. 2017 Apr;28:239-62.

[62] Jimson S, Prakash CA, Balachandran C, Raman M. Oral myiasis: case report. Indian journal of dental research : official publication of Indian Society for Dental Research. 2013;24:750-2.

[63] Sharma A. Oral Myiasis is a Potential Risk in Patients with Special Health Care Needs. Journal of global infectious diseases. 2012 Jan;4:60-1.

[64] Candamourty R, Venkatachalam S, Yuvaraj V, Sujee C. Oral myiasis in an adult associated with filariasis and Hansen's disease. Journal of natural science, biology, and medicine. 2013 Jan;4:259-62.

[65] Shikha S, Prasad Guru R, Ashutoshdutt P, Meenakshi S. Oral Myiasis: A Rare Case Report and Literature Review. Journal of dentistry (Tehran, Iran). 2015 Jun;12:456-9.

[66] Kumar P, Singh V. Oral myiasis: case report and review of literature. Oral and maxillofacial surgery. 2014 Mar;18:25-9.

[67] Droma EB, Wilamowski A, Schnur H, Yarom N, Scheuer E, Schwartz E. Oral myiasis: a case report and literature review. Oral surgery, oral medicine, oral pathology, oral radiology, and endodontics. 2007 Jan;103:92-6.

[68] Avula JK, Avula H, Arora N, Manchukonda UK, Vivekavardhan Reddy N. Orofacial myiasis of the gingiva and nasal cavity: a report of two cases and general review. Journal of periodontology. 2011 Sep;82:1383-8.

[69] Mengji AK, Yaga US, Gollamudi N, Prakash B, Rajashekar E. Mucormycosis in a surgical defect masquerading as osteomyelitis: a case report and review of literature. The Pan African medical journal. 2016;23:16.

[70] Hua F, He H, Ngan P, Bouzid W. Prevalence of peg-shaped maxillary permanent lateral incisors: A meta-analysis. American Journal of Orthodontics and Dentofacial Orthopedics. 2013;144(1):97-109.

[71] Al Shethri S. The prevalence of the Carabelli cusp in selected Saudi population. King Saud University Journal of Dental Sciences. 2011;2(1-2):13-6.

[72] Hobœk A. Fibrous Dysplasia – Fibro-Osteoma – Osteoma of the Facial Bones and the Skull. Acta Radiologica. 1951;os-36(2):97-113. Available from: https://doi.org/10.1177/028418515103600203.

[73] Drettner B, Herberts G. Fibroosteoma of the maxillary region. Acta oto-laryngologica. 1957 Sep;48:183-92.

[74] Billing L, Ringertz N. Fibro-Osteoma: A Pathologico-anatomical and Roentgenological Study. Acta Radiologica. 1946;27(2):129. Available from: https://doi.org/10.3109/00016925109176978.

[75] Cardesa A, Slootweg PJ, Gale N, Franchi A. Pathology of the Head and Neck. Springer; 2017.

[76] Jain A, Shetty DC, Juneja S, Narwal N. Molecular Characterization of Clear Cell Lesions of Head and Neck. Journal of clinical and diagnostic research : JCDR. 2016 May;10:ZE18-23.

[77] Rekhtman N, Baine MK, Bishop JA. Quick Reference Handbook for Surgical Pathologists. 2nd ed. Springer; 2019. Available from: http://dx.doi.org/10.1007/978-3-319-97508-5_13.

[78] Jezierska M, Stefanowicz J, Romanowicz G, Kosiak W, Lange M. Langerhans cell histiocytosis in children– a disease with many faces. Recent advances in pathogenesis, diagnostic examinations and treatment. Advances in Dermatology and Allergology/Postepy Dermatologii i Alergologii. 2018;35(1):6.

[79] Semwal S, Joshi D, Gupta V, Kapoor N. Cartilaginous choristoma of tongue: A rare case report. Journal of Oral and Maxillofacial Pathology: JOMFP. 2019;23(Suppl 1):40.

[80] Fletcher C. Diagnostic histopathology of tumors. 4th ed. Elsevier, Saunders; 2013.

[81] Chou L, Hansen LS, Daniels TE. Choristomas of the oral cavity: a review. Oral surgery, oral medicine, oral pathology. 1991;72(5):584-93.

[82] Batra R. The pathogenesis of oral choristomas. Journal of Oral and Maxillofacial Surgery, Medicine, and Pathology. 2012;24(2):110-4.

[83] Deshmukh S, Prashanth S. Ectodermal dysplasia: a genetic review. International journal of clinical pediatric dentistry. 2012;5(3):197.

[84] Fernández González F, Vázquez Álvarez R, Reboiras López D, Gándara Vila P, García García A, Gándara Rey JM. Histopathological findings in oral lichen planus and their correlation with the clinical manifestations. Med Oral Patol Oral Cir Bucal. 2011 Aug;(1;16(5):e641-6.).

[85] Antonini LG, Luder HU. Discoloration of teeth from tetracyclines-even today? Schweizer Monatsschrift für Zahnmedizin SMfZ. 2011;121(5):414-31.

Made in United States
Orlando, FL
04 November 2026

90207392R00265